# Precision Radiation Oncology

# Precision Radiation Oncology

*Edited by* **Bruce G. Haffty**
**and Sharad Goyal**

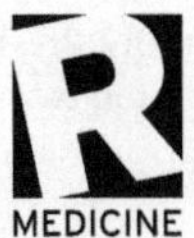

**Rutgers University Press Medicine**

*New Brunswick, Camden, and Newark, New Jersey, and London*

A Cataloging-in-Publication record for this book is available from the Library of Congress.

A British Cataloging-in-Publication record for this book is available from the British Library.

978-0-8135-8596-3
978-0-8135-9254-1
978-0-8135-9255-8
978-0-8135-9256-5



♾ The paper used in this publication meets the requirements of the American National Standard for Information Sciences—Permanence of Paper for Printed Library Materials, ANSI Z39.48-1992.

www.rutgersuniversitypress.org

Manufactured in the United States of America

# CONTENTS

# CONTRIBUTORS

**Sanjay Aneja, MD**
*Resident Physician*
Department of Therapeutic Radiology
Yale School of Medicine
New Haven, Connecticut

**John Byun, MD**
*Resident Physician*
Department of Radiation Oncology
Robert Wood Johnson Medical
    School
Rutgers Cancer Institute of
    New Jersey
Rutgers, The State University of
    New Jersey
New Brunswick, New Jersey

**Joseph M. Caster, MD**
*Resident Physician*
Department of Radiation Oncology
University of North Carolina
    Hospitals
Chapel Hill, North Carolina

**Brian G. Czito, MD**
*Gary Hock and Lyn Proctor Associate
    Professor of Radiation Oncology*
Department of Radiation Oncology
Duke University School of Medicine
Durham, North Carolina

**George Farha, MD**
*Clinical Fellow*
Department of Radiation Oncology
Sunnybrook Odette Cancer
    Centre
University of Toronto
Toronto, Ontario, Canada

**Sharad Goyal, MD**
*Professor & Division Chief*
Radiation Oncology
George Washington University
    School of Medicine and Health
    Sciences
George Washington University
    Cancer Center
Washington, DC

**Bruce G. Haffty, MD**
*Chief of Staff*
Rutgers Cancer Institute of
    New Jersey
*Professor and Chair*
Department of Radiation Oncology
Robert Wood Johnson Medical
    School
Rutgers, The State University of
    New Jersey
New Brunswick, New Jersey

**Salma K. Jabbour, MD**
*Professor*
*Director of Education*
Department of Radiation Oncology
Robert Wood Johnson Medical
    School
Rutgers Cancer Institute of
    New Jersey
Rutgers, The State University of
    New Jersey
New Brunswick, New Jersey

**Sachin Jhawar, MD**
*Resident Physician*
Department of Radiation Oncology
Robert Wood Johnson Medical School
Rutgers Cancer Institute of New Jersey
Rutgers, The State University of
    New Jersey
New Brunswick, New Jersey

**Atif J. Khan, MD**
*Associate Attending*
Department of Radiation Oncology
Memorial Sloan Kettering Cancer
    Center
New York, New York

**Randall J. Kimple, MD, PhD**
*Assistant Professor*
Departments of Human Oncology
    and Medical Physics
Carbone Comprehensive Cancer
    Center
University of Wisconsin School
    of Medicine and Public Health
Madison, Wisconsin

**Omar Mahmoud, MD**
*Assistant Professor*
Department of Radiation Oncology
Robert Wood Johnson Medical School

Rutgers Cancer Institute of New Jersey
Rutgers, The State University of
    New Jersey
New Brunswick, New Jersey

**Dodul Mondal, MBBS**
*Fellow*
Department of Radiation Oncology
Robert Wood Johnson Medical School
Rutgers Cancer Institute of New Jersey
Rutgers, The State University of
    New Jersey
New Brunswick, New Jersey

**Zachary S. Morris, MD, PhD**
*Assistant Professor*
Department of Human Oncology
Carbone Comprehensive Cancer
    Center
University of Wisconsin School of
    Medicine and Public Health
Madison, Wisconsin

**Nichole J. Newman**
Department of Radiation Oncology
University of North Carolina at
    Chapel Hill
Chapel Hill, North Carolina

**Ke Nie, PhD**
*Assistant Professor*
Department of Radiation Oncology
Robert Wood Johnson Medical School
Rutgers, The State University of
    New Jersey
New Brunswick, New Jersey

**John L. Nosher, MD**
*Clinical Professor and Chair of Radiology*
*Chief of Vascular and Interventional
    Radiology*
Robert Wood Johnson Medical School
Rutgers Cancer Institute of New Jersey

Rutgers, The State University of
New Jersey
New Brunswick, New Jersey

**Manisha Palta, MD**
*Assistant Professor*
Department of Radiation Oncology
Duke University School of Medicine
Durham, North Carolina

**Rahul R. Parikh, MD**
*Medical Director, Proton Beam Therapy*
Department of Radiation Oncology
Rutgers Cancer Institute of New Jersey
*Assistant Professor of Radiation
Oncology*
Robert Wood Johnson Medical School
New Brunswick, New Jersey

**Artish N. Patel**
Department of Radiation Oncology
University of North Carolina at
Chapel Hill
Chapel Hill, North Carolina

**Ryan Rhome, MD, PhD**
Department of Radiation Oncology
Icahn School of Medicine at Mount
Sinai
New York, New York

**Stephen A. Rosenberg, MD, MS**
Department of Human Oncology
University of Wisconsin School of
Medicine and Public Health
Madison, Wisconsin

**Barry S. Rosenstein, MD, PhD**
*Associate Professor*
Department of Radiation Oncology
Icahn School of Medicine at
Mount Sinai
New York, New York

**Mark Ruschin, PhD, MCCPM**
*Assistant Professor*
Department of Radiation Oncology
Sunnybrook Odette Cancer Centre
University of Toronto
Toronto, Ontario, Canada

**Arjun Sahgal, MD, FRCPC**
*Associate Professor*
Sunnybrook Odette Cancer Centre
University of Toronto
Toronto, Ontario, Canada

**Joseph K. Salama, MD**
*Associate Professor*
*Chief, Radiation Oncology Clinical
Services*
*Radiation Oncologist*
Department of Radiation Oncology
Duke University School of
Medicine
Durham, North Carolina

**Arman Sarfehnia, MSc, PhD**
*Assistant Professor*
Department of Radiation Oncology
Sunnybrook Odette Cancer Centre
University of Toronto
Toronto, Ontario, Canada

**David Schlesinger, PhD**
*Associate Professor, Medical Physicist*
Department of Radiation Oncology
University of Virginia School of
Medicine
Charlottesville, Virginia

**Ann W. Silk, MD, MS**
*Assistant Professor of Medicine*
Division of Medical Oncology, Solid
Tumor Section
Robert Wood Johnson Medical School
Rutgers Cancer Institute of New Jersey

Rutgers, The State University of
New Jersey
New Brunswick, New Jersey

**Charles B. Simone II, MD**
*Medical Director*
Maryland Proton Treatment
Center
*Director*
Stereotactic Radiosurgery and
Radiotherapy
*Fellowship Director*
Advanced Radiation Modalities
Fellowship
Department of Radiation Oncology
University of Maryland Medical
Center
Baltimore, Maryland

**Min-Ying Lydia Su, PhD**
*Director*
John Tu & Thomas Yuen Center for
Functional Onco-Imaging
*Professor*
Department of Radiological
Sciences
University of California, Irvine
Irvine, California

**Daniel J. Tandberg, MD**
*Resident Physician*
Department of Radiation Oncology
Duke University School of
Medicine
Durham, North Carolina

**Neil K. Taunk, MD, MS**
*Assistant Professor*
Department of Radiation Oncology
University of Pennsylvania
Philadelphia, Pennsylvania

**Jordan A. Torok, MD**
*Medical Instructor*
*Radiation Oncologist*
Department of Radiation Oncology
Duke University School of Medicine
Durham, North Carolina

**Vivek Verma, MD**
*Resident Physician*
Department of Radiation Oncology
College of Medicine
University of Nebraska
Omaha, Nebraska

**Andrew Z. Wang, MD**
*Associate Professor*
Department of Radiation Oncology
University of North Carolina at
Chapel Hill
Chapel Hill, North Carolina

**Christopher G. Willett, MD**
*Chair*
Department of Radiation Oncology
Duke University School of Medicine
Durham, North Carolina

**James B. Yu, MD, MHS**
*Associate Professor*
Department of Therapeutic Radiology
*Director*
Prostate and Genitourinary Cancer
Program
Yale School of Medicine
New Haven, Connecticut

**Tian Zhang, MD**
*Assistant Professor of Medicine*
Department of Hematology and
Oncology
Duke University School of Medicine
Durham, North Carolina

# Precision Radiation Oncology

## AN INTRODUCTION

*Sharad Goyal, Sachin Jhawar, and Bruce G. Haffty*

The concept of precision radiation oncology involves much more than a mastery of technology. The definition of *precision* is more sophisticated and involves a deeper understanding of the underlying biological foundation of cancer, which can then be targeted with strategic interventions. Rather than treating many to benefit a few, precision radiation oncology aims to (a) maximize the antitumor effect (eg, determine whether a patient should be treated, whether the ionizing radiation dose might be escalated, or whether other antineoplastic drugs should be combined) and (b) avoid unnecessary toxicity without jeopardizing the patient's outcome (eg, decide whether to decrease the dose or the volume). Either the technology-driven improvement of radiation delivery to the defined target volume or novel biological strategies for personalized treatment may achieve these goals.

## TECHNOLOGY-DRIVEN ADVANCES TOWARD PRECISION RADIATION ONCOLOGY

After the golden era of advanced three-dimensional conformal treatment, modern radiation oncology has been mainly driven by the rapid adoption of intensity-modulated radiation therapy (IMRT) techniques with image guidance (image-guided radiation therapy [IGRT]), which now represents the gold standard treatment option in most industrialized countries. These treatments are typically delivered using clinical linear accelerators (LINACs) and utilize real-time, in-room imaging for improved accuracy. Moreover, the implementation of IGRT and IMRT has paved the way to the concept of *focal therapy*; for small target volumes, stereotactic radiotherapy applies a large number of radiation fields or multiple radiation arcs to produce a very steep dose fall off outside the target volume. This often enables very high, ablative doses to be prescribed in one to five treatments. One of the primary challenges in radiation oncology today is to select and delineate the target volume. Once this volume is defined, the limitations to accurate delivery come from uncertainties in the daily patient setup and the determination of the positions of both the tumor and the surrounding normal tissues, which patient or organ motion can complicate. Technologies are now available to mitigate patient motion and to track target motion to ensure conformal treatment.

A particularly exciting technology being explored for clinical applications is particle therapy with protons or heavy ions—another advance toward precision radiation oncology. Particle therapy can deposit energy at or around the target with no exit dose beyond the target, a phenomenon known as the *Bragg peak* (1). In contrast, photons deliver radiation that gradually deposits the dose through tissue both on the way toward and distal to the target tumor, with the maximum dose close to the skin's surface. This means that particle beams have relatively lower doses in the entrance channel in front of the tumor, and tissues behind the tumor receive little to none of the radiation dose. Two main benefits of particle therapy are that normal tissues are significantly less exposed to intermediate and low doses compared with photon therapy, and in cases in which crucial normal tissues are located in direct proximity to the tumor, particle therapy may be able to deliver the necessary curative radiation dose, compared to photon radiotherapy.

## BIOLOGY-DRIVEN ADVANCES TOWARD PRECISION RADIATION ONCOLOGY

Classically, the "four *R*'s" of radiotherapy describe the radiobiological mechanisms that determine one's sensitivity or resistance to radiotherapy; these include the repair of DNA damage caused by radiotherapy, reoxygenation during treatment, repopulation between radiotherapy fractions, and the redistribution of surviving, cycling cells after a radiation–induced cell cycle blockade (2). Today, a large proportion of patients treated with radiotherapy receive combined modality treatment, with cytotoxic drugs, molecular targeted agents, immunotherapeutic approaches, or antihormonal therapy. The addition of these systemic therapies can affect and alter the radiobiology of both the tumor and normal tissue.

Notable progress has been made in gaining knowledge of the biological factors of radiation response and their underlying molecular basis, and these advances have created a plethora of potential biomarkers. Theoretically, the concept of precision radiation oncology should target those most (or least) likely to benefit from radiotherapy. Biology-driven precision radiation oncology, which tailors treatments to individual patients based on the biological features of the tumor or normal tissues beyond anatomical information, is still in its infancy. It is well recognized that substantial heterogeneity of radiation response in normal tissues and tumors exists between and within individual patients, as well as tumors of the same histology (3). For example, different regions even within the same tumor can have varying levels of radiosensitivity, dependent on the tumor microenvironment; the heterogenous distribution of cancer stem cells; or possibly, specific genetic or molecular alterations. Thus, biomarker assays that predict the treatment outcome are clearly needed[3]. Furthermore, two objectives should be achieved before routinely integrating biomarkers to radiation treatments: rigorous validation and easy implementation. These tools could then help to identify favorable patient cohorts in order to de-escalate treatments or select unfavorable patient cohorts to create new treatments with different regimens or radiosensitizing targeted therapies. Anatomically individualized treatment plans may allow one to implement precision strategies that to a large extent work with different radiation doses or fractionation schedules. Therefore, radiation oncology has considerable potential for showcasing personalized precision oncology.

## CONCLUSIONS

Over the past two decades, the paradigm of radiation oncology has moved away from the obsolete principle of exclusively radical "one-size-fits-all" treatments. Currently, precision radiation oncology aims to combine maximal oncological efficacy with minimal impact on a patient's quality of life and functionality. A deeper knowledge of anatomy and cancer biology coupled with better diagnostic instruments will allow us to improve indications for radiotherapy, to optimize radiation treatment planning, and to tailor the delivery of radiotherapy to each patient. We have entered an era of precision radiation oncology, and further clinical and translational research is needed to address many unmet needs and to fully realize the potential of this field.

### References


1. Jiang GL. Particle therapy for cancers: a new weapon in radiation therapy. *Front Med.* 2012;6(2):165–172.
2. Pajonk F, Vlashi E, McBride WH. Radiation resistance of cancer stem cells: the 4 R's of radiobiology revisited. *Stem Cells.* 2010;28(4):639–648.
3. Baumann M, Krause M, Overgaard J, et al. Radiation oncology in the era of precision medicine. *Nat Rev Cancer.* 2016;16(4):234–249.

# Combining Cytotoxic Chemotherapy and Radiation Therapy

*Vivek Verma and Charles B. Simone II*

## THE CONCEPT AND RATIONALE OF COMBINED MODALITY THERAPY

A foremost principle explaining the potential benefits of chemoradiation (CRT) administration involves mechanistic themes. Most generally, because radiation therapy (RT) acts locally and chemotherapy (CT) is distributed throughout the body, combined CRT attempts to control both locoregional disease and potential distant micrometastatic spread, a notion known as *spatial interaction*. When delving into molecular mechanisms, however, RT is known to cause damage to neoplastic cells largely by free radical–mediated DNA double-strand breaks. Various CT agents, on the other hand, act via several different pathways. Many commonly utilized CT drugs act directly or indirectly on DNA. Alkylators/ linkers of DNA, such as cyclophosphamide or cisplatin, directly modify DNA to create crosslinks, which can result in additional DNA damage beyond what RT causes. Indirect DNA agents act on proteins that themselves directly act on DNA; for instance, the anthracycline doxorubicin stabilizes the complex between topoisomerase II and DNA, thus preventing the reconnection of temporary DNA strand breaks that normally provide mechanical relief from the torsional forces caused by DNA unwinding. The commonly used compounds paclitaxel and vincristine act on microtubules, most of which are prominently involved in cytostructure and intracellular communication, whereas the antimetabolite methotrexate prevents the collection and use of folates needed for purine and certain amino acid synthesis. In part owing to these diverse mechanisms, combined-modality therapy (CMT) is radiobiologically favorable and may also promote cell cycle synchronization, DNA damage repair inhibition, hypoxic cell sensitization, and the impedance of rapid cellular repopulation.

Seminal clinical trials are often prime examples of these oncologic principles supporting CRT. In 2005 a landmark publication demonstrated the biological superiority of adding the DNA alkylator temozolomide concurrently and adjuvantly to RT alone (60 Gy/30 fractions) for patients with glioblastoma (1). In this randomized trial of 573 patients, most of whom had undergone surgery, the 2-year overall survival (OS) increased from 10.4% with RT alone to 26.5% with CRT. This highlights the appeal of CMT for biologically aggressive neoplasms. Many such tumors are associated with various degrees of radioresistance, owing to inherent (eg, genetic profiles of cancer stem cells) or acquired (eg, from hypoxia) reasons. Because these neoplasms have a higher risk of recurrence if unimodality therapy is performed, adding another agent may indeed improve outcomes; this was recently corroborated in a randomized trial of melanoma, a similarly aggressive and relatively radioresistant tumor, when the addition of RT to the surgical resection of lymph nodes demonstrated enhanced tumor control with CMT (2).

Some aggressive tumors for which there is a strong rationale for CMT lack or have less-convincing data for CMT. In these circumstances, although unimodality therapy is prevalent, CMT offers the opportunity to utilize a complete oncologic arsenal. Although overtreatment is a concern and more intensive (and potentially more morbid) treatment cannot be standard without compelling supportive data, undertreatment may compromise patient outcomes in diseases for which randomized trials have not been feasible or have not demonstrated clear results. A similar situation occurred regarding the optimal treatment of esophageal cancer; prior randomized trials between neoadjuvant CRT and surgery versus surgery alone were criticized and included no convincing numerical OS improvement. As a result, many patients received unimodality therapy. In 2012 the randomized Chemoradiotherapy for Oesophageal Cancer Followed by Surgery Study (CROSS) trial of neoadjuvant CRT (carboplatin/paclitaxel + 41.4 Gy in 23 fractions of RT) followed by surgery, versus surgery alone, demonstrated a doubling of OS, from 24.0 months in the surgery-only arm to 49.4 months in the CMT arm (3). Thereafter, combined CRT followed by surgical resection has emerged as the standard of care in virtually all patients meeting trial eligibility criteria.

Combining CT and RT, when delivered sequentially, can also assist in determining the response to one modality and potentially tailoring the other modality according to this initial response. For instance, cases of locally advanced breast cancer can benefit from neoadjuvant CT prior to surgery, largely for debulking purposes (eg, maintaining appropriate cosmesis and/or decreasing the risk of positive surgical margins). A retrospective analysis of 3,088 patients from two prospective breast cancer trials found that the extent of residual disease is a strong predictor of outcome (regardless of the type or extent of surgery) (4). Residual disease after neoadjuvant therapy is likely a marker for more aggressive biology and hence can result in changes in the management of postoperative RT. Although far from a consensus, the lack of an appropriate outcome after neoadjuvant CT may lead some radiation oncologists to administer slightly higher RT doses and/or electively treat certain nodal volumes owing to the proven higher risk of relapse.

Regarding head and neck malignancies, it has been proven advantageous to deliver CRT in patients with clinicopathologic characteristics portending a higher risk of failure. Two randomized trials from the Radiation Therapy Oncology Group (RTOG) and the European Organization for the Research and Treatment of Cancer (EORTC) demonstrated an OS benefit when adding CT to RT in high-risk head and neck cancers (5–6). Whereas the RTOG trial strictly included patients with extranodal extension, positive surgical margins, and/or two or more regional nodes, the EORTC trial also included pathologic T3 and T4 disease. Although both trials observed an improvement in locoregional control (LRC) and disease-free survival (DFS), only the EORTC trial showed an OS benefit. In a pooled analysis of both trials, the greatest benefit of adding CT to postoperative RT was exhibited in cases with positive margins and extranodal extension, and CRT is now routinely administered in these subgroups (7).

Lastly, an emerging area of combined CT and RT utilization is to prophylactically address cellular clones potentially resistant to standard therapies. Metastatic prostate cancer is often characterized by neoplastic cells that are resistant to hormonal (androgen deprivation) therapy (HT) and hence termed castrate-resistant prostate cancer. Therefore, there is biological rationale to suggest that this phenomenon can occur in high-risk prostate cancer and that prophylactically treating androgen- (and possibly radio-) resistant clones may be of benefit. The maturing RTOG 0521 trial addressed this question and randomized 562 patients between RT/HT and RT/HT/CT (docetaxel) (8). Preliminary results suggest a statistically significant improvement in 4-year OS, from 89% to 93%. Although a longer follow-up is needed, this trial may lead to a novel paradigm shift toward CMT in the management of select patients at higher risk of developing resistance to standard treatment options.

The usage of combined CT and RT continues to expand. With the growth of personalized medicine and the conception of precision radiotherapy, a pivotal effect of evidence-driven oncology has been the attempt to delineate specific subpopulations in which CMT is optimal. It is important to recognize that this entity remains ever changing, with future advances highly likely to revise and refine the current standards.

## TECHNIQUES

This section will discuss the two primary methods for administering combined CRT: sequentially (Table 1.1) and concurrently (Table 1.2). The existence of high-level evidence regarding outcomes and expected treatment toxicities largely drives the clinical decision making for either technique. For some cancer types, but not for others, the synergy between CT and RT has been proven; radiosensitization has been well documented for many CT compounds (eg, platinum compounds, fluoropyrimidines/capecitabine, and gemcitabine). Although enhanced neoplastic destruction is the ultimate goal of oncologic management, these potential gains must be weighed against the toxicities that often amplify when CT and RT are given together. Seminal trials have quantified not only the magnitude of outcome benefits but also the increase in various toxicities

**TABLE 1.1** Comparison of the advantages and disadvantages of *sequential* chemoradiotherapy over radiotherapy alone

| Pros | Cons |
| --- | --- |
| • Control of both primary disease and potential micrometastases | • Increased toxicities over unimodality therapy alone |
| • Tailor second modality treatment to the response of the first | • Suboptimal tolerance of first treatment may impair complete receipt of secondary therapy |
| • Debulking of large tumor mass, possibly resulting in increased efficacy of the second modality | • Could promote the development of clones resistant to the initial therapy that are more difficult to treat with the second modality |

**TABLE 1.2** Comparison of the advantages and disadvantages of *concurrent* chemoradiotherapy over radiotherapy alone

| Pros | Cons |
| --- | --- |
| • Simultaneous treatment of both primary disease and potential micrometastases | • Increased toxicities over unimodality therapy alone |
| • Potential radiosensitization, possibly leading to increased local control | • Possibility of not receiving a complete course of either treatment |
| • Possibly associated with needing lower doses of either modality or smaller radiotherapy fields | • No ability to cytoreduce the tumor burden |

with concurrent CRT. Hence, although various tumor types and clinical circumstances may lend themselves to CMT, clinicians must first decide whether a given patient is a candidate for it. Subsequently, they must determine, based on available evidence as well as several patient-specific factors, whether the expected benefits of concurrent CRT outweigh its potentially increased toxicity risks. These decisions may be best made, when possible, in a multidisciplinary fashion and on a case-by-case basis.

## Sequential Chemoradiation

As previously mentioned, the goal of combining CT and RT—regardless of timing or technique—is to control both the primary disease and potential micrometastases. It is important to understand that each malignancy has a certain risk of metastatic spread that is influenced by several factors not limited to tumor histology, differentiation, genetics, location, and stage. Patient factors such as cancer history, prior RT and/or CT, and immune system status are also important to consider. The oncologist's goal is to holistically estimate the risk of metastasis outside the primary site or the likelihood of local tumor control with and without CMT and add CT accordingly. Breast cancer, for which gene panels have been clinically validated to correlate with the risks of lymphatic and distant spread, is the most ubiquitous example of this concept (9). Hence, quantification of this risk has resulted in the administration of CT after RT in patients with genetics portending metastasis. Nevertheless, this section will elaborate on the advantages of sequencing RT before or after CT.

Two important rationales for the administration of CT followed by RT can be illustrated using the example of non-Hodgkin's lymphoma. The Southwestern Oncology Group (SWOG) 8736 trial randomized 401 patients to eight cycles of CHOP (cyclophosphamide, doxorubicin, vincristine, and prednisone) CT versus three cycles plus involved-field RT (40–55 Gy) (10). The addition of RT to CT resulted in a significant increase in 5-year progression-free survival (PFS) from 64% to 77% and a corresponding OS benefit from 72% to 82%. The first concept demonstrated in this trial was that the addition of RT allowed for a shorter CT course. Although often extrapolated to signify decreased CT doses if RT will be delivered, either method may result in fewer toxicities. Indeed, in the SWOG trial, there was a trend toward decreased life-threatening toxicities in the CMT group. Therefore, in patients who may not be able to tolerate a full course or dose of CT, CMT may be advantageous. Second, the evolution of RT for lymphoma has now moved to involved-site RT as the standard of care. The administration of CT prior to RT is therefore helpful to radiation oncologists to decrease treatment volumes, more sharply define the major foci of disease, and even reduce total RT doses.

Conversely, certain situations are best suited for the delivery of RT prior to CT. The central nervous system poses a challenge to the penetration of CT agents; therefore, it has historically been advocated to treat newly diagnosed brain metastases (especially if symptomatic) with RT (or surgery) prior to commencing CT for metastatic disease. This can be conceptualized by examining a subset of pediatric medulloblastomas treated as part of a prospective randomized trial in Germany (11). The study randomized 127 patients from multiple risk groups to immediate postoperative RT (35.2 Gy/16 fractions followed by a 20-Gy/10 fraction boost to the posterior fossa) followed by CT (intravenous ifosfamide, etoposide, methotrexate, cisplatin, and cytarabine) versus CT followed by RT. Relapse-free survival at 3 years statistically favored the RT before CT group over the CT before RT group (78% vs. 65%). Multiple factors can potentially explain this. First, bone marrow toxicity initiated by CT and exacerbated by craniospinal RT often resulted in treatment delays and prolongation of the overall treatment time. Next, RT might act directly without impedance by the blood–brain barrier. Overall, however, anatomic circumstances, such as those of the central nervous system, often necessitate sequential RT followed by CT for optimal disease control.

## Concurrent Chemoradiation

Concurrent CRT can be delivered for various reasons, but it is commonly believed that the effects of both CT and RT can be greater than either alone, or even when delivered sequentially. It is important to first answer whether prospective studies have demonstrated a local control benefit of concurrent CRT over RT alone. Although strong supporting data for CRT exist for many disease sites, concurrent CRT is often given in various other settings without optimal evidence (eg, select cases of locoregionally recurrent disease). These decisions are largely at the discretion of the treating oncologists; a factor to consider is that concurrent CRT may result in decreased doses of CT, RT, or both. This may assist in shortening the treatment course and preventing major toxicities. Two major advantages of concurrent CRT will be expounded upon hereafter: radiosensitization and controlling disease progression to allow surgical resection.

One instance of true radiosensitization from concurrent CRT leading to improved survival was described in a phase III trial from the United Kingdom (12). This trial randomized 585 locally advanced anal cancer patients between RT alone (45 Gy + 15–25-Gy brachytherapy boost depending on response) and RT with the continuous infusion of 5-fluorouracil and mitomycin C. This study demonstrated a statistically significant improvement in local control from 41% to 64% with the addition of concurrent CT. This corresponded to improved outcomes; although OS was not statistically different, 3-year cancer-specific survival improved from 61% to 72%. This paradigm has also been demonstrated to be efficacious in several other malignancies, including lung cancer. Among patients with locally advanced non–small cell lung cancer (NSCLC), the benefit of concurrent CRT over sequential CT followed by RT in a meta-analysis was limited to an improvement in locoregional progression with no difference in distant progression. The 6.1% improvement in locoregional progression at 5 years (35.0% vs. 28.9%) drove a 4.5% survival benefit with concurrent CRT (15.1% vs. 10.6%) at 5 years (13). A current area of active investigation is assessing whether clinically apparent radiosensitization is achieved with targeted therapies. If proven, these therapies would be important in neoplasms that are relatively radioresistant and to patients who may not be able to tolerate RT with concurrent cytotoxic CT.

Another emerging application of concurrent CRT is to control disease progression enough to perform surgery—exemplified by the rise of concurrent neoadjuvant CRT for pancreatic cancer (14). Pancreatic adenocarcinoma is a highly aggressive neoplasm with a very poor survival rate, and disease progression is nearly inevitable. Surgical resection offers the greatest OS benefit, but most patients are either unresectable or borderline resectable. Although the majority of initially unresectable patients do not undergo resection, borderline resectable disease (abutting but not invading/encircling key arteries such as the celiac, common hepatic, or superior mesenteric) is a different scenario. The goal of CRT in these patients is twofold: first, neoadjuvant therapy must halt disease progression, ideally both locally (which could result in worsening involvement of the arterial vasculature) and distantly. Second, although achieving a clinical (or pathologic) complete response to neoadjuvant CRT is unlikely, decreasing the disease burden even slightly near the vasculature may greatly assist in the technical aspects of surgical resection. Theoretically, the rate of positive margins (eg, on the vasculature) could be decreased as well with this approach. The benefits of local control for pancreatic adenocarcinoma are being further assessed with ongoing prospective trials using stereotactic body radiation therapy.

## TIMING

Concurrent CRT has many advantages in oncologic therapy. However, regarding the third pillar of cancer care, surgery, the temporally based placement of CRT relative to surgery becomes a major factor. The implications of CRT timing include differential CT and RT doses, RT volumes, and opportunities for salvage therapy. Although the timing of CT and/or RT has been justified through high-volume clinical trials in most neoplasms, it is less certain in other

**TABLE 1.3**  Benefits of definitive, neoadjuvant, and adjuvant chemoradiotherapy

| Definitive | Adjuvant | Neoadjuvant |
|---|---|---|
| • Avoids the morbidity of surgical procedures<br>• Addresses areas of micrometastasis that surgery does not<br>• Allows for organ preservation<br>• Potentially allows for salvage options with surgery | • Information from surgical pathology may be useful for subsequent therapy<br>• May not directly cause potential surgical complications<br>• Sterilizes microscopic disease after resection, including elective irradiation | • Well-defined radiotherapy volumes and lower doses<br>• Avoids postoperative hypoxia and potential radioresistance<br>• Can allow for tumor debulking to possibly make surgery safer and/or less extensive |

cancers (eg, pancreatic cancer, as mentioned previously). This section will discuss the concepts and the principles behind definitive, adjuvant, and neoadjuvant CRT, most often in the concurrent setting (Table 1.3).

### Definitive Chemoradiation

Definitive CRT is generally delivered with a goal of curing the patient, without surgery as an immediate management option. In this circumstance the goal of CRT is to sterilize the entire bulk of disease, as well as address possible micrometastases. Because surgery is often not expected to address all possible high-risk areas of metastasis (eg, regional lymphatics), the radiation oncologist is correspondingly expected to judiciously treat these areas. Whereas in the past, the data for some neoplasms supported definitive RT or CRT over surgical-based options (as demonstrated in bulky cervical cancer [15]), for other malignancies recent paradigms are reintroducing surgery for conditions in which it was previously not standard (eg, ongoing clinical trials of transoral resection in p16+ oropharyngeal squamous cell carcinoma). The subsequent discussion of definitive CRT presents examples of nonoperative circumstances and organ preservation.

The most ubiquitous use of definitive CRT is for nonoperative conditions, which encompass medical inoperability, technical/surgical inoperability, synchronous diseases necessitating immediate treatment, and/or patient refusal. For instance, many locally advanced NSCLC patients are not surgical candidates, largely owing to poor cardiopulmonary function from an extensive smoking history. A randomized trial of 155 nonoperative stage III NSCLC patients receiving cisplatin/vinblastine followed by RT (60 Gy/30 fractions) versus RT alone was published in 1990 (16). The authors were able to discern a statistically significant OS benefit with combined therapy (13.8 months vs. 9.7 months). A randomized trial of 610 nonoperative stage III NSCLC patients subsequently demonstrated concurrent CRT to be superior to the sequential treatment (17). The median OS statistically improved from 14.6 months to 17.0 months with concurrent CRT, which has now become the standard, definitive treatment for nonoperative NSCLC.

In addition to its analog in many laryngeal cancer cases, definitive CRT is now the chief rationale for bladder-preservation therapy in appropriate instances of muscle-invasive (T2–T4) bladder cancer. Although no randomized trials have been conducted comparing radical cystectomy to bladder preservation, an early report in the mid–1980s by the Danish National Bladder Cancer Group demonstrated no differences in OS between neoadjuvant RT (40 Gy/20 fractions) followed by cystectomy versus definitive RT (60 Gy/30 fractions) (18). This randomized trial of 183 patients, despite showing that surgery substantially improved pelvic control rates (35% vs. 7%), did not reveal an OS benefit. Retrospective data demonstrating no discernible differences in 10-year OS with either definitive RT or cystectomy have backed this up (19). In 2012 a prospective 360-patient study showed that RT alone (55 Gy/20 fractions or 64 Gy/ 32 fractions) was inferior to CRT (with a continuous infusion of 5-fluorouracil and mitomycin C) (20). Although OS was numerically improved in the CRT arm (48% vs. 35%), it did not reach statistical significance. However, 2-year locoregional disease-free survival was statistically higher in the CRT arm (67% vs. 54%), indicating potential radiosensitization. Furthermore, although a secondary end point of salvage cystectomy rates was underpowered, there was a trend toward increased salvage cystectomies in the RT-only group (17% vs. 11%). Overall, these and other data have resulted in national recommendations for select (eg, unifocal T2–T4, <5 cm, and good bladder function without hydronephrosis or hydroureter) patients to undergo concurrent CRT as part of bladder-preservation therapy.

## Adjuvant Chemoradiation

Adjuvant CRT poses unique challenges to the radiation oncologist. RT doses are generally higher than those of preoperative RT (particularly with certain surgical findings such as close/positive surgical margins or concerning histological features), which may result in increased toxicities. These may in turn escalate if concurrent CRT (as opposed to sequential) is delivered. Furthermore, some patients recovering from surgery may also tolerate CRT less well or be more susceptible to toxicities (ie, radiation pneumonitis in patients receiving RT after thoracic surgery) than surgery-naïve patients. In terms of RT treatment planning, treatment volumes are less well defined, including (provided optimally performed surgery) no gross tumor volume, resulting in a subjective definition of high-risk targets. Owing to surgery, tissue architecture (eg, natural anatomic boundaries or fat planes) is distorted, which may result in differential dose-volume distributions that may not have occurred before surgery or large RT volumes necessary to attempt to control microscopic disease or sites of potential spread from surgical tracking (ie, sarcoma or mesothelioma). Moreover, the relatively hypoxic tissue state postoperatively may be radiobiologically unfavorable because hypoxia has been extensively linked to radioresistance. Although the clinician must be aware of the risks associated with adjuvant CRT, its relatively common use has proven efficacious and will continue to be used in several neoplasms. Hereafter, two advantages of adjuvant CRT will be noted: as a postoperative effort to sterilize microscopic disease in aggressive neoplasms and as an addition in the event of worrisome surgical findings.

One use of adjuvant CRT is to sterilize as much microscopic disease as possible after resection, even with negative surgical margins. This is especially true of malignancies with high rates of regional nodal metastases, for which adjuvant RT can attempt to sterilize nodal spread, or for highly malignant neoplasms such as mesothelioma, for which CRT is often delivered after extrapleural pneumonectomy. This malignancy, which usually carries a very poor prognosis, was associated with encouraging outcomes when investigators at Harvard treated 183 patients with adjuvant RT (30 Gy/20 fractions followed by a boost to 50.4 Gy) and concurrent paclitaxel followed by subsequent paclitaxel (21). In patients with epithelial histology, no extra-pleural lymph nodes, and negative surgical margins, , 5-year survival was reported to be 46%. Additionally, intriguing phase II results were published by Italian investigators who administered postoperative intrapleural epidoxorubicin and interleukin-2 along with subsequent RT (30 Gy), followed by systemic cisplatin/gemcitabine, as well as long-term interleukin-2 (22). Of 49 patients receiving this multimodality regimen, 13 were alive at a median follow-up of nearly 5 years, resulting in a 5-year survival of 23%, along with a corresponding median OS of 26 months. Hence, aggressive postoperative multimodality therapy may be useful to eliminate potential foci of microscopic disease in an equally aggressive tumor.

The necessity of adjuvant CRT depending on surgical findings, similar to that illustrated with head and neck cancers with positive surgical margins and/or extracapsular extension, is well delineated in carcinoma of the cervix, as shown in the Gynecologic Oncology Group 109 (RTOG 9112) study (23). This randomized trial included 243 patients with stages IB/IIA and IA2 cervical cancer after radical hysterectomy and pelvic lymphadenectomy with positive nodes, surgical margins, and/or parametrial extension. Two arms were compared: RT alone (49.3 Gy/29 fractions) versus concurrent RT and cisplatin/5-fluorouracil CT. There was a substantial improvement with the addition of CT to RT in both PFS (80% vs. 63%) and OS (81% vs. 71%) at 4 years. Although toxicities (hematologic and gastrointestinal) increased in the CRT group, administering CRT to these high-risk patients is now the standard of care based on surgical and pathologic findings.

## Neoadjuvant Chemoradiation

As discussed previously, neoadjuvant CRT offers many advantages in oncologic care, including more defined treatment volumes (partially as a result of intact tissue architecture), lower doses, and no frank hypoxia in the microenvironment from surgery. The timing of neoadjuvant therapy also has salient risks and benefits; although neoadjuvant CRT may offer early management of possible micro-metastases, delays in surgery could be a risk with this method. Additionally, a principal goal of neoadjuvant therapy (especially CRT) is to decrease the disease burden to make resection more feasible, potentially including increased rates of pathologic complete response, negative resection margins, and a decreased risk of resecting critical/semicritical structures. However, receiving a full course of CRT, especially when delivered concurrently, may make surgical resection logistically or technically difficult to perform and could be associated with greater surgical morbidities and mortality. An example of this phenomenon (without the contribution of CT) is the more common use of salvage irradiation to treat postprostatectomy relapsed disease but largely a lack of salvage surgery after full-dose prostatic irradiation and subsequent relapse. Taken together, although neoadjuvant therapy, like adjuvant therapy, provides many notable benefits, these are very often not without notable risks. The next section will elaborate upon two concepts that support the use of neoadjuvant CRT: treatment adherence/surgical downstaging and organ preservation.

A classic randomized trial demonstrating the prominent benefits of neoadjuvant CRT was published by German investigators in 2004, randomizing 823 patients with locally advanced rectal cancer to preoperative or postoperative CRT (24). The CT used in the trial was 5-fluorouracil, and RT was delivered to a total dose of 50.4 Gy/28 fractions preoperatively versus 55.8 Gy/31 fractions postoperatively. First, intuitively, there were no differences in major outcomes between groups, including disease-free survival, distant metastases, or OS at 5 years. There was, however, a significant local control benefit to neoadjuvant therapy (local recurrence was 6% vs. 13%); this is possibly related to downstaging from neoadjuvant therapy, although only 8% of patients experienced a pathologic complete response. A potentially more likely reason is that whereas 92% of preoperatively treated patients received the full RT dose, this was true for only 54% of postoperative cases. This highlights a major advantage of neoadjuvant therapy, during which physiologic conditions are less impaired by surgical manipulation, and CRT tolerance may be higher. It follows that both acute (27% vs. 40%) and late (14% vs. 24%) toxicities were decreased with neoadjuvant therapy without a statistically significant increase in postoperative complications. Although the study did not examine the rates of positive surgical margins with either approach, neoadjuvant CRT for esophageal cancer has been shown to decrease such incidences (3). Arguably, the most important point is that among patients initially suspected to be eligible for sphincter-preserving surgery, preoperative therapy was associated with a twofold increase in the completion of sphincter-preserving surgeries (39% vs. 19%). This important phase III trial highlights the fact that neoadjuvant therapy is often associated with fewer toxicities and treatment breaks or delays, along with a decreased necessity to surgically remove important structures (eg, the anal sphincter).

This notion of neoadjuvant CRT attenuating the neoplastic burden enough to perform less extensive surgery provides another significant rationale for preoperative CRT. Although level I, randomized evidence for using neoadjuvant CRT to spare limbs in the treatment of sarcoma is currently lacking, it is very common to perform preoperative CRT not only to increase the chances for limb preservation but also to avoid the surgical removal of structures such as nerves, bone, and some vasculature. The largest recent neoadjuvant CRT series, from Poland, describes 100 synovial sarcoma cases (20 Gy/5 fractions and ifosfamide/cisplatin/doxorubicin). Of these patients, 89% were able to undergo limb-sparing surgery (25). The 5-year OS was 76%, and 38% of patients developed wound complications—a number similar to the 35% seen in phase III data on preoperative RT (26). Although it can be problematic to compare data between studies, no evidence suggests that the addition of CT to neoadjuvant RT increases these complications. Therefore, although phase III data comparing preoperative CRT to RT alone are not available, CRT may benefit patients with high-risk disease, such as large, deeply situated, and/or high-grade tumors, in the efforts to promote limb preservation.

## MANAGEMENT OF TOXICITIES

Adverse effects from CRT can occur for several reasons; based on the mechanisms of CT and RT of killing actively cycling cells, it is intuitive that administering both in succession—and especially together—could damage a larger volume of normal tissues to a greater degree. Much of the aforementioned prospective clinical data on CRT (particularly concurrent CRT) have demonstrated numerically or statistically significantly greater toxicities with CRT. These have in turn increased in both the frequency and severity of toxicities. Because toxicities are often categorized as *acute* or *late*, CRT may incur adverse effects long after the cessation of treatment. Although late RT toxicities are thought to pertain to the surrounding organs exposed to irradiation, late CT toxicities can resemble and amplify some RT toxicities. Examples include chronic fatigue, premature aging, cognitive dysfunction, cardiac dysfunction, infertility, and secondary malignancies (most commonly leukemias or myelodysplasias). Hence, multidisciplinary oncologists are expected to closely monitor patients undergoing CRT for acute toxicities, but additional longer-term follow-up in these patients is also warranted. The next section will thematically evaluate several strategies to reduce toxicities from CRT: patient selection, CT and RT factors, RT modalities, and supportive care.

## Patient Selection

Depending on the primary neoplasm, adverse effects from treatment may occur to different degrees in various subpopulations and scenarios. The presence of important patient variables such as age, performance status, and pre-existing comorbidities plays a large role in selecting patients fit for CRT. Specifically, many medical oncologists may hesitate to administer CT to patients with a poor performance status due to their expected low tolerance of the treatment. Although RT can often be better tolerated than CT, performance status may have an impact on the ability to deliver RT or the extent to which RT is delivered. Age is often used as a binary cut off, with data on some (eg, head and neck) cancers demonstrating no benefit to using CT in "elderly" patients (27). However, age and performance status should ideally be used hand in hand to determine the appropriateness of CRT; quantitative measures such as the Comprehensive Geriatric Assessment, which takes into account several medical, functional, and psychosocial factors, are often useful to assess tolerance to CRT. Because several elements play into a patient's tolerance of CRT, studies that assess the tolerance and efficacy of CT and/or RT regimens in vulnerable populations must examine not only specific subgroups (eg, based on age, performance status, comorbidities, etc) but also other end points aside from crude toxicity (eg, hospitalization rates and treatment compliance).

Clinical scenarios that may signal poor CRT tolerance include reirradiation and treatment designed for curative versus palliative intent. Reirradiation is challenging and presents difficult decisions for the radiation oncologist regarding doses, volumes, and treatment logistics. Although a longer interval is preferred between RT courses, this may not be feasible in aggressive, locally recurrent malignancies. In many cases, therefore, the multidisciplinary management and balancing of doses and schedules of RT versus CT may be quite important. Similarly, RT doses are generally lower in palliative circumstances compared to curative purposes. Often in practice, however, the line between both is blurred with so-called aggressive palliation approaches in which the patient's prognosis is poor, but delivered RT doses exceed those required for traditional palliative circumstances. This is perhaps most notable in patients with stage IV oligometastatic disease who are treated with definitive doses of RT in an attempt to achieve durable local control, improve progression-free survival, delay the next line of systemic therapy until needed, and in select cases possibly lengthen OS. Although the location of irradiation plays a large role in tolerating these increased doses, toxicities may occur at nearly any anatomical location. Oncologists must recognize the specific clinical scenario calling for potential CRT, which in addition to the variables already discussed can assist in the modification of treatment regimens and logistics to minimize toxicity.

A burgeoning area of patient selection for CMT that is expected to become increasingly crucial in the future is related to molecular/genetic analysis. Using advanced techniques and biomarkers, researchers hope to develop molecular signatures, stratifying patients into those who may need escalated or de-escalated therapies. This was elegantly illustrated in the EORTC 26951 randomized study of 368 anaplastic oligodendrogliomas receiving RT (59.4 Gy/33 fractions) with or without adjuvant CT (procarbazine, lomustine, and vincristine) (28). Although a benefit with CMT was indicated in all patients, tumors with the 1p/19q codeletion exhibited a strong trend toward increased OS with CMT (median OS not reached vs. 112 months). Those without the codeletion showed statistically insignificant differences in median OS (25 months vs. 21 months). These molecular/genetic stratifications of randomized trials are needed to examine which patients could benefit from de-escalated therapies and hence potentially decreased toxicities. In addition to microRNA sequencing for prognostic purposes, this paradigm is being actively emulated in ongoing clinical trials of p16+ oropharyngeal squamous cell carcinoma at certain stages by evaluating decreased RT doses and/or decreasing, replacing, or omitting CT doses.

## Chemotherapy Factors

CT alterations during therapy are designed to relieve toxicities that could affect further CT/CRT adherence. Owing to their structural similarity, several CT agents (eg, cisplatin and carboplatin) are often used interchangeably for oncotoxic purposes, yet they can display strikingly different toxicity profiles. CT doses and intervals of administration are also commonly adjusted due to toxicity concerns. The modality of CT administration (eg, bolus vs. continuous infusion) can also be modified. Lastly, if toxicities persist, sequential CRT (preferably without RT interruption) may be the best option if CMT is in the best interests of the patient. It should be noted, however, that head–to–head data indicating the superiority of a CT approach (eg, dose, frequency, modality, and timing) may or may not be available for each tumor type. Accordingly, although modifying CT treatments may be associated with poorer outcomes, oncological medicine's goal has always been to balance tumoricidal benefits and toxicities. If, as judged by the treating physician, a patient is experiencing severe toxicities that threaten the baseline health state or the ability to complete oncologic therapy, CT modification may be required despite the known impact.

Systemic therapy has undergone revolutionary changes in recent years, with targeted therapies (TT) and immunotherapy purported to be "the next frontier" of cancer therapy. TT, discussed in more detail in a subsequent chapter, are most commonly small-molecule inhibitors or humanized antibodies that can provide immense potential to relieve toxicities when compared with existing "nonspecific" CT. This is largely a result of a very specific mechanism of action that often targets a certain subsite of an individual receptor isoform. TT may fit into several paradigms of cancer treatment. First, the addition of TT to existing CT/RT/CRT is a major question that needs to be addressed; specifically, whether additive or synergistic effects are shown with multimodality therapy. The ramifications for radiosensitization and chemosensitization by TT, if proven, would be immense and may necessitate revising current dogmatic therapeutic approaches. Second, replacing CT with TT is a pragmatic option, which if proven successful could result in a significant drop in toxicities from systemic therapy. It may enable patients unfit for CT to receive systemic therapy or allow patients at risk of developing toxicities with CMT to still receive multimodality therapy (albeit in a different form).

One of the first randomized trials utilizing TT was designed for patients with head and neck cancers who may not be able to receive CMT. That trial randomized 424 patients to RT alone (three possible dose/fractionation regimens) versus RT with the epidermal growth factor receptor–inhibiting antibody cetuximab (29). The in vitro radiosensitizing properties of cetuximab were supported by increased locoregional control in the CMT arm (24 months vs. 15 months), and this corresponded to not only a statistical increase in PFS but an OS benefit as well (49 months vs. 29 months). And importantly, with the exception of acneiform rash and infusion reactions, toxicities were no different between groups. In a population prone to treatment breaks, treatment delays, and morbidities (eg, anorexia or feeding tube placement) from radiation mucositis, these results were compelling. Ongoing clinical trials in multiple other tumors are aiming to assess the efficacy of cetuximab and other TT either in lieu of CT or in addition to CT.

## Radiation Therapy Factors

RT doses and volumes may be modified to curb toxicities during treatment. Although many tumor types and clinical scenarios may warrant certain "minimal doses" for optimal tumor control—either from radiobiological principles and/or clinical trials—prescribed doses are often larger. For instance, despite the dose of 41.4 Gy used in the CROSS trial (3) of neoadjuvant concurrent CRT for esophageal cancer, many clinicians opt to treat to 45 or 50.4 Gy. In stage III NSCLC treated with definitive concurrent CRT, the superior arm of the recent RTOG 0617 trial used a treatment of 60 Gy and not the dose-escalated arm to 74 Gy, and yet it is commonplace for these patients to receive 63–66 Gy (30). Although there will likely never be randomized trials of two dose levels in such proximity, consideration should be given to decreasing absolute doses in patients with a poor performance status or who may have more difficulty tolerating CMT.

Next, the role of RT volumes is controversial and is largely dependent on physician preference or based on a clinical protocol. However, with the rapid increase in image-guided platforms, decreasing planning target volume margins (and thus the treatment volume) has been a major subject of investigation across numerous disease sites. The increase in metallic fiducials and electromagnetic transponders for several different tumors has necessitated dealing with this issue on a case-by-case basis, including the type and precision of image guidance, to provide high-fidelity RT delivery. However, for the purposes of this section, the modification of margins does remain an understudied facet of reducing irradiated volumes and hence potentially decreasing toxicity risks.

Consequently, RT fractionation is an important consideration for the radiation oncologist. Hypofractionated RT, delivering larger doses per fraction than conventional RT (generally 1.8–2.0 Gy per fraction), can lead to treatment toxicities (acute and late)—especially late toxicities to organs at risk (OAR) at anatomically adjacent areas. The decision to hypofractionate should be guided by consulting the available literature and clinically judging the toxicity risk of each patient. For example, stereotactic body radiotherapy for pancreatic head adenocarcinomas prompted a revision from the initially used single fraction (25 Gy/1 fraction) to a multifraction regimen (largely institution dependent) owing to substantial late toxicities with single-fraction delivery (31).

Conversely, late toxicities can often be reduced by greater fractionation, but acute toxicities are amplified with hyperfractionated RT. This was best demonstrated in a randomized study of 417 patients with limited-stage small cell lung cancer treated with concurrent CRT (cisplatin/etoposide) in a hyperfractionated (45 Gy in 30 twice-daily fractions) or conventionally fractionated

(45 Gy in 25 once-daily fractions) manner (32). Although the hyperfractionated arm showed a statistically significant OS improvement (23 months vs. 19 months), acute grade 3 esophageal toxicity occurred in 27% of patients, compared with 11% in the conventionally fractionated arm. Despite the OS improvement, many centers opt to treat these patients with conventional fractionation, either due to concerns about toxicity or because of patient and/or facility difficulties in delivering twice daily irradiation with fractions at least 6 hours apart. Taken together, both hypofractionation and hyperfractionation offer a balance of risks and benefits, and these pros and cons must especially be weighed in the context of CMT. Accordingly, RT dose, fractionation, and treatment volumes must be tailored on a case-by-case basis to ensure proper treatment completion and control of toxicities.

## Radiation Therapy Modalities

The applicability of many clinical trials from the past is to some extent limited, owing to the present ubiquity of more conformal RT techniques, and thus toxicity profiles and toxicity-related mortality from older studies may not be representative of modern RT. The development of three-dimensional conformal radiotherapy (3DCRT), using high-quality three-dimensional anatomical definition of targets and OAR, has allowed for high-quality target localization and more precisely controlled RT doses to nearby OAR. The advent of inverse-planned algorithms has given IMRT increased target conformality and dosimetric accuracy over 3DCRT planning. IMRT has been proven to offer clinically superior toxicity profiles over 3DCRT for several tumor types, most prominently those that involve the close apposition of target volumes and OAR. Thus, when performing concurrent CRT, highly conformal RT techniques, such as IMRT, may be preferable in many cases.

Stereotactic radiotherapy (SRT), the focus of a subsequent chapter, has also revolutionized the treatment of several disease sites. The shortened treatment course, which allows for optimal patient convenience and improved cost-effectiveness, makes SRT an attractive option to treat a wide area of anatomic sites in a variety of clinical settings (eg, localized and metastatic disease, primary RT and reirradiation). The high conformality of SRT is at the crux of its potential in minimizing doses to surrounding OAR, especially at anatomically vulnerable areas. However, because SRT is most commonly performed in five or fewer fractions, it has a small overlap with CT administration, and therefore potential radiosensitization is more challenging. Nevertheless, its application for patients with substantial comorbidities is especially noteworthy, and it is the standard of care in nonoperative early-stage NSCLC. There is rapidly growing evidence that the extreme hypofractionated nature of its delivery results in substantially greater tumor control than conventionally fractionated RT (33). An intriguing combination of certain cancers treated with SRT and immunotherapy could be a logical next step to further reduce toxicities from traditional CRT.

The most recent technology to rise rapidly in radiation oncology care is proton beam therapy (PBT), which when delivered via several advanced techniques and approaches (eg, pencil-beam scanned PBT or intensity-modulated proton therapy) augments dosimetric advantages even greater than passively scattered proton therapy methods. A fundamental principle of PBT is the ability to place the location of maximal dose deposition (the Bragg peak) and provide essentially no exit dose distal to the target volume of interest. Doing so decreases the overall integral dose to patients and decreases numerical doses to surrounding OAR. However, a substantial knowledge gap exists regarding whether dosimetric gains translate to clinically reduced toxicities and if so, in which patients PBT proves most useful. Other issues associated with PBT need convincing resolution as well, including range uncertainties due to unforeseen heterodensities in the beam path and the economic sustainability of PBT centers. Additionally, the conformality of PBT may lend itself to dose-escalation strategies, but toxicities in those scenarios (especially as part of CMT) may be a concern and warrant further study. Although a complete discussion of PBT is beyond the scope of this chapter, multiple prospective trials are determining the safety and efficacy of PBT for a wide variety of neoplasms. Three open phase III studies (prostate, lung, and breast cancers) are currently examining the efficacy and toxicities of PBT versus photon-based RT. When mature, these trials will provide the highest level of evidence to date in determining whether PBT can enhance the therapeutic ratio over photon-based RT, along with analyzing several secondary end points such as quality of life and cost-effectiveness. The results of these trials will have major implications, including whether adding PBT to concurrent CRT is safe and feasible.

## Supportive Care

The value of proper ancillary care cannot be understated in any form of oncologic therapy. This extends not only to those individuals close to the patient but also to hospital-based teams. With regard to a multidisciplinary oncologic care team, the assistance of social workers, nurses, psychologists, counselors, therapists, and nutritionists, among others, is essential. All members of the oncologic team should ideally be able to recognize common toxicities and conditions (eg, depression) in all patients—including quickly identifying those at higher risk of developing such symptoms—and respond with early and effective interventions. Despite the often disappointing randomized trial results of radioprotectors in patients undergoing concurrent CRT (34), the liberal use of supportive medications given concurrently with RT—or even prophylactically—is often beneficial. The early institution of palliative care is highly recommended in appropriate patients, owing to improved reported mood and quality of life (35). Although mood and quality of life are quantifiable, they are often dismissed as "subjective measures." However, the symptoms of a cancer patient, regardless of the receipt of CRT, are often labeled as both physical and mental; pain, for instance, is known to be a neurological perception. The perception of toxicities and their amelioration is a grossly understudied topic in oncological medicine. A randomized study of 235 women with metastatic breast cancer demonstrated that the "perception of pain" improved in women receiving supportive-expressive group therapy for 90 minutes per week (36). Such results, although not as often quoted as clinical outcome measures, are prime examples that patients' oncologic battles are mental as well as physical. These results have intuitive applications in patients suffering toxicities from CRT as well, and cancer care teams are encouraged to resourcefully address the patient as a whole instead of addressing just the neoplasm itself.

## CONCLUSIONS

As medicine transitions into a new era of personalized care, oncology faces a multitude of challenges and unanswered questions but also potentially paradigm-changing discoveries. Although one must look to future goals, recalling the lessons of the past is essential. CT and RT have both progressed substantially just in the last 10 years, and the dogmatic definition of combining CT and RT will likely undergo rapid continued evolution in the decades to come. A chief goal of these advancements will be to alleviate iatrogenic toxicities through increased precision at the cellular, molecular, and atomic levels. If successful, it is certainly possible that these "advancements" of precision can one day be hailed as the standard of care in multidisciplinary oncologic therapy.

## References


1. Stupp R, Mason WP, van den Bent MJ, et al. Radiotherapy plus concomitant and adjuvant temozolomide for glioblastoma. *N Engl J Med*. 2005;352(10):987–996.
2. Henderson MA, Burmeister BH, Ainslie J, et al. Adjuvant lymph-node field radiotherapy versus observation only in patients with melanoma at high risk of further lymph-node field relapse after lymphadenectomy (ANZMTG 01.02/TROG 02.01): 6-year follow-up of a phase 3, randomised controlled trial. *Lancet Oncol*. 2015;16(9):1049–1060.
3. van Hagen P, Hulshof MC, van Lanschot JJ, et al. Preoperative chemoradiotherapy for esophageal or junctional cancer. *N Engl J Med*. 2012;366(22):2074–2084.

4. Mamounas EP, Anderson SJ, Dignam JJ, et al. Predictors of locoregional recurrence after neoadjuvant chemotherapy: results from combined analysis of National Surgical Adjuvant Breast and Bowel Project B-18 and B-27. *J Clin Oncol.* 2012;20(32):3960–3966.

5. Cooper JS, Pajak TF, Forastiere AA, et al. Postoperative concurrent radiotherapy and chemotherapy for high-risk squamous-cell carcinoma of the head and neck. *N Engl J Med.* 2004;350(19):1937–1944.

6. Bernier J, Domenge C, Ozsahin M, et al. Postoperative irradiation with or without concomitant chemotherapy for locally advanced head and neck cancer. *N Engl J Med.* 2004;350(19):1945–1952.

7. Bernier J, Cooper JS, Pajak TF, et al. Defining risk levels in locally advanced head and neck cancers: a comparative analysis of concurrent postoperative radiation plus chemotherapy trials of the EORTC (#22931) and RTOG (#9501). *Head Neck.* 2005;27(10):843–850.

8. Sandler HM, Hu C, Rosenthal SA, et al. A phase III protocol of androgen suppression (AS) and 3DCRT/IMRT versus AS and 3DCRT/IMRT followed by chemotherapy (CT) with docetaxel and prednisone for localized, high-risk prostate cancer (RTOG 0521) [abstract LBA5002]. *J Clin Oncol.* 2015;33(suppl).

9. Sparano JA, Gray RJ, Makower DF, et al. Prospective validation of a 21-gene expression array in breast cancer. *N Engl J Med.* 2015;373(21):2005–2014.

10. Miller TP, Dahlberg S, Cassady JR, et al. Chemotherapy alone compared with chemotherapy plus radiotherapy for localized intermediate- and high-grade non-Hodgkin's lymphoma. *N Engl J Med.* 1998;339(1):21–26.

11. Kortmann RD, Kuhl J, Timmermann B, et al. Postoperative neoadjuvant chemotherapy before radiotherapy as compared to immediate radiotherapy followed by maintenance chemotherapy in the treatment of medulloblastoma in childhood: results of the German prospective randomized trial HIT '91. *Int J Radiat Oncol Biol Phys.* 2000;46(2):269–279.

12. UKCCCR Anal Cancer Working Party. Epidermoid anal cancer: results from the UKCCCR randomised trial of radiotherapy alone versus radiotherapy, 5-fluorouracil, and mitomycin. *Lancet.* 1996;348(9034):1049–1054.

13. Auperin A, Le Pechoux C, Rolland E, et al. Meta-analysis of concomitant versus sequential radiochemotherapy in locally advanced non-small-cell lung cancer. *J Clin Oncol.* 2010;28(13):2181–2190.

14. Winner M, Goff SL, Chabot JA. Neoadjuvant therapy for non-metastatic pancreatic ductal adenocarcinoma. *Semin Oncol.* 2015;42(1):86–97.

15. Landoni F, Maneo A, Colombo A, et al. Randomised study of radical surgery versus radiotherapy for stage Ib-IIa cervical cancer. *Lancet.* 1997;350(9077):535–540.

16. Dillman RO, Seagren SL, Propert KJ, et al. A randomized trial of induction chemotherapy plus high-dose radiation versus radiation alone in stage III non-small-cell lung cancer. *N Engl J Med.* 1990;323(14):940–945.

17. Curran WJ Jr, Paulus R, Langer CJ, et al. Sequential vs. concurrent chemoradiation for stage III non-small cell lung cancer: randomized phase III trial RTOG 9410. *J Natl Cancer Inst.* 2011;103(19):1452–1460.

18. Sell A, Jakobsen A, Nerstrom B, et al. Treatment of advanced bladder cancer category T2 T3 and T4a. A randomized multicenter study of preoperative irradiation and cystectomy versus radical irradiation and early salvage cystectomy for residual tumor. DAVECA protocol 8201. Danish Vesical Cancer Group. *Scand J Urol Nephrol.* 1991;138(suppl): 193–201.

19. Munro NP, Sundaram SK, Weston PM, et al. A 10-year retrospective review of a non-randomized cohort of 458 patients undergoing radical radiotherapy or cystectomy in Yorkshire, UK. *Int J Radiat Oncol Biol Phys.* 2010;77(1):119–124.

20. James ND, Hussain SA, Hall E, et al. Radiotherapy with or without chemotherapy in muscle-invasive bladder cancer. *N Engl J Med.* 2012;366(16):1477–1488.

21. Sugarbaker DJ, Flores RM, Jaklitsch MT, et al. Resection margins, extrapleural nodal status, and cell type determine postoperative long-term survival in trimodality therapy of malignant pleural mesothelioma: results in 183 patients. *J Thorac Cardiovasc Surg.* 1999;117(1):54–63.

22. Lucchi M, Chella A, Melfi F, et al. Four-modality therapy in malignant pleural mesothelioma: a phase II study. *J Thorac Oncol.* 2007;2(3):237–242.

23. Peters WA III, Liu PY, Barrett RJ II, et al. Concurrent chemotherapy and pelvic radiation therapy compared with pelvic radiation therapy alone as adjuvant therapy after radical surgery in high-risk early-stage cancer of the cervix. *J Clin Oncol.* 2000;18(8):1606–1613.

24. Sauer R, Becker H, Hohenberger W, et al. Preoperative versus postoperative chemoradiotherapy for rectal cancer. *N Engl J Med.* 2004;351(17):1731–1740.

25. Ruka W, Rutkowski P, Falkowski S, et al. Aggressive combined treatment of synovial sarcoma patients (pts) without distant metastases—single-center experience. *J Clin Oncol.* 2004;22(suppl 14):9018.

26. O'Sullivan B, Davis AM, Turcotte R, et al. Preoperative versus postoperative radiotherapy in soft-tissue sarcoma of the limbs: a randomised trial. *Lancet.* 2002;359(9325): 2235–2241.

27. Pignon JP, le Maitre A, Maillard E, et al. Meta-analysis of chemotherapy in head and neck cancer (MACH-NC): an update on 93 randomised trials and 17,346 patients. *Radiother Oncol.* 2009;92(1):4–14.

28. van den Bent MJ, Brandes AA, Taphoorn MJ, et al. Adjuvant procarbazine, lomustine, and vincristine chemotherapy in newly diagnosed anaplastic oligodendroglioma: long-term follow-up of EORTC brain tumor group study 26951. *J Clin Oncol.* 2013;31(3): 344–350.

29. Bonner JA, Harari PM, Giralt J, et al. Radiotherapy plus cetuximab for squamous-cell carcinoma of the head and neck. *N Engl J Med.* 2006;354(6):567–578.

30. Bradley JD, Paulus R, Komaki R, et al. Standard-dose versus high-dose conformal radiotherapy with concurrent and consolidation carboplatin plus paclitaxel with or without cetuximab for patients with stage IIIA or IIIB non-small-cell lung cancer (RTOG 0617): a randomised, two-by-two factorial phase 3 study. *Lancet Oncol.* 2015;16(2):187–199.

31. Schellenberg D, Goodman KA, Lee F, et al. Gemcitabine chemotherapy and single-fraction stereotactic body radiotherapy for locally advanced pancreatic cancer. *Int J Radiat Oncol Biol Phys.* 2008;72(3):678–686.

32. Turrisi AT III, Kim K, Blum R, et al. Twice-daily compared with once-daily thoracic radiotherapy in limited small-cell lung cancer treated concurrently with cisplatin and etoposide. *N Engl J Med.* 1999;340(4):265–271.

33. Grutters JP, Kessels AG, Pijls-Johannesma M, et al. Comparison of the effectiveness of radiotherapy with photons, protons, and carbon-ions for non-small cell lung cancer: a meta-analysis. *Radiother Oncol.* 2009;95(1):32–40.

34. Buentzel J, Micke O, Adamietz IA, et al. Intravenous amifostine during chemoradiotherapy for head-and-neck cancer: a randomized placebo-controlled phase III study. *Int J Radiat Oncol Biol Phys.* 2006;64(3):684–691.

35. Temel JS, Greer JA, Muzikansky A, et al. Early palliative care for patients with metastatic non-small-cell lung cancer. *N Engl J Med.* 2010;363(8):733–742.

36. Goodwin PJ, Leszcz M, Ennis M, et al. The effect of group psychosocial support on survival in metastatic breast cancer. *N Engl J Med.* 2001;345(24):1719–1726.

# Molecular Targeted Therapy and Radiation 2

*Stephen A. Rosenberg, Zachary S. Morris, and Randall J. Kimple*

---

## List of Abbreviations

| | |
|---|---|
| DCIS | ductal carcinoma in situ |
| ECOG | Eastern Oncology Cooperative Group |
| EGFR | epidermal growth factor receptor |
| ERK | extracellular signal-regulated kinase |
| FGF | fibroblast growth factor |
| HDAC | histone deacetylase |
| HER2 | human epidermal growth factor receptor family 2 |
| HGF | hepatocyte growth factor |
| HIF | hypoxia-inducible factor |
| HR | homologous recombination |
| MAPK | mitogen-activated protein kinase |
| MEK | MAPK/ERK kinase |
| MET | MET protooncogene, receptor tyrosine kinase |
| mTOR | mammalian target of rapamycin |
| NSABP | National Surgical Adjuvant Breast and Bowel Project |
| NSCLC | non–small cell lung cancer |
| OS | overall survival |
| PARP | poly(ADP-ribose) polymerase 1 |
| PDGF | platelet-derived growth factor |
| PI3K | phosphoinositide 3-kinase |
| PRDR | pulsed reduced dose rate |
| RTOG | Radiation Therapy Oncology Group |
| SBRT | stereotactic body radiotherapy |
| VEGF | vascular endothelial growth factor |

## INTRODUCTION

The past decade has seen radiation oncologists make significant strides in improving the delivery of conformal and ablative doses of radiotherapy. Advances in imaging, motion management, and dose modulation have led to significant improvements in the conformality of radiation dose distributions and have resulted in the possibility of escalating the dose while still sparing adjacent normal tissue. For example, stereotactic body radiotherapy (SBRT) significantly improves outcomes over conventionally fractionated treatment doses across various disease sites (1,2). Although our technical ability to deliver radiation continues to improve, it remains unlikely that any single modality will be able to provide both local and systemic control of tumors.

During the early 20th century, Paul Ehrlich conceptualized molecular targeted therapeutics when he postulated the existence of selective receptors on microorganisms that could be targeted by organic molecules for therapeutic effect. Half a century later, the earliest broad-spectrum cytotoxic chemotherapies including nitrogen mustard and aminopterin were pursued with the intent of targeting molecules such as DNA or the pathway of folic acid synthesis (3). The specificity of the molecular targeted therapies with lower toxicity profiles remains one of the core advantages of targeted treatment. In the early 1970s, George Steel postulated multiple mechanisms by which combined modality treatment could improve clinical outcomes (4). The notion of independent toxicities was a crucial part of this hypothesis: combinations of drugs with incompletely overlapping adverse effects allow for increased therapeutic intensity without prohibitive toxicity, thus widening the therapeutic window compared to increasing the intensity of a single treatment modality (5).

The unique mechanism of action of a given targeted therapy often results in a toxicity profile with minimal overlap with radiation-induced toxicities. Combining molecularly targeted drugs and radiation may enhance the therapeutic ratio without significantly increasing side-effect profiles. Molecular targeted drugs were not fully imagined in the 1970s, and a modernization of the Steel hypothesis has been proposed to afford continued utility in describing the exploitable interactions of radiation and cancer drugs (6). Antibody-directed targeted therapeutics were not developed until Levy and colleagues introduced the monoclonal platform in 1981 (7). The ability to rapidly target cell surface receptors led to significant insight into signal transduction cascades, as well as a better understanding of tyrosine kinase receptor signaling and cell growth and development (ie, epidermal growth factor receptor [EGFR] and human epidermal growth factor receptor family 2 [HER2]). The last two decades have seen a large advancement in the promise of molecular therapies and an ever-expanding list of targets and candidate molecules (8,9). These small molecule

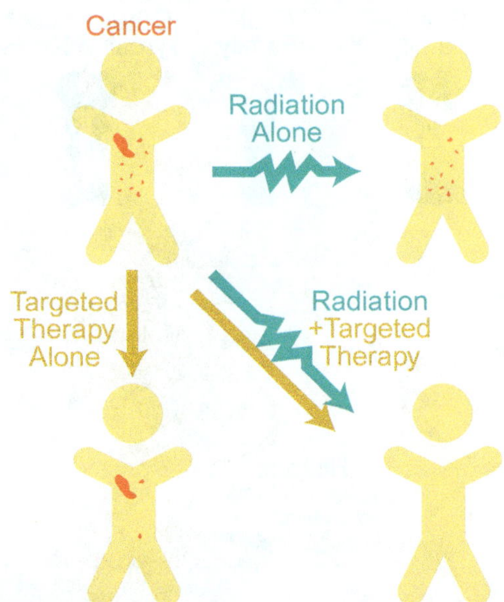


**FIGURE 2.1**  Spatiotemporal and cytotoxic cooperation
Combining molecular targeted therapy and radiation may lead to improved tumor responses. Radiation is effective at eliminating high-volume, localized disease, while chemotherapy is better at controlling low-volume distributed cancers. Treating a localized cancer with radiation does not treat potential micrometastatic disease. Chemotherapy alone is unable to control gross tumors. The combination of radiation and chemotherapy may result in the eradication of both local disease and systemic disease, thus rendering a patient cancer-free.

inhibitors block pathways regulating cell survival, apoptosis, senescence, and autophagy, among other critical cellular functions.

The modern era of molecular targeting in oncology has followed from the early clinical success of the anti–HER2 antibody, trastuzumab, and the small molecule inhibitors. As will be discussed, clinical trials demonstrate the therapeutic efficacy of drugs targeting EGFR (cetuximab and panitumumab), BCR-ABL fusion protein (imatinib), B-RAF (vemurafenib), and vascular endothelial growth factor (VEGF [bevacizumab]). This chapter explores the rationale and evidence that these drugs have the ability to improve outcomes when combined with radiotherapy. Utilizing Steel's revised framework, radiation and molecular targeted agents may interact to improve clinical outcomes via both spatiotemporal modulation and cytotoxic cooperation (Figure 2.1). This may allow for temporal and/or biological modulation, enabling the killing of tumor cells that may otherwise be resistant to radiation. It is important to remember that increasing the efficacy of radiotherapy by even 10% per fraction can result in a significant increase in tumor control probability when multiplied over many fractions (10–12).

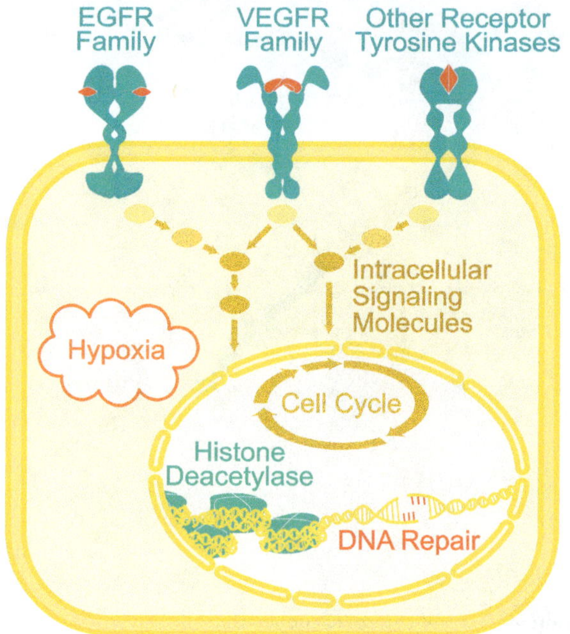


**FIGURE 2.2** Molecular targets of radiosensitizers

Molecular therapies may interact with radiation through a myriad of mechanisms involving a wide array of cellular targets. Illustrated here are the cellular targets that molecular therapeutics most commonly pinpoint.

This chapter provides a broad overview of the rationale for combining molecular targeted therapy with radiation. We illustrate this through both preclinical and clinical examples of combinatorial therapy. The examples provided focus on agents that modulate receptor tyrosine kinases, hypoxia, intracellular signaling pathways, DNA damage repair, and histone deacetylases (Figure 2.2). These agents represent the most commonly used molecularly targeted radiosensitizers. Although a significant number of other compounds are in various phases of development, they will only be peripherally discussed. The translation of these small molecular targeted therapies into the clinic remains an ongoing opportunity to exploit cooperative cell killing while sparing normal tissues.

## THE COMBINATION OF RADIATION AND MOLECULAR AGENTS TARGETING GROWTH FACTOR RECEPTORS

The EGFR is a tyrosine kinase receptor implicated in a variety of cellular processes regulating cell survival, growth, proliferation, intrinsic radiosensitivity, and DNA damage response. Nearly 50% of tumors overexpress EGFR or have an activating mutation in the EGFR receptor. The overexpression and/or mutation of EGFR has been connected to a worse prognosis and resistance to chemoradiation across various disease sites (13,14). Multiple experiments have shown that clinically relevant doses of radiation (ie, 2 Gy/fraction) activate EGFR activity, even in the absence of ligand binding. The exact mechanism underlying this activation remains unclear. The activation of EGFR has significant implications because it can lead to prosurvival PI3K/MAPK signaling and may promote resistance to radiation. Inhibiting EGFR signaling has been a prime target for molecular therapy in combination with radiation for nearly 20 years (15–17).

Sato and Mendelsohn were the first to identify EGFR as an important molecular target (18). Extensive preclinical validation begat early-phase clinical studies that demonstrated the safety and efficacy of EGFR inhibition with a human-mouse chimeric anti-EGFR antibody later named *cetuximab*. The initial Food and Drug Administration (FDA) approval of cetuximab followed a demonstration of improved median survival in patients with refractory metastatic colorectal cancer whose tumors expressed EGFR (19,20). Preclinical studies showed that the combination of EGFR inhibition synergized with radiation by enhancing apoptosis, attenuating DNA damage response, affecting cell cycle distribution, and inhibiting accelerated repopulation (17,21,22). Buoyed by promising preclinical studies, clinical trials were initiated to explore the combination of radiation and cetuximab in head and neck cancer patients (23). Based, in part, on high rates of complete response in these early trials, a phase III study was designed to evaluate the combination of radiotherapy with or without cetuximab. The results from this study demonstrated a 10% improvement in overall survival (OS) and a doubling of the median survival (24,25). The development of cetuximab shows the potential benefit of combining molecular targeted agents and radiotherapy, with an absolute survival benefit to patients undergoing curative treatment.

Around the same time Bonner et al were completing the randomized trial proving the efficacy of cetuximab as a radiosensitizer in head and neck cancer, several trials were reported that changed the standard of care for patients with locally advanced head and neck cancer from radiotherapy alone to radiotherapy with concurrent cisplatin (26). These advances led to the development of the Radiation Therapy Oncology Group (RTOG) 0522, a randomized study that examined the potential benefit of adding cetuximab to concurrent platinum-based chemoradiation. The results of this trial demonstrated no benefit in OS or progression-free survival from trimodality therapy (27). This suggests that cetuximab does not offer an additional therapeutic advantage when added to platinum-based chemoradiation. An alternative, fully humanized inhibitory anti-EGFR antibody, or panitumumab, has also been studied in conjunction with radiotherapy for head and neck cancer. Results from the CONCERT-1 and -2 studies demonstrated that panitumumab cannot replace cisplatin in head and neck cancer and, consistent with RTOG 0522, confirmed that EGFR inhibition offers no additional benefit when added to platinum-based therapy (28,29).

The aforementioned studies in the definitive treatment of head and neck cancer led to RTOG 0234, a recently reported phase II clinical trial that illustrated the feasibility and safety of combining EGFR inhibition with either docetaxel or cisplatin in the high-risk postoperative setting (30). The results from this study provided the evidence and rationale for initiating RTOG 1216, a randomized study that will evaluate the optimal concurrent therapy in the adjuvant treatment of high-risk postoperative head and neck cancer patients. These patients will be randomized to chemoradiation with cisplatin versus docetaxel versus docetaxel plus cetuximab. This trial highlights a likely approach across different disease sites by incorporating molecular therapy with surgery, chemotherapy, and radiotherapy.

Multiple trials have shown that non–small cell lung cancer (NSCLC) patients with specific EGFR mutations can benefit from agents targeting these mutations (31). Despite nearly a decade of work in these cancers, the combination of radiation therapy and EGFR inhibition in NSCLC has only recently been investigated in multiple early-phase studies (32). The success of EGFR inhibition in metastatic NSCLC and in head and neck cancer led to the development of RTOG 0617, a phase III study that examined both radiation dose escalation and the addition of cetuximab to standard cytotoxic chemotherapy. This study failed to demonstrate any advantage to either regimen (33). Several early-phase studies have suggested that EGFR inhibition combined with radiotherapy leads to higher rates of pneumonitis in NSCLC (34,35). The utility of EGFR inhibition with radiation therapy has yet to be defined in lung cancer.

Early studies suggested a potential benefit for cetuximab combined with radiotherapy in esophageal cancer. This led to the development of RTOG 0436, a phase III trial that randomized patients to neoadjuvant cisplatin, paclitaxel, and radiation with or without cetuximab. During an early analysis in 2012, this study failed to meet a prespecified end point of improved clinical disease response and was closed to further enrollment (36). An abstract reporting results from the REAL-3 (epirubicin, oxaliplatin, and capecitabine with or without panitumumab for patients with previously untreated advanced oseophagogastric cancer) study in 2012 indicated worse survival for patients with metastatic esophageal cancer receiving multiagent chemotherapy plus panitumumab, although the peer-reviewed publication remained unpublished as of 2016 (37). Similarly presented in abstract form only, the phase III SCOPE1 (chemoradiotherapy with or without cetuximab in patients with esophageal cancer) trial from the United Kingdom, which evaluated the benefit of EGFR inhibition in patients with advanced esophageal cancer, demonstrated worse survival with the addition of cetuximab. These results have appropriately decreased enthusiasm for using EGFR inhibition in these patients, and the regimen of concurrent chemoradiation and EGFR inhibition in esophageal cancer is not recommended.

The role of EGFR inhibition has also been investigated in other types of cancer. In rectal cancer, the phase II EXPERT-C trial (neoadjuvant oxaliplatin, capecitabine, and preoperative radiotherapy with or without cetuximab followed by total mesorectal excision in patients with high-risk rectal cancer) examined the effect of adding cetuximab to induction chemotherapy and concurrent chemoradiation. This study showed that cetuximab improved the rates of radiographic response and OS in patients with wild-type KRAS/BRAF but did not meet its primary end point of improved complete response rates (38). EGFR inhibitors have also been studied with radiation in early-phase trials for patients with high-grade glioma. Despite demonstrating reasonable safety, these studies have not clearly shown improved efficacy (39).

HER2 is a membrane-spanning receptor tyrosine kinase closely related to EGFR. HER2 amplification is observed in some breast cancer tumors. Clinically approved drugs that target HER2 include the monoclonal antibody trastuzumab and the small molecule dual EGFR/HER2 tyrosine kinase inhibitor lapatinib. Trastuzumab is used in women with HER2-expressing breast cancer and is routinely given concurrently with adjuvant radiotherapy. There is scant data studying the combination of radiation and trastuzumab in breast cancer patients. Phase II data from a multicenter French study suggested a potential for cardiac toxicity with the concurrent administration of trastuzumab and radiation (40). This result was not duplicated in a subsequent phase II study that failed to reproduce such toxicity and also indicated a potential for radiosensitization (41). The National Surgical Adjuvant Breast and Bowel Project (NSABP) B-43 is currently enrolling patients with high-risk, HER2-positive ductal carcinoma in situ (DCIS) and comparing whole breast irradiation with or without concurrent trastuzumab. Early toxicity results from this study show that radiotherapy with trastuzumab is well tolerated (42). Kimple and colleagues have also reported on a phase I study of lapatinib and radiation for women with locoregionally recurrent breast cancer (43). The combination therapy was well tolerated with only expected toxicities identified. The overexpression of HER2 is also seen in gastrointestinal cancers treated with radiotherapy. Early-phase clinical trials in esophageal cancer have demonstrated reasonable safety and encouraging results from the addition of trastuzumab (36). RTOG 1010 is an ongoing phase III trial investigating the addition of trastuzumab concurrent with carboplatin, paclitaxel, and radiation as a neoadjuvant regimen for patients with locally advanced HER2/neu-positive esophageal tumors. Multiple additional ongoing early-phase studies are investigating the use of agents targeting the ERbB/HER family given concurrent with radiotherapy.

c-MET (MET protooncogene, receptor tyrosine kinase, or hepatocyte growth factor receptor) is a tyrosine kinase receptor implicated in cell proliferation and resistance to apoptosis. The hepatocyte growth factor (HGF) binds to c-MET and causes receptor dimerization, phosphorylation, and downstream kinase activation (44). The activation of the c-MET signaling pathway is associated with significant cross talk with EGFR and PI3K/MAPK signaling (45). This activation of the c-MET pathway can occur due to activating mutations, overexpression, or radiation (46,47). The inhibition of c-MET signaling is associated with significant tumor radiosensitization, which may occur through decreased DNA damage repair, although the exact mechanism remains unclear (48). Inappropriate c-MET activation is seen in a variety of malignancies treated with radiotherapy (eg, head, neck, and lung cancer), suggesting that blocking this pathway could be beneficial. Crizotinib, a small molecule ALK inhibitor, also inhibits c-MET, leading to a growing clinical interest in combining crizotinib with radiotherapy. Although some preclinical studies have failed to demonstrate a benefit to combining crizotinib with radiotherapy in c-MET-expressing cells, other studies have shown promising results with this approach (49,50).

## THE COMBINATION OF RADIATION AND MOLECULAR AGENTS TARGETING HYPOXIA AND ANGIOGENESIS

Early studies of cancer identified disorganized vasculature and significant areas of hypoxia that arose during tumor growth (51). Regions of hypoxia within tumors are often resistant to radiotherapy for a variety of reasons. Ionizing radiation requires the presence of oxygen to form reactive oxygen species, which are a prime mode of DNA damage. Hypoxia also activates prosurvival mechanisms that can lead to resistance to the effects of radiotherapy. The development of hypoxic cell radiosensitizers has been (and continues to be) the subject of significant preclinical work (52,53). Nimorazole is a hypoxic cell radiosensitizer that improves tumor control when combined with radiotherapy (54).

In response to hypoxic growth conditions, cancer cells increase HIF1α (hypoxia-inducible factor) signaling, which increases the production and release of the proangiogenic factors: fibroblast growth factor (bFGF), platelet-derived growth factor (PDGF), and vascular endothelial growth factor (VEGF) (55). These receptors have partially overlapping biological functions in angiogenesis and as progrowth receptor tyrosine kinases. Targeting angiogenesis for therapeutic effect in cancer was initially postulated as a means of depriving tumors of oxygen and nutrients. Careful study has revealed that the inhibition of angiogenesis may actually result in vascular normalization and enhanced perfusion, thus counteracting the intended effect (56). Enhancing oxygenation at the time of radiation makes VEGF inhibitors attractive candidates for combinatorial treatment by increasing the ability of a radiation dose to circumvent the relative resistance of hypoxic tumors to radiation.

One of the first antiangiogenic agents, the anti-VEGF antibody bevacizumab, received FDA approval in 2004 for the treatment of metastatic colon cancer (57). Multiple early-phase studies have investigated enhanced tumor response with the combination of radiation and bevacizumab in esophageal, rectal, head and neck, prostate, and pancreatic cancer; high-grade glioma; and soft tissue sarcoma (58,59). Unfortunately, reports on the use of bevacizumab and radiation in the treatment of NSCLC raised concern about increased esophageal toxicity—a finding that has not been replicated in a phase II study of bevacizumab plus chemoradiation for patients with esophageal cancer (60–62). In a trial of patients with high-risk prostate cancer treated with radiotherapy, androgen deprivation, and bevacizumab, late toxicities were increased compared to historical controls, but no change in acute toxicities was seen (63). A study of twice-daily radiotherapy combined with bevacizumab in locally advanced head and neck cancer resulted in disappointing local control (64). In contrast to the aforementioned results, other early reports on the use of conventional chemoradiation with bevacizumab show promising safety and efficacy data (65,66). Similar conflicting results have been seen in studies investigating the combination of radiation and bevacizumab in pancreatic cancer: potential duodenal toxicity in one study and a lack of excess toxicity in another (67,68). A phase II study combining bevacizumab and cisplatin-based definitive chemoradiation in locally advanced cervical cancer also indicated both feasibility and safety (69).

With regard to high-grade glioma, bevacizumab plays an important role, particularly in the recurrent setting. Multiple phase II studies in high-grade glioma have demonstrated both the safety and feasibility of combining bevacizumab with definitive radiation. Both the phase III AVAglio and RTOG 0825 studies showed improvement in progression-free survival but not OS with these approaches (70,71). Our institution is currently pursuing reirradiation with pulsed reduced dose-rate (PRDR) radiotherapy in combination with bevacizumab for recurrent high-grade glioma (clinicaltrials.gov ID: NCT01743950). This study is based on our institutional experience suggesting improved outcomes compared to historical controls in patients treated with PRDR radiation in conjunction after the disease has progressed (72).

## THE COMBINATION OF RADIATION AND INTRACELLULAR SIGNALING KINASE INHIBITION

Over the last 15 years, significant development efforts have gone into designing inhibitors of the intracellular kinases implicated in oncogenesis. Despite these efforts, relatively few small molecule tyrosine kinase inhibitors have advanced to phase III clinical trials in combination with radiation (Table 2.1). One potential reason for these agents' lack of efficacy in early clinical trials is the activation of feedback loops and molecular cross talk, which render single-agent targeting ineffective. Alternative strategies are now being explored that focus on compounds that simultaneously target multiple kinases. The combination of radiotherapy with these drugs may lead to synergy by overwhelming the cancer cells and preventing the development of molecular resistance.

Molecular targeted therapy has changed the landscape of treating tumors harboring RAS/BRAF signaling pathway mutations (73,74). RAS/BRAF pathway mutations often contribute to cell growth and survival. Mutations in RAS

**TABLE 2.1**  Molecular targeted agents currently under investigation in phase III study in combination with radiation therapy

| Drug | Target | Class of inhibitor | Site(s) |
| --- | --- | --- | --- |
| Bevacizumab | VEGF | Antibody | Recurrent high-grade gliomas |
| Cetuximab | EGFR | Antibody | HNSCC, NSCLC, esophageal/gastroesophageal junction |
| Endostatin | Angiogenesis | Peptide | Nasopharynx |
| Gefitinib | EGFR | Small molecule | NSCLC |
| Lapatinib | EGFR and HER2 | Small molecule | HNSCC |
| Rituximab | CD20 | Antibody | Lymphoma |
| Sorafenib | Multiple kinases | Small molecule | Liver |
| Trastuzumab | HER2 | Antibody | Breast, esophageal/gastroesophageal junction |
| Vorinostat | HDAC | Small molecule | Pediatric high-grade glioma |
| Monoclonal antibody 17-1A | Epcam | Antibody | Rectal |

*Note:* EGFR, epidermal growth factor receptor; HDAC, histone deacetylase; HER2, human epidermal growth factor receptor family 2; HNSCC, head and neck squamous cell carcinoma; NSCLC, non–small cell lung cancer; VEGF, vascular endothelial growth factor.

or BRAF are typically mutually exclusive because they both converge on common downstream effectors such as the mitogen-activated protein kinase kinase 1 (MEK)-ERK (extracellular signal-regulated kinase) signaling cascade. Approximately 50% of melanoma tumors harbor mutations in BRAF (most commonly V600E) (74). High rates of RAS/BRAF pathway aberrations are also seen in thyroid, lung, gastrointestinal stromal, colorectal, and other tumors (75,76). Mutations in RAS are predictive of a poor response to cetuximab in colon cancer, although the importance of BRAF mutations remains an area of active study in this disease (77). Multiple compounds that target signaling proteins located downstream of BRAF have been developed over the last decade. The inhibition of both B-Raf and downstream signaling proteins, such as MEK, results in radiosensitization (78). Radiosensitization has also been described in other cell lines (ie, colorectal) harboring BRAF mutations but not in BRAF$^{wt}$ cells (79). Inhibiting the MEK/ERK kinases can also increase radiation sensitivity; a result that may be due to effects on DNA damage repair (80,81). These effects have led to clinical trials investigating MEK inhibition in combination with concurrent radiotherapy in NSCLC (the MEKRT-MEK Inhibitor and Thoracic Radiotherapy Trial) and in rectal cancer (ClinicalTrials.gov ID: NCT01146756).

A cautionary note is appropriate, however, as the combination of B-Raf/MEK inhibition with radiation has been associated with pulmonary, dermatologic, neurologic, and bowel toxicity. Interestingly, targeted therapy combined with central nervous system (CNS) irradiation has shown a relatively safe combinational profile (82). It is generally recommended that BRAF and MEK inhibition be held at least 3 days before and after fractionated radiotherapy and at least 1 day before stereotactic radiosurgery (SRS) outside the setting of a clinical trial (83). The increased normal tissue toxicity associated with B-Raf inhibition has been postulated to be due to the transactivation of RAF dimers and the activation of ERK signaling in B-RAF$^{wt}$ normal tissue, but further studies are needed to assess this possibility (84).

Numerous malignancies depend on PI3K pathway signaling through either *PTEN* loss (glioblastoma and prostate cancer) or PI3K/Akt activation (breast cancer and ovarian cancer) (85). Therapies targeting the PI3K pathway remain an active focus of ongoing drug development. Early preclinical models have suggested that mutations in *PIK3CA* or loss of PTEN correlated with higher rates of response to PI3K inhibitors or rapalog treatment (86–89). Clinical studies utilizing drugs targeting the PI3K pathway inhibition as a monotherapy have generally been disappointing (90–92). Numerous experiments have shown that inhibition of the PI3K axis leads to feedback-loop activation of MAPK signaling—and ultimately to tumor progression. Rapamycin remains a prime example of this phenomenon as multiple studies have shown that mTOR inhibition leads to MAPK activation as a mechanism of cell escape and survival (93–95). It is hoped that an improved understanding of these feedback loops will aid in the development of rational drug combinations. For example, preclinical studies of glioblastoma multiforme demonstrated that the combined inhibition of MEK and mTOR causes a significant cell cycle arrest at the $G_1$ to S transition and leaves cells in a relatively radiosensitive state (96). Future work such as this may provide a rationale for improved drug combinations and identify potential mechanisms by which these compounds can synergize with radiation.

Once a pariah of kinase inhibitor development, drugs with multitarget effects are now finding renewed interest due to their ability to overcome feedback-loop activation. Beyond their potential use as single agents, these compounds may be significant radiosensitizers. Treatment with radiation and the dual PI3K/mTOR inhibitor BEZ235 leads to impaired DNA double-strand break repair (97,98). Early-phase trials have investigated the multikinase inhibitors sorafenib and sunitinib in various tumors. The wide target range of these molecules can lead to an increase in side effects but may also block the potential feedback-loop activation seen with more specific drugs. Sorafenib, a multikinase inhibitor, is being studied in combination with SBRT for patients with hepatocellular carcinoma (99). Understanding the molecular consequences of these compounds may allow us to overcome resistance and better radiosensitize cells.

Molecular targeted therapies are traditionally thought of as less toxic than chemotherapy. However, it is vital to understand that these targeted therapies have systemic effects and may have unanticipated and important side effects. These effects may be augmented when used in combination with radiotherapy, or they may make radiotherapy less effective. For example, rapalogs can result in immunosuppression and have been associated with an increased infection risk (100). Other chapters of this book highlight the importance of the immune system and its connection to treatment response with radiotherapy. Numerous early-phase clinical trials are underway to evaluate the combination of radiation with inhibitory antibodies targeting coregulatory T-cell checkpoint receptors or other immunologic targets (101). With this in mind, a targeted therapy that causes immunosuppression may lead to the decreased effectiveness of radiation in vivo. Taking into account the other effects of targeted therapy and its interactions with radiation will continue to be important.

## EPIGENETIC MODIFICATION COMBINED WITH RADIOTHERAPY

Histones help organize DNA into regular repeating units of chromatin. The acetylation of histones modulates DNA/chromatin structure, resulting in altered patterns of gene expression. Altered histone acetylation contributes to oncogenesis and is the target of histone deacetylase (HDAC) inhibitors (102). HDAC inhibitors have been studied in the preclinical setting (eg, valproic acid and vorinostat) and have been found to exert their effects on cell cycles, apoptosis, and DNA repair through both histone and nonhistone proteins (ie, p21, p53, and Ku70) (102–105). HDAC inhibitors are radiosensitizers in multiple preclinical studies across diverse tumors, including prostate cancer and gliomas (102,106). Emerging preclinical data show that certain HDAC inhibitors may also protect normal cells from radiation (107). This possibility raises the specter that HDAC inhibitors may significantly improve the therapeutic window, enabling their use in the treatment of patients. Numerous phase II trials with HDAC inhibitors have been attempted, with mixed results, but overall this therapy appears to be well tolerated. A few reports have been published studying the combination of HDAC inhibitors and radiotherapy (108–110). Ongoing studies are looking at the combination of vorinostat and radiation in diffuse pontine gliomas (clinicaltrials.gov ID:NCT01189266). In the fall of 2016, a search of clinicaltrials.gov for "histone deacetylase and radiation" identified eight actively recruiting trials.

## PROTEASOME OR AUTOPHAGY INHIBITION COMBINED WITH RADIOTHERAPY

The cellular proteasome is a large multiprotein complex responsible for degrading unneeded and damaged proteins from a cell. This is a highly regulated process that depends on cyclin, cyclin-dependent kinases, and other antiapoptotic factors (Bax and Bcl-2). Multiple preclinical studies have found that interrupting appropriate proteolysis with targeted therapies increases apoptosis across various cancer cell lines. Several groups have shown that the use of a proteasome inhibitor (eg, bortezomib, MG-132, and nelfinavir) increases radiation sensitivity across multiple cell lines such as prostate cancer, colorectal cancer, pancreatic cancer, or NSCLC (111–114). Recently reported data from the phase II Eastern Oncology Cooperative Group (ECOG) E1304 examining bortezomib combined with irinotecan in the recurrent head and neck cancer setting showed minimal antitumor activity (115). Multiple clinical trials combining proteasome inhibition with radiation are ongoing.

*Autophagy* is an important cellular process that allows for the recycling and degradation of cellular components. Preclinical models show that the irradiation of tumor cells induces a stress response and the induction of autophagy (116,117). Multiple preclinical studies have demonstrated that the inhibition of autophagy can radiosensitize cancer cell lines in vitro. However, most of the compounds used in these studies are not specific autophagy inhibitors, and the story is further complicated by data indicating that autophagy may play a role in regulating the immunogenic properties of tumors in conjunction with radiotherapy (118).

## POLY(ADP-RIBOSE) POLYMERASE INHIBITION COMBINED WITH RADIOTHERAPY

Single-strand DNA (ssDNA) breaks are preferentially detected and repaired by poly(ADP-ribose) polymerase (PARP) 1. PARP1 also participates in cell cycle and transcriptional regulation. PARP inhibitors initially cause the accumulation of single-strand breaks, which build up and result in double-strand DNA breaks. These double-strand breaks are preferentially repaired by homologous recombination (HR), and this has provided the rationale for using PARP inhibitors in tumors with mutations in HR-involved proteins such as BRCA1 and BRCA2. Normal cells are proficient in HR and can repair double-strand breaks, while tumor cells deficient in HR are unable to repair the accumulated damage, leading to cell death. This "synthetic lethality" has been demonstrated across a range of BRCA-deficient tumor models (119,120). Radiation's ability to cause DNA breaks has led to several groups testing PARP inhibitors in combination with radiation. Preclinical models show that the irradiation of tumor cells treated with PARP inhibitors results in synergistic cell killing in multiple cell lines (121,122). Although treatment with single-agent PARP inhibitors has been met with modest results, these compounds are currently being studied in combination with radiation (123,124). Multiple phase I clinical trials in esophageal and pancreatic cancer are currently in development. A phase II study of veliparib, a blood–brain barrier permeable PARP inhibitor, in combination with whole-brain radiotherapy in patients with brain metastasis from NSCLC, was recently reported. In this small study, no improvement in intracranial response rate, time to progression, or OS was noted with this regimen (125).

Further clinical studies will be needed to determine the potential utility of combining PARP inhibitors with radiation.

## FUTURE DIRECTIONS IN COMBINING RADIATION AND MOLECULAR TARGETED THERAPEUTICS

After more than 100 years of use in the treatment of malignancy, radiation remains an important pillar of therapy for cancer patients. As oncologists' ability to control micrometastatic disease with new chemotherapy treatments improves, the importance of local control of primary tumors will only increase.

Molecular targeted therapy has the ability to play an important role in improving local therapy when combined with radiotherapy. Although many of these drugs have been disappointing when used as single modalities, preliminary data suggests that combining them with radiotherapy may potentially reveal their important roles in the care of cancer patients (126,127). It is crucial to remember that small differences in radiosensitivity, when multiplied over numerous fractions, can lead to significant improvements in tumor control (see Figure 2.2) (10–12).

Combining multiple molecular targeted therapies has also emerged as a promising arena of study (eg, B-Raf and MEK inhibition) as highlighted by improved outcomes in melanoma patients treated with multiple targeted therapies (128,129). How these agents should be combined with radiotherapy remains a clinical challenge. As of 2009 only 36 phase III studies had examined the use of radiation together with any single molecular targeted agent (130). Since that time, few phase III studies with newer drugs have been started, much less completed (131). Multiple groups continue to encourage the development of clinical trials that incorporate both radiotherapy and targeted molecular therapy as exemplified by trial RTOG 1216, which incorporates molecular targeted therapy, chemotherapy, and radiotherapy (5).

Several steps can be taken to increase the use of molecular therapeutics in combination with radiotherapy. Preclinical studies investigating molecular targeted therapies must be performed with standard-of-care chemoradiation. Local control end points, rather than tumor growth delay, should be utilized when conducting in vivo studies. In vitro and in vivo radiation should be conducted on multiple model systems using irradiators with known, validated dosimetry. Clinical trials should be carefully designed to allow for the significant rate of grade 3 or greater toxicity seen with the many standard-of-care chemoradiation combinations currently used. This would avoid the "failure" of studies due to toxicities expected from standard treatment alone. Finally, we should consider using a "basket trial" approach (accruing patients by mutational status rather than histology) to study molecular targeted agents in the cancers most likely to benefit from additional therapy. Determining how to design and recruit patients to these trials, as well as select robust clinical end points, remains a challenge. End points to consider in this context include improved patient-reported toxicity, pathological complete response, and/or changes in the natural history of disease (5). Radiation oncologists must play a key role in this process because they understand the side effect profiles to be expected with standard therapy. It is imperative that they develop and maintain collaborations with industry and medical oncology colleagues. Ultimately, the success of personalized medicine depends upon demonstrable advances in our ability to cure individual patients.

Combining molecular targeted therapies with radiation offers significant opportunities to improve cancer patients' quality of life and outcomes.

## References


1. Iyengar P, Timmerman RD. Stereotactic ablative radiotherapy for non-small cell lung cancer: rationale and outcomes. *J Nat Compr Canc Netw.* 2012;10:1514–1520.
2. Rusthoven KE, Kavanagh BD, Cardenes H, et al. Multi-institutional phase I/II trial of stereotactic body radiation therapy for liver metastases. *J Clin Oncol.* 2009;27:1572–1578.
3. Mendelsohn J. Personalizing oncology: perspectives and prospects. *J Clin Oncol.* 2013;31:1904–1911.
4. Steel GG. Terminology in the description of drug-radiation interactions. *Int J Rad Oncol Biol Phys.* 1979;5:1145–1150.
5. Sharma RA, Plummer R, Stock JK, et al. Clinical development of new drug-radiotherapy combinations. *Nat Rev Clin Oncol.* 2016;13:627–642.
6. Bentzen SM, Harari PM, Bernier J. Exploitable mechanisms for combining drugs with radiation: concepts, achievements and future directions. *Nat Clin Pract Oncol.* 2007;4: 172–180.
7. Miller RA, Maloney DG, Warnke R, et al. Treatment of B-cell lymphoma with monoclonal anti-idiotype antibody. *New Engl J Med.* 1982;306:517–522.
8. Roskoski R. A historical overview of protein kinases and their targeted small molecule inhibitors. *Pharmacol Res.* 2015;100:1–23.
9. Subbiah IM, Gonzalez-Angulo AM. Advances and future directions in the targeting of HER2-positive breast cancer: implications for the future. *Curr Treat Options Oncol.* 2014;15:41–54.
10. Bentzen SM. Radiobiological considerations in the design of clinical trials. *Radiother Oncol.* 1994;32:1–11.
11. Diez P, Vogelius IS, Bentzen SM. A new method for synthesizing radiation dose-response data from multiple trials applied to prostate cancer. *Int J Radiat Oncol Biol Phys.* 2010; 77:1066–1071.
12. Williams SG. A new method for synthesizing radiation dose-response data from multiple trials applied to prostate cancer: in regard to Diez P, et al. (Int J Radiat Oncol Biol Phys 2010;77:1066–1071). *Int J Radiat Oncol Biol Phys.* 2011;80:639; author reply, 40.
13. Ang KK, Berkey BA, Tu X, et al. Impact of epidermal growth factor receptor expression on survival and pattern of relapse in patients with advanced head and neck carcinoma. *Cancer Res.* 2002;62:7350–7356.
14. Gupta A, Raina V. Geftinib. *J Cancer Res Ther.* 2010;6:249–254.
15. Dent P, Yacoub A, Contessa J, et al. Stress and radiation-induced activation of multiple intracellular signaling pathways. *Radiat Res.* 2003;159:283–300.
16. Yacoub A, McKinstry R, Hinman D, et al. Epidermal growth factor and ionizing radiation up-regulate the DNA repair genes XRCC1 and ERCC1 in DU145 and LNCaP prostate carcinoma through MAPK signaling. *Radiat Res.* 2003;159:439–452.
17. Huang SM, Bock JM, Harari PM. Epidermal growth factor receptor blockade with C225 modulates proliferation, apoptosis, and radiosensitivity in squamous cell carcinomas of the head and neck. *Cancer Res.* 1999;59:1935–1340.
18. Kawamoto T, Sato JD, Le A, et al. Growth stimulation of A431 cells by epidermal growth factor: identification of high-affinity receptors for epidermal growth factor by an anti-receptor monoclonal antibody. *Proc Natl Acad Sci USA.* 1983;80:1337–1341.

19. Cunningham D, Humblet Y, Siena S, et al. Cetuximab monotherapy and cetuximab plus irinotecan in irinotecan-refractory metastatic colorectal cancer. *New Eng J Med* 2004;351: 337–345.

20. Jonker DJ, O'Callaghan CJ, Karapetis CS, et al. Cetuximab for the treatment of colorectal cancer. *New Engl J Med*. 2007;357:2040–2048.

21. Huang SM, Harari PM. Modulation of radiation response after epidermal growth factor receptor blockade in squamous cell carcinomas: inhibition of damage repair, cell cycle kinetics, and tumor angiogenesis. *Clin Cancer Res*. 2000;6:2166–2174.

22. Saleh MN, Raisch KP, Stackhouse MA, et al. Combined modality therapy of A431 human epidermoid cancer using anti-EGFr antibody C225 and radiation. *Cancer Biother Radiopharm*. 1999;14:451–463.

23. Robert F, Ezekiel MP, Spencer SA, et al. Phase I study of anti-epidermal growth factor receptor antibody cetuximab in combination with radiation therapy in patients with advanced head and neck cancer. *J Clin Oncol*. 2001;19:3234–3243.

24. Bonner JA, Harari PM, Giralt J, et al. Radiotherapy plus cetuximab for squamous-cell carcinoma of the head and neck. *New Engl J Med*. 2006;354:567–578.

25. Bonner JA, Harari PM, Giralt J, et al. Radiotherapy plus cetuximab for locoregionally advanced head and neck cancer: 5-year survival data from a phase 3 randomised trial, and relation between cetuximab-induced rash and survival. *Lancet Oncol*. 2010;11: 21–28.

26. Forastiere AA, Zhang Q, Weber RS, et al. Long-term results of RTOG 91-11: a comparison of three nonsurgical treatment strategies to preserve the larynx in patients with locally advanced larynx cancer. *J Clin Oncol*. 2013;31:845–852.

27. Ang KK, Zhang QE, Rosenthal DI, et al. A randomized phase III trial (RTOG 0522) of concurrent accelerated radiation plus cisplatin with or without cetuximab for stage III-IV head and neck squamous cell carcinomas (HNC) [ASCO Annual Meeting Proceedings abstract 5500]. *J Clin Oncol*. 2011;29:(May 20 suppl).

28. Giralt J, Trigo J, Nuyts S, et al. Panitumumab plus radiotherapy versus chemoradiotherapy in patients with unresected, locally advanced squamous-cell carcinoma of the head and neck (CONCERT-2): a randomised, controlled, open-label phase 2 trial. *Lancet Oncol*. 2015;16:221–32.

29. Mesía R, Henke M, Fortin A, et al. Chemoradiotherapy with or without panitumumab in patients with unresected, locally advanced squamous-cell carcinoma of the head and neck (CONCERT-1): a randomised, controlled, open-label phase 2 trial. *Lancet Oncol*. 2015;16:208–20.

30. Harari PM, Harris J, Kies MS, et al. Postoperative chemoradiotherapy and cetuximab for high-risk squamous cell carcinoma of the head and neck (RTOG 0234). *J Clin Oncol*. 2014; In press.

31. Russo A, Franchina T, Ricciardi GR, et al. A decade of EGFR inhibition in EGFR-mutated non small cell lung cancer (NSCLC): old successes and future perspectives. *Oncotarget*. 2015;6:26814–26825.

32. Koh PK, Faivre-Finn C, Blackhall FH, et al. Targeted agents in non-small cell lung cancer (NSCLC): clinical developments and rationale for the combination with thoracic radiotherapy. *Cancer Treatmen Rev*. 2012;38:626–640.

33. Bradley JD, Paulus R, Komaki R, et al. Standard-dose versus high-dose conformal radiotherapy with concurrent and consolidation carboplatin plus paclitaxel with or without cetuximab for patients with stage IIIA or IIIB non-small-cell lung cancer (RTOG 0617): a randomised, two-by-two factorial phase 3 study. *Lancet Oncol*. 2015;16: 187–199.

34. Okamoto I, Takahashi T, Okamoto H, et al. Single-agent gefitinib with concurrent radiotherapy for locally advanced non-small cell lung cancer harboring mutations of the epidermal growth factor receptor. *Lung Cancer.* 2011;72:199–204.

35. Wan J, Cohen V, Agulnik J, et al. Unexpected high lung toxicity from radiation pneumonitis in a phase I/II trial of concurrent erlotinib with limited field radiation for intermediate prognosis patients with stage III or inoperable stage IIb non-small cell lung cancer (NSCLC). *Int J Radiat Oncol Biol Phys.* 2009;75:S110.

36. Hong TS, Wo JY, Kwak EL. Targeted therapies with chemoradiation in esophageal cancer: development and future directions. *Sem Radiat Oncol.* 2013;23:31–37.

37. Waddell TS, Chau I, Barbachano Y, et al. A randomized multicenter trial of epirubicin, oxaliplatin, and capecitabine (EOC) plus panitumumab in advanced esophagogastric cancer (REAL3). *J Clin Oncol.* 2012;30:LBA4000.

38. Dewdney A, Cunningham D, Tabernero J, et al. Multicenter randomized phase II clinical trial comparing neoadjuvant oxaliplatin, capecitabine, and preoperative radiotherapy with or without cetuximab followed by total mesorectal excision in patients with high-risk rectal cancer (EXPERT-C). *J Clin Oncol.* 2012;30:1620–1627.

39. Karpel-Massler G, Schmidt U, Unterberg A, et al. Therapeutic inhibition of the epidermal growth factor receptor in high-grade gliomas: where do we stand? *Mol Cancer Res.* 2009;7:1000–1012.

40. Belkacemi Y, Gligorov J, Ozsahin M, et al. Concurrent trastuzumab with adjuvant radiotherapy in HER2-positive breast cancer patients: acute toxicity analyses from the French multicentric study. *Ann Oncol.* 2008;19:1110–1116.

41. Horton JK, Halle J, Ferraro M, et al. Radiosensitization of chemotherapy-refractory, locally advanced or locally recurrent breast cancer with trastuzumab: a phase II trial. *Int J Rad Oncol Biol Phys.* 2010;76:998–1004.

42. Siziopikou KP, Anderson SJ, Cobleigh MA, et al. Preliminary results of centralized HER2 testing in ductal carcinoma in situ (DCIS): NSABP B-43. *Breast Cancer Res Treat.* 2013;142:415–421.

43. Kimple RJ, Horton JK, Livasy CA, et al. Phase I study and biomarker analysis of lapatinib and concurrent radiation for locally advanced breast cancer. *Oncologist.* 2012;17:1496–503.

44. Maulik G, Kijima T, Ma PC, et al. Modulation of the c-Met/hepatocyte growth factor pathway in small cell lung cancer. *Clin Cancer Res.* 2002;8:620–627.

45. Organ SL, Tsao MS. An overview of the c-MET signaling pathway. *Ther Adv Med Oncol.* 2011;3:S7-S19.

46. Sierra JR, Tsao MS. c-MET as a potential therapeutic target and biomarker in cancer. *Ther Adv Med Oncol.* 2011;3:S21-S35.

47. De Bacco F, Luraghi P, Medico E, et al. Induction of MET by ionizing radiation and its role in radioresistance and invasive growth of cancer. *J Natl Cancer Inst.* 2011;103:645–661.

48. Bhardwaj V, Zhan Y, Cortez MA, et al. C-Met inhibitor MK-8003 radiosensitizes c-Met-expressing non-small-cell lung cancer cells with radiation-induced c-Met-expression. *J Thorac Oncol.* 2012;7:1211–1217.

49. Baschnagel AM, Galoforo S, Thibodeau BJ, et al. Crizotinib fails to enhance the effect of radiation in head and neck squamous cell carcinoma xenografts. *Anticancer Res.* 2015;35:5973–5982.

50. De Bacco F, D'Ambrosio A, Casanova E, et al. MET inhibition overcomes radiation resistance of glioblastoma stem-like cells. *EMBO Mol Med.* 2016;8:550–668.

51. Niu G, Chen X. Vascular endothelial growth factor as an anti-angiogenic target for cancer therapy. *Curr Drug Targets.* 2010;11:1000–1017.

52. Kimple RJ. Strategizing the clone wars: pharmacological control of cellular sensitivity to radiation. *Mol Interv.* 2010;10:341–353.
53. Denny WA, Wilson WR. Tirapazamine: a bioreductive anticancer drug that exploits tumour hypoxia. *Expert Opin Investig Drugs.* 2000;9:2889–2901.
54. Overgaard J, Hansen HS, Specht L, et al. Five compared with six fractions per week of conventional radiotherapy of squamous-cell carcinoma of head and neck: DAHANCA 6 and 7 randomised controlled trial. *Lancet.* 2003;362:933–940.
55. Begg AC, Stewart FA, Vens C. Strategies to improve radiotherapy with targeted drugs. *Nat Rev Cancer.* 2011;11:239–253.
56. Carmeliet P, Jain RK. Principles and mechanisms of vessel normalization for cancer and other angiogenic diseases. *Nat Rev Drug Disc.* 2011;10:417–427.
57. Hurwitz H, Fehrenbacher L, Novotny W, et al. Bevacizumab plus irinotecan, fluorouracil, and leucovorin for metastatic colorectal cancer. *New Engl J Med.* 2004;350: 2335–2342.
58. Kleibeuker EA, Griffioen AW, Verheul HM, et al. Combining angiogenesis inhibition and radiotherapy: a double-edged sword. *Drug Resist Updat.* 2012;15:173–182.
59. Wadlow RC, Ryan DP. The role of targeted agents in preoperative chemoradiation for rectal cancer. *Cancer.* 2010;116:3537–3548.
60. Socinski MA, Stinchcombe TE, Moore DT, et al. Incorporating bevacizumab and erlotinib in the combined-modality treatment of stage III non-small-cell lung cancer: results of a phase I/II trial. *J Clin Oncol.* 2012;30:3953–3959.
61. Spigel DR, Hainsworth JD, Yardley DA, et al. Tracheoesophageal fistula formation in patients with lung cancer treated with chemoradiation and bevacizumab. *J Clin Oncol.* 2010;28:43–48.
62. Bendell JC, Meluch A, Peyton J, et al. A phase II trial of preoperative concurrent chemotherapy/radiation therapy plus bevacizumab/erlotinib in the treatment of localized esophageal cancer. *Clin Adv Hem Oncol.* 2012;10:430–437.
63. Vuky J, Pham HT, Warren S, et al. Phase II study of long-term androgen suppression with bevacizumab and intensity-modulated radiation therapy (IMRT) in high-risk prostate cancer. *Int J Rad Oncol Biol Phys.* 2012;82:e609-e615.
64. Salama JK, Haraf DJ, Stenson KM, et al. A randomized phase II study of 5-fluorouracil, hydroxyurea, and twice-daily radiotherapy compared with bevacizumab plus 5-fluorouracil, hydroxyurea, and twice-daily radiotherapy for intermediate-stage and T4N0-1 head and neck cancers. *Ann Oncol.* 2011;22:2304–2309.
65. Fury MG, Lee NY, Sherman E, et al. A phase 2 study of bevacizumab with cisplatin plus intensity-modulated radiation therapy for stage III/IVB head and neck squamous cell cancer. *Cancer.* 2012;118:5008–5014.
66. Lee NY, Zhang Q, Pfister DG, et al. Addition of bevacizumab to standard chemoradiation for locoregionally advanced nasopharyngeal carcinoma (RTOG 0615): a phase 2 multi-institutional trial. *Lancet Oncol.* 2012;13:172–180.
67. Crane CH, Winter K, Regine WF, et al. Phase II study of bevacizumab with concurrent capecitabine and radiation followed by maintenance gemcitabine and bevacizumab for locally advanced pancreatic cancer: Radiation Therapy Oncology Group RTOG 0411. *J Clin Oncol.* 2009;27:4096–4102.
68. Small W Jr, Mulcahy MF, Rademaker A, et al. Phase II trial of full-dose gemcitabine and bevacizumab in combination with attenuated three-dimensional conformal radiotherapy in patients with localized pancreatic cancer. *Int J Rad Oncol Biol Phys.* 2011; 80:476–482.
69. Schefter TE, Winter K, Kwon JS, et al. A phase II study of bevacizumab in combination with definitive radiotherapy and cisplatin chemotherapy in untreated patients with locally

advanced cervical carcinoma: preliminary results of RTOG 0417. *Int J Rad Oncol Biol Phys.* 2012;83:1179–1184.

70. Henriksson R, Bottomley A, Mason W, et al. Progression-free survival (PFS) and health-related quality of life (HRQoL) in AVAglio, a phase III study of bevacizumab (Bv), temozolomide (T), and radiotherapy (RT) in newly diagnosed glioblastoma (GBM). *J Clin Oncol.* 2013;31:2005.

71. Gilbert MR, Dignam J, Won M, et al. RTOG 0825: phase III double-blind placebo-controlled trial evaluating bevacizumab (Bev) in patients (Pts) with newly diagnosed glioblastoma (GBM). *J Clin Oncol.* 2013;31:1.

72. Magnuson W, Ian Robins H, Mohindra P, et al. Large volume reirradiation as salvage therapy for glioblastoma after progression on bevacizumab. *J Neurooncol.* 2014;117:133–139.

73. Wilhelm SM, Carter C, Tang L, et al. BAY 43-9006 exhibits broad spectrum oral anti-tumor activity and targets the RAF/MEK/ERK pathway and receptor tyrosine kinases involved in tumor progression and angiogenesis. *Cancer Res.* 2004;64:7099–7109.

74. Solit DB, Garraway LA, Pratilas CA, et al. BRAF mutation predicts sensitivity to MEK inhibition. *Nature.* 2006;439:358–362.

75. Prior IA, Lewis PD, Mattos C. A comprehensive survey of Ras mutations in cancer. *Cancer Res.* 2012;72:2457–2467.

76. Kebebew E, Weng J, Bauer J, et al. The prevalence and prognostic value of BRAF mutation in thyroid cancer. *Ann Surg.* 2007;246:466–470; discussion 70–71.

77. Barras D. BRAF mutation in colorectal cancer: an update. *Biomark Cancer.* 2015;7:9–12.

78. Sambade MJ, Peters EC, Thomas NE, et al. Melanoma cells show a heterogeneous range of sensitivity to ionizing radiation and are radiosensitized by inhibition of B-RAF with PLX-4032. *Radiother Oncol.* 2011;98:394–399.

79. Dasgupta T, Haas-Kogan DA, Yang X, et al. Genotype-dependent cooperation of ionizing radiation with BRAF inhibition in BRAF V600E-mutated carcinomas. *Invest New Drugs.* 2013;31:1136–1141.

80. Marampon F, Gravina GL, Di Rocco A, et al. MEK/ERK inhibitor U0126 increases the radiosensitivity of rhabdomyosarcoma cells in vitro and in vivo by downregulating growth and DNA repair signals. *Mol Cancer Ther.* 2011;10:159–168.

81. Yacoub A, Park JS, Qiao L, et al. MAPK dependence of DNA damage repair: ionizing radiation and the induction of expression of the DNA repair genes XRCC1 and ERCC1 in DU145 human prostate carcinoma cells in a MEK1/2 dependent fashion. *Int J Radiat Biol.* 2001;77:1067–1078.

82. Xu Z, Lee CC, Ramesh A, et al. BRAF V600E mutation and BRAF kinase inhibitors in conjunction with stereotactic radiosurgery for intracranial melanoma metastases. *J Neurosurg.* 2016:126:1–9.

83. Anker CJ, Grossmann KF, Atkins MB, et al. Avoiding severe toxicity from combined BRAF inhibitor and radiation treatment: consensus guidelines from the Eastern Cooperative Oncology Group (ECOG). *Int J Radiat Oncol Biol Phys.* 2016;95:632–646.

84. Poulikakos PI, Zhang C, Bollag G, et al. RAF inhibitors transactivate RAF dimers and ERK signalling in cells with wild-type BRAF. *Nature.* 2010;464:427–430.

85. Sawyers CL. Will mTOR inhibitors make it as cancer drugs? *Cancer Cell.* 2003;4:343–8.

86. Ihle NT, Lemos R, Wipf P, et al. Mutations in the phosphatidylinositol-3-kinase pathway predict for antitumor activity of the inhibitor PX-866 whereas oncogenic Ras is a dominant predictor for resistance. *Cancer Res.* 2009;69:143–150.

87. Janku F, Tsimberidou AM, Garrido-Laguna I, et al. PIK3CA mutations in patients with advanced cancers treated with PI3K/AKT/mTOR axis inhibitors. *Mol Cancer Ther.* 2011;10:558–565.

88. Moroney JW, Schlumbrecht MP, Helgason T, et al. A phase I trial of liposomal doxorubicin, bevacizumab, and temsirolimus in patients with advanced gynecologic and breast malignancies. *Clin Cancer Res.* 2011;17:6840–6846.

89. Shi Y, Gera J, Hu L, et al. Enhanced sensitivity of multiple myeloma cells containing PTEN mutations to CCI-779. *Cancer Res.* 2002;62:5027–5034.

90. Galanis E, Buckner JC, Maurer MJ, et al. Phase II trial of temsirolimus (CCI-779) in recurrent glioblastoma multiforme: a North Central Cancer Treatment Group Study. *J Clin Oncol.* 2005;23:5294–5304.

91. Wolff AC, Lazar AA, Bondarenko I, et al. Randomized phase III placebo-controlled trial of letrozole plus oral temsirolimus as first-line endocrine therapy in postmenopausal women with locally advanced or metastatic breast cancer. *J Clin Oncol.* 2013;31:195–202.

92. Armstrong AJ, Shen T, Halabi S, et al. A phase II trial of temsirolimus in men with castration-resistant metastatic prostate cancer. *Clin Genitourin Cancer.* 2013;11:397–406.

93. Carracedo A, Ma L, Teruya-Feldstein J, et al. Inhibition of mTORC1 leads to MAPK pathway activation through a PI3K-dependent feedback loop in human cancer. *J Clin Invest.* 2008;118:3065–3074.

94. Laplante M, Sabatini DM. mTOR signaling in growth control and disease. *Cell.* 2012;149:274–293.

95. Martini M, Ciraolo E, Gulluni F, et al. Targeting PI3K in cancer: any good news? *Front Oncol.* 2013;3:108.

96. Paternot S, Roger PP. Combined inhibition of MEK and mammalian target of rapamycin abolishes phosphorylation of cyclin-dependent kinase 4 in glioblastoma cell lines and prevents their proliferation. *Cancer Res.* 2009;69:4577–4581.

97. Gil del Alcazar CR, Hardebeck MC, Mukherjee B, et al. Inhibition of DNA double-strand break repair by the dual PI3K/mTOR inhibitor NVP-BEZ235 as a strategy for radiosensitization of glioblastoma. *Clin Cancer Res.* 2014;20:1235–1248.

98. Mukherjee B, Tomimatsu N, Amancherla K, et al. The dual PI3K/mTOR inhibitor NVP-BEZ235 is a potent inhibitor of ATM- and DNA-PKCs-mediated DNA damage responses. *Neoplasia.* 2012;14:34–43.

99. Ibrahim N, Yu Y, Walsh WR, et al. Molecular targeted therapies for cancer: sorafenib mono-therapy and its combination with other therapies (review). *Oncol Rep.* 2012;27:1303–1311.

100. Sarkaria JN, Galanis E, Wu W, et al. Combination of temsirolimus (CCI-779) with chemoradiation in newly diagnosed glioblastoma multiforme (GBM) (NCCTG trial N027D) is associated with increased infectious risks. *Clin Cancer Res.* 2010;16:5573–5580.

101. Formenti SC, Demaria S. Combining radiotherapy and cancer immunotherapy: a paradigm shift. *J Nat Cancer.* 2013;105:256–265.

102. Chinnaiyan P, Cerna D, Burgan WE, et al. Postradiation sensitization of the histone deacetylase inhibitor valproic acid. *Clin Cancer Res.* 2008;14:5410–5415.

103. Shabason JE, Tofilon PJ, Camphausen K. Grand rounds at the National Institutes of Health: HDAC inhibitors as radiation modifiers, from bench to clinic. *J Cell Mol Med.* 2011;15:2735–2744.

104. Margueron R, Duong V, Castet A, et al. Histone deacetylase inhibition and estrogen signalling in human breast cancer cells. *Biochem Pharmacol.* 2004;68:1239–1246.

105. Frew AJ, Johnstone RW, Bolden JE. Enhancing the apoptotic and therapeutic effects of HDAC inhibitors. *Cancer Lett.* 2009;280:125–133.

106. Xiao W, Graham PH, Hao J, et al. Combination therapy with the histone deacetylase inhibitor LBH589 and radiation is an effective regimen for prostate cancer cells. *PLoS One.* 2013;8:e74253.

107. Konsoula Z, Velena A, Lee R, et al. Histone deacetylase inhibitor: antineoplastic agent and radiation modulator. *Adv Exp Med Biol.* 2011;720:171–179.

108. Ree AH, Dueland S, Folkvord S, et al. Vorinostat, a histone deacetylase inhibitor, combined with pelvic palliative radiotherapy for gastrointestinal carcinoma: the Pelvic Radiation and Vorinostat (PRAVO) phase 1 study. *Lancet Oncol.* 2010;11:459–464.

109. Noguchi H, Yamashita H, Murakami T, et al. Successful treatment of anaplastic thyroid carcinoma with a combination of oral valproic acid, chemotherapy, radiation and surgery. *Endocr J.* 2009;56:245–249.

110. Wagner JM, Hackanson B, Lübbert M, et al. Histone deacetylase (HDAC) inhibitors in recent clinical trials for cancer therapy. *Clin Epigenetics.* 2010;1:117–136.

111. Goktas S, Baran Y, Ural AU, et al. Proteasome inhibitor bortezomib increases radiation sensitivity in androgen independent human prostate cancer cells. *Urology.* 2010;75: 793–798.

112. Cacan E, Spring AM, Kumari A, et al. Combination treatment with sublethal ionizing radiation and the proteasome inhibitor, bortezomib, enhances death-receptor mediated apoptosis and anti-tumor immune attack. *Int J Mol Sci.* 2015;16:30405–30421.

113. Grimes KR, Daosukho C, Zhao Y, et al. Proteasome inhibition improves fractionated radiation treatment against non-small cell lung cancer: an antioxidant connection. *Int J Oncol.* 2005;27:1047–1052.

114. Kimple RJ, Vaseva AV, Cox AD, et al. Radiosensitization of epidermal growth factor receptor/HER2-positive pancreatic cancer is mediated by inhibition of Akt independent of ras mutational status. *Clin Cancer Res.* 2010;16:912–923.

115. Gilbert J, Lee JW, Argiris A, et al. Phase II 2-arm trial of the proteasome inhibitor, PS-341 (bortezomib) in combination with irinotecan or PS-341 alone followed by the addition of irinotecan at time of progression in patients with locally recurrent or metastatic squamous cell carcinoma of the head and neck (E1304): a trial of the Eastern Cooperative Oncology Group. *Head Neck.* 2013;35:942–948.

116. Chaurasia M, Bhatt AN, Das A, et al. Radiation-induced autophagy: mechanisms and consequences. *Free Radic Res.* 2016;50:273–290.

117. Zois CE, Koukourakis MI. Radiation-induced autophagy in normal and cancer cells: towards novel cytoprotection and radio-sensitization policies? *Autophagy.* 2009;5: 442–450.

118. Ko A, Kanehisa A, Martins I, et al. Autophagy inhibition radiosensitizes in vitro, yet reduces radioresponses in vivo due to deficient immunogenic signalling. *Cell Death Differ.* 2014;21:92–99.

119. Bryant HE, Helleday T. Poly(ADP-ribose) polymerase inhibitors as potential chemotherapeutic agents. *Biochem Soc Trans.* 2004;32:959–961.

120. Bryant HE, Schultz N, Thomas HD, et al. Specific killing of BRCA2-deficient tumours with inhibitors of poly(ADP-ribose) polymerase. *Nature.* 2005;434:913–917.

121. Albert JM, Cao C, Kim KW, et al. Inhibition of poly(ADP-ribose) polymerase enhances cell death and improves tumor growth delay in irradiated lung cancer models. *Clin Cancer Res.* 2007;13:3033–3042.

122. Barreto-Andrade JC, Efimova EV, Mauceri HJ, et al. Response of human prostate cancer cells and tumors to combining PARP inhibition with ionizing radiation. *Mol Cancer Ther.* 2011;10:1185–1193.

123. Tutt A, Robson M, Garber JE, et al. Oral poly(ADP-ribose) polymerase inhibitor olaparib in patients with BRCA1 or BRCA2 mutations and advanced breast cancer: a proof-of-concept trial. *Lancet.* 2010;376:235–244.

124. Benafif S, Hall M. An update on PARP inhibitors for the treatment of cancer. *Onco Targets Ther.* 2015;8:519–528.

125. Chabot P, Hsia TC, Ryu JS, et al. Veliparib in combination with whole-brain radiation therapy for patients with brain metastases from non-small cell lung cancer: results of a randomized, global, placebo-controlled study. *J Neurooncol.* 2016: 131:105–115.

126. Margolin K, Longmate J, Baratta T, et al. CCI-779 in metastatic melanoma: a phase II trial of the California Cancer Consortium. *Cancer.* 2005;104:1045–1048.

127. Flaherty KT. The future of tyrosine kinase inhibitors: single agent or combination? *Curr Oncol Rep.* 2008;10:264–270.

128. Flaherty KT, Infante JR, Daud A, et al. Combined BRAF and MEK inhibition in melanoma with BRAF V600 mutations. *New Engl J Med.* 2012;367:1694–1703.

129. Long GV, Stroyakovskiy D, Gogas H, et al. Combined BRAF and MEK inhibition versus BRAF inhibition alone in melanoma. *New Engl J Med.* 2014;371:1877–1888.

130. Ataman OU, Sambrook SJ, Wilks C, et al. The clinical development of molecularly targeted agents in combination with radiation therapy: a pharmaceutical perspective. *Int J Rad Oncol Biol Phys.* 2012;84:e447–e454.

131. Morris ZS, Harari PM. Interaction of radiation therapy with molecular targeted agents. *J Clin Oncol.* 2014;32:2886–2893.

# Current State of the Art in Intracranial Stereotactic Radiosurgery Technology

## ACCURACY, PRECISION, AND CLINICAL IMPACT

*George Farha, David Schlesinger, Arman Sarfehnia,*
*Arjun Sahgal, and Mark Ruschin*

---

**Highlights and Take-Home Messages:**

- Review of the various factors affecting accuracy and precision in radiosurgery.
- Dose falloff depends on multiple factors, and multicenter prospective trials must determine if any system confers dosimetric advantages.
- Clinical outcomes are similar between different systems.
- Hypofractionation is an emerging technique especially for the treatment of large or recurrent disease.

---

## DEFINITION OF STEREOTACTIC RADIOSURGERY

In the context of radiotherapy and radiosurgery, the term *stereotactic* defines the three-dimensional localization of a point in space by a unique set of coordinates that corresponds to a fixed, external reference frame. Neurosurgeons were the first to develop the technique of stereotactic radiosurgery (SRS), which was based on narrow beams of cobalt 60 gamma rays (the Gamma Knife) focused on a small target within the brain. With the advent of linear accelerators (LINAC), SRS became available in radiation therapy centers and gained further expansion in terms of clinical utilization. Lars Leksell defined SRS as a single-session treatment of surgically affixing an invasive metallic frame to the patient's skull; this concept of frame-based stereotaxy went unchallenged for 50 years. The development of image-guided radiation therapy (IGRT) facilitated frameless SRS, which has been demonstrated to have accuracy equivalent to that achieved with a stereotactic frame, and also allowed SRS to be delivered in more than one fraction. The American Association of Neurological Surgeons (AANS) has recently redefined SRS as a stereotactically targeted, image-guided treatment of one to five sessions.

## FACTORS AFFECTING ACCURACY AND PRECISION IN RADIOSURGERY

In this chapter we discuss accuracy, precision, and clinical impact. The term *accuracy* refers to how closely the intended radiation dose distribution matches that delivered. The term *precision* refers to how conformal the entire distribution is around the target; the more compact the distribution, the greater the precision. Table 3.1 summarizes some of the relevant factors discussed here and how they contribute to accuracy, precision, and clinical impact. The clinical success of SRS hinges on understanding what role each factor plays and how to account for it. The treatment of brain metastases with SRS is becoming more complex. For example, it is becoming acceptable to treat 10 or more brain metastases in a single session; patients are frequently returning for further SRS to new metastases and avoiding whole brain radiotherapy (WBRT) because of improvements in systemic treatments; and the role of hypofractionation for large or recurrent disease, including postoperative cavities, is also increasing. Given this increased complexity, more stringent demands on technical accuracy and precision are required to maximally spare healthy tissue and more importantly, understand the linkage between clinical outcomes and radiation dose in this rapidly evolving field.

The following briefly describes some major factors contributing to accuracy and precision, each of which will be expanded upon.

### Patient Setup and Irradiation

How well the patient is positioned and immobilized with respect to the machine isocenter is a major factor affecting the accuracy of SRS. If treating with one fraction, any displacement of the patient from the intended position results in a systematic shift of the entire distribution, leading to potential geographical misses and the overdosing of normal tissue. Historically, rigid invasive frames have been the gold standard for localization in SRS, but there has been a recent push toward frameless treatments and the reliance on image guidance to ensure adequate localization.

### Reference Dosimetry

*Reference dosimetry* refers to measuring the absorbed dose to water at a reference point under reference conditions using a detector that has a calibration factor

**TABLE 3.1** Brief summary of factors discussed in this chapter that affect accuracy and precision

| Factors affecting accuracy | Effect on dose distribution | Clinical impact | Effect of dose distribution[§] |
|---|---|---|---|
| Reference dosimetry | • Systematic increase or decrease of the entire dose distribution for all field sizes | • Overdose normal tissue<br>• Underdose target | 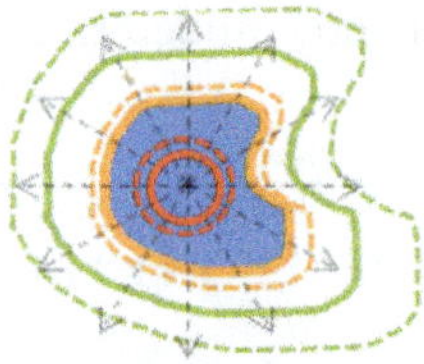 |
| Relative dosimetry | • Systematic increase or decrease of the entire dose distribution for specific field sizes | • Overdose normal tissue<br>• Underdose target | |
| Dose calculation in treatment planning | • Systematic increase or decrease of entire dose distribution for specific field sizes<br>• Nonuniform changes in dose distribution near boundaries | • Overdose normal tissue<br>• Underdose target | 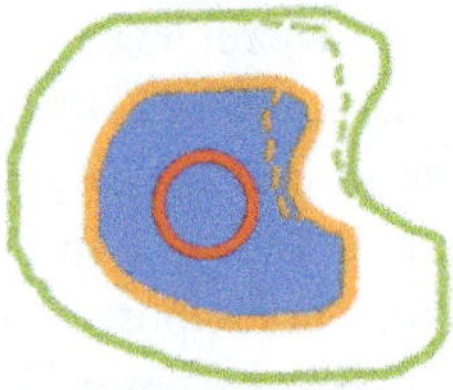 |
| Patient positioning and immobilization | • Systematic shift of entire distribution | • Geographic miss<br>• Use of PTV increases normal tissue dose | 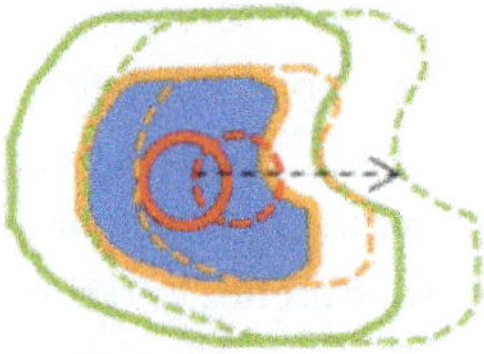 |
| System makeup (collimation, source size, etc) | • Dose falloff<br>• Integral dose | • V12Gy for single-fraction: brain necrosis<br>• Unknown for hypofractionated<br>• Retreatments | 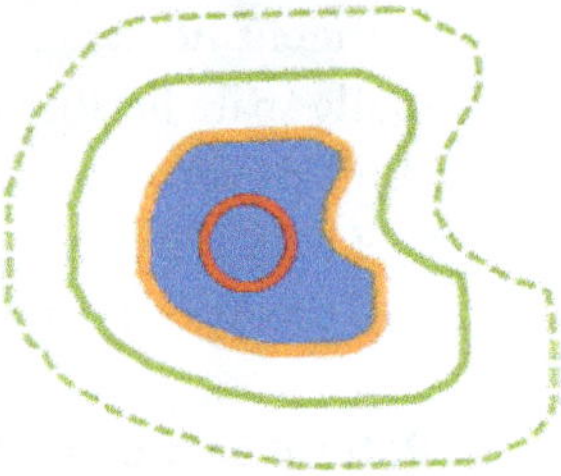 |
| Treatment technique (eg, conformal or VMAT, number of arcs, inverse planning) | • Dose falloff<br>• Dose heterogeneity | • V12Gy for single-fraction: brain necrosis<br>• Unknown for hypofractionated<br>• Retreatments | |
| Patient positioning and immobilization | • Random errors blur distribution and decrease dose falloff | • Unknown | 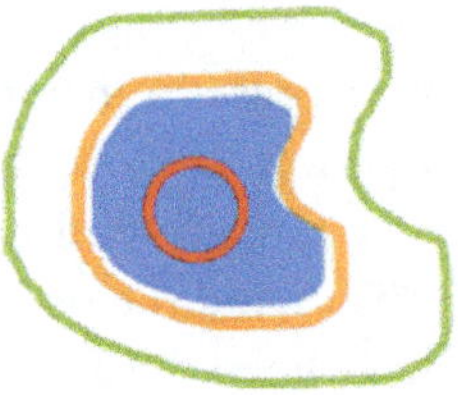 |
| Hypofractionation | • Lower dose per fraction<br>• Prescribed to a PTV to account for daily setup error | • Enables safe irradiation of larger or recurrent disease | |

§ Blue shaded area = GTV. Solid lines represent nominal isodose lines (orange = prescription, red = hot spot, green = 50%). Dashed lines represent change in isodose lines by the factor indicated. For "Hypofractionation," the orange solid line is prescribed to the GTV + margin to account for daily setup error.

*Note:* GTV, gross tumor volume; PTV, planning target volume; VMAT, volumetric modulated arc therapy.

traceable to national standard laboratories. Most protocols involve measuring the dose in a $10 \times 10$ cm$^2$ field at a 10-cm distance and a 10-cm depth in water. For machines such as the Gamma Knife and the CyberKnife, these reference conditions are not achievable, and other approaches and recommendations are being developed. Regardless of the protocol, miscalibration at the level of reference dosimetry would translate to a systematic error in the entire dose distribution, and therefore special attention will be given to how this is performed, particularly for non–LINAC devices.

## Relative Dosimetry

*Relative dosimetry* refers to measuring the dose at all other points of interest under nonreference conditions, thus relating the dose throughout a volume to the reference condition. The challenge in SRS is in measuring the dose at "small fields" because if performed improperly it would translate to systematic errors in dose distributions for those specific field sizes or conditions.

## Dose Calculation for Treatment Planning

The treatment-planning system incorporates reference and relative dosimetry measurements and models how the dose is calculated in patient anatomy. For brain SRS the anatomy is fairly uniform, and simple dose calculation algorithms, such as the Gamma Knife's tissue maximum ratio (TMR) method, fare reasonably well compared to the state-of-the-art convolution or Monte Carlo, except around regions of heterogeneity (the sinuses and the skull). The effect of tissue heterogeneities will cause local, nonuniform distortions of the dose distribution and are more clinically significant if the treated tumor is situated in the vicinity.

## System Design and Treatment Technique

Each device is a complex system consisting of one or more radiation sources and collimation systems. As such each will have its own dosimetric characteristics that describe, for example, beam penumbra, leakage/transmission, and scatter dose. All will ultimately factor into how precise a dose distribution can be around a target; that is, how conformal lower isodose lines are around the target or how fast the dose falls off. Furthermore, for any given system, the treatment technique itself (eg, conformal arc vs. volumetric modulated arc therapy [VMAT]) can influence precision. In general, the physics of the device dictate dose falloff, but one can artificially enhance the dose falloff by using techniques such as modulation. Usually, the latter strategy comes at a cost of higher monitor units and a more heterogeneous dose distribution reflected by hotter doses within the target volume.

## Hypofractionation

A special mention of hypofractionation is made because by design it is less precise than the single-fraction SRS technique since daily setup errors are introduced, frameless systems are needed, and the machine fluctuates daily. However, this reduced precision has actually facilitated a safe and effective treatment for larger or recurrent disease, with clinical outcomes and toxicity at rates equivalent to or better than single-fraction SRS.

## Other Factors

Other factors related to imaging, image fusion, and delineation can also affect how accurately the dose is delivered. Although not discussed here for brevity, knowledge of the entire SRS chain is recommended. Advanced imaging for assessing biological function or response is an exciting field that will play a larger role in SRS treatments in the near future.

# TECHNOLOGICAL DEVELOPMENTS FOR RADIOSURGERY

## Immobilization and Positioning Devices

The systems used to position and immobilize patients for SRS can be broadly categorized into two groups: (a) frame-based systems, which often involve the surgical attachment of a rigid frame to the patient's skull; or (b) frameless systems, which involve affixing the device to the patient via a bite-block system, a thermoplastic, or some combination of the two. Frame-based systems have historically served as both positioner and immobilizer, whereas more recent frameless devices rely more heavily on image guidance for positioning, and some imaging systems provide real or nearly real-time monitoring for motion. The term *frame* can be confusing, as bite-block systems often consist of a frame-based support, but such systems are considered "frameless" because they rely on image guidance, not the stereotactic coordinate system. In this chapter we refer to frame-based systems as relying solely on stereotactic localization and "frameless" systems as those relying on image-based localization. We will also give a brief description of immobilization devices and how well they perform.

## Frame-Based Systems

Some examples of neurosurgical frames that remain the most reliable and stable include the Cosman-Roberts-Wells (CRW) frame and the Leksell frame. Accurate fixation of the stereotactic frame to the patient's head is achieved by means of three to four steel pins screwed into the outer table of the patient's skull. A local anesthetic and a neurosurgeon are required for both frame placement and removal.

The original Brown-Roberts-Wells (BRW) system designed in the 1970s consisted of a skull base ring with carbon epoxy head posts. The frame ring is attached to the patient with screws that are tightened into the skull. Target coordinates are established by identifying the axial slice that best features the lesion. The x and y coordinates for each of nine fiducial rods are identified on the CT or MRI, as are the x and y coordinates for the target. All coordinates are then converted to coordinates in stereotactic space. In the 1980s Wells and Cosman simplified and improved the BRW by designing an arc guidance frame similar to the Leksell frame. The resulting CRW system included the introduction of MRI-compatible frames and localizers and versatility in arc-to-frame applications that enabled inferior trajectories into the posterior cranial fossa or lateral routes into the temporal lobe. In one study (1), the BRW was compared to the PinPoint® system using the Vision RT surface-matching system. On average, for 11 patients (19 lesions) the mean three-dimensional intrafraction translational and rotational motions were observed to be 0.3 mm and 0.2°, respectively, for both systems. In terms of immobilization performance, Ramakrishna et al measured a mean three-dimensional intrafraction motion of $0.40 \pm 0.30$ mm with the invasive BRW head frame (2).

The Leksell Coordinate Frame G, made of titanium, is fixed to the patient's head using four self-tapping screws, which keep the frame firmly and accurately in place. It is lighter than the CRW frame and fully MR compatible. The model G base frame is rectangular and measures 190 mm by 210 mm. A straight or curved front piece can be used, as it allows for airway access in emergencies. The Leksell frame is supported by many treatment-planning systems, but it is the only frame currently in clinical use with the Leksell Gamma Knife® (LGK) system (Figure 3.1).

The Gill-Thomas-Cosman (GTC) frame consists of an aluminum alloy base ring attached to a treatment couch for rigid immobilization, a dental plate/oral appliance, an occipital headrest pad, and Velcro straps. To enable daily setup reproducibility, the Velcro strap lengths can be marked at each side, and a clear plastic hemispherical dome with fixed holes or portals, called a *depth confirmation helmet*, can be used. The depth confirmation helmet is placed over the head ring, and a rod with a millimeter scale is inserted into each hole to measure the distance to the cranial surface. The distance readings from each hole can be compared to the readings obtained at the time of CT simulation to ensure that the frame has been accurately placed. The GTC frame is a relocatable head frame that was adapted for compatibility with the BRW stereotactic coordinate system. Its design was originally based on the Gill-Thomas frame (3,4). The daily relocation error of the GTC frame has been reported to be $1.03 \pm 0.34$ mm (5).

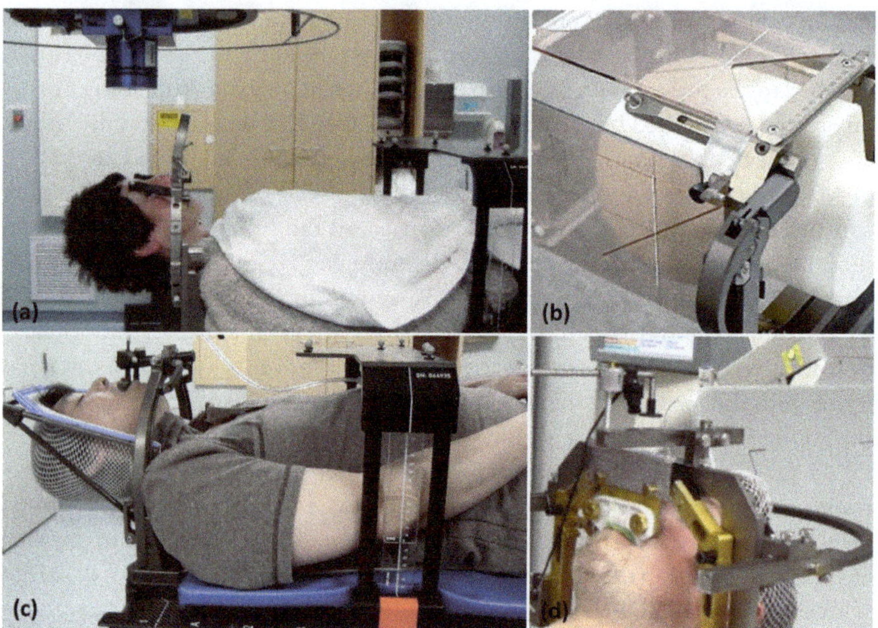

**FIGURE 3.1** Photos of some of the immobilization devices discussed in Chapter 3 (A) is the Cosman–Roberts–Wells frame; (B) is the Leksell frame; (C) is the Aktina Pin-Point system; (D) is the Gill–Thomas–Cosman frame.

## Frameless Systems

To compensate for the loss of rigid immobilization associated with invasive head frames, image guidance is a major component of all frameless systems. Imaging at the time of treatment is used to directly determine the position of the target and to correct for any patient movement and/or positioning errors. As a result, an accurate correlation between patient anatomy and the immobilization device, which is key to the frame-based stereotactic approach, is no longer essential. Optical video methods based on fixed geometry wall-mounted cameras in the treatment room and reflective markers on the patient can be used (Figure 3.2). For frameless positioning, treatment room image-guided systems must include onboard cone-beam CT (CBCT), onboard megavoltage electronic portal imaging devices (MV EPID), or onboard kilovolt images and/or kilovolt x-ray systems mounted on the ceiling and floor (Figure 3.3). Some commercially available noninvasive frameless systems include the Extend frame, PinPoint frame, optically guided bite block, and Brainlab frameless system.

The Extend frame system (Elekta, Stockholm, Sweden)—also referred to as Fraxion—is a noninvasive vacuum bite-block repositioning head frame for cra-

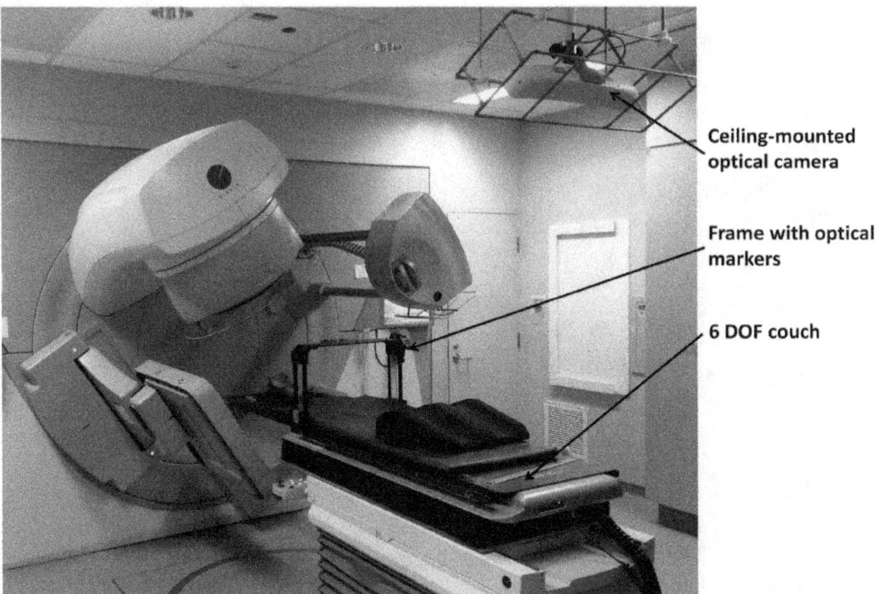


**FIGURE 3.2** Modern LINAC with orthogonal kV CBCT imaging system and 6DOF robotic couch

An optical camera mounted on the ceiling (shown inside a protective cage) picks up optical markers on the indexed frame on the couch for fine adjustments of translation and rotation.

*Note:* 6DOF, 6 degrees of freedom; CBCT, cone-beam CT; LINAC, linear accelerator.

nial immobilization. Its main components include a carbon fiber frame body that is attached to the treatment couch, a headrest, and a mouthpiece that is affixed to the frame body using a frontpiece (6). A vacuum device is used to suction the custom bite block to the patient's upper hard palate. To verify that the patient's head is accurately positioned within the Extend frame, a spring-loaded digital dial gauge is inserted through slotted holes in a repositioning check tool (RCT) attached to the frame. The distance between the frame and the patient's head is measured and compared to reference values taken on the initial day of treatment. The patient can then be repositioned at the time of setup if the difference exceeds a predefined tolerance (eg, 1 mm). In one study that evaluated four patients immobilized with the Extend frame and treated on a Gamma Knife machine (Perfexion™, Elekta Instruments AB, Stockholm, Sweden), the mean radial positioning error was found to be between 0.33 and 0.84 mm (7). Using CBCT, Ruschin et al reported the mean three-dimensional intrafraction motion to be $0.4 \pm 0.3$ mm (6).

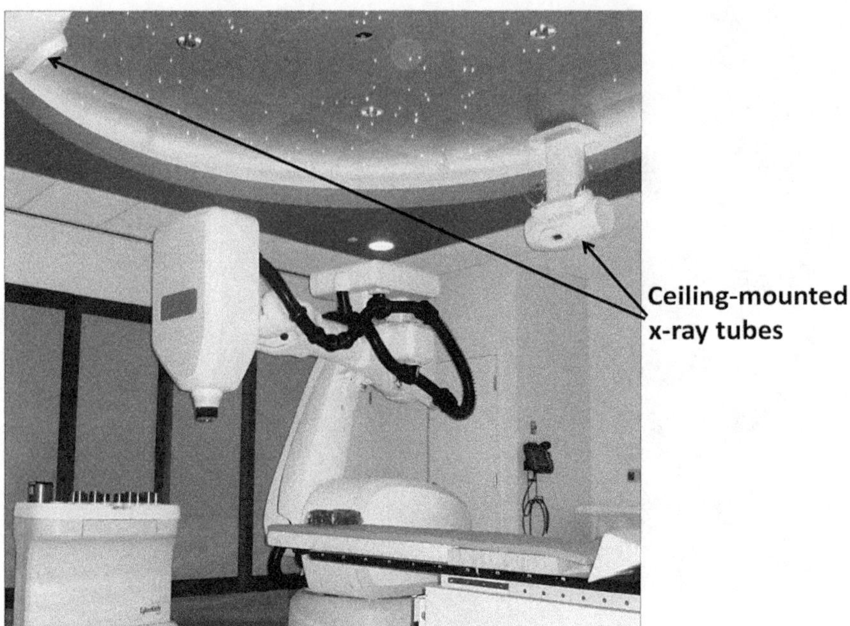


**FIGURE 3.3**  Photo of a CyberKnife system
Two flat-panel detectors in the floor process X-ray exposures of the isocenter, which are used for patient positioning and to verify patient motion during treatment.

Similar in design to the Extend frame, the PinPoint (Aktina Medical, Congers, NY) is a noninvasive frameless system equipped with a vacuum fixation bite-block device for patient localization and immobilization. A gentle vacuum suction is applied between the dental mouthpiece and the upper hard palate to assure tight contact. A patient-specific head support is formed by creating an impression of the back of the skull. Once the patient is immobilized in the PinPoint frame, the patient's head cannot move without losing suction. One study evaluated the PinPoint frameless system and its ability to immobilize patients and restrict head motion. Based on two hypofractionated (SRT) and two single-fraction (SRS) patients (10 treatment fractions in total), the mean translations and rotations were $0.3 \pm 0.2$ mm and $0.2° \pm 0.1°$, respectively (1). These values were found to be consistent with the magnitude of motion quantified with the BRW head frame.

The Brainlab frameless thermoplastic mask (Brainlab AG, Feldkirchen, Germany) is a system strengthened with a custom-made mouthpiece and three reinforcing straps attached under the mask that cover the forehead, chin, and the area below the nose (8). For localization and real-time tracking, six infrared markers are placed on top of the thermoplastic mask and are detected by an infrared camera system (ExacTrac) mounted to the ceiling. In conjunction with this optical guidance system, stereoscopic, planar kilovolt x-ray images (Novalis Body) are taken and registered in 6 degrees of freedom (6DOF) with the digitally reconstructed radiographs (DRRs) from the planning CT images. Once the registration is accepted, any departures from the treatment isocenter are determined. Translational and rotational positioning errors in 6DOF can be corrected for with the treatment couch and a robotic tilt module underneath the tabletop (9,10). Gevaert et al investigated the setup errors and the intrafraction motion of 40 patients immobilized with the Brainlab frameless mask system. The mean three-dimensional intrafractional motion was $0.58 \pm 0.42$ mm, and the mean intrafractional rotations in all directions were within $\pm 0.03°$.

## Technology for Image-Guided Localization
### Onboard Cone-Beam CT

CBCT (11–13) has become nearly ubiquitous in commercially available SRS-equipped LINACS. The key advantage of CBCT is the acquisition of high-quality kilovoltage three-dimensional images that can be used to localize the targeted tumor and determine the difference between its positions at the time of patient setup to the planned tumor position. The coregistration of CBCT to CT images has been quoted to be submillimeter in terms of accuracy. Proper quality assurance and calibration procedures must be performed for CBCT to ensure accuracy between the actual LINAC treatment isocenter and that of the CBCT system. The transformation between the CBCT and the CT relative to the isocenter can be corrected through automatic couch translations and rotations. The residual error associated with the CBCT image-guidance process has typically been quoted to be about one millimeter or less.

### 6 Degrees-of-Freedom Couch

Correcting rotational misalignment has a limited utility for small spherical targets that are readily localized at the treatment isocenter. However, rotational misalignment can have substantial dosimetric consequences for targets that (a) are complex in shape, such as paraspinal lesions that are impinging upon a critical organ; (b) do not have nearby localization anatomy, such as targets in the center of the skull; or (c) are nonisocentric, such as multiple intracranial targets treated using a single isocenter.

To mitigate this uncertainty, more advanced system corrections can be made in 6DOF. 6DOF systems comprise a pitch-and-roll stage that is sandwiched between the couch translation stage and the couch top.

## Technology for Intratreatment Positional Monitoring
### Stereoscopic Imaging

Stereoscopic x-ray imagers use a pair of x-ray sources and corresponding flat-panel detectors mounted in the treatment room. The central rays of the sources intersect at the machine isocenter and are separated by an angle sufficient for the stereoscopic visualization of patient anatomy (10). Stereoscopic systems are capable of submillimeter accuracy (10), comparable to a stereotactic frame (8). One advantage of room-fixed stereoimaging systems relative to gantry-mounted systems is that images can be obtained over a wider range of gantry and couch positions. During treatment, stereoscopic x-ray images can also be acquired several times per minute to ensure that the patient's position remains stable. Stereoscopic images are processed via automatic registration software and coregistered to the DRRs generated from the treatment- planning CT. If deviations in position are detected beyond tolerance, the patient's position is adjusted via couch shifts.

### Intrafraction Motion Monitoring

Intrafraction motion-monitoring systems have been developed to oversee patient position during treatment, eliminating the need for a frame to maintain targeting accuracy. Using the CyberKnife system, one group studied intrafraction motion for intracranial targets and showed that 95% of displacements were less than 1.6 mm over a 15-minute interval (14). They recommended repeat imaging and patient setup correction at 5-minute intervals and suggested a 0.6 mm margin to account for residual motion. Similarly, another study found that intrafraction motion in the skull typically stayed within 0.8 mm over 1- to 5-minute intervals and concluded that a tracking interval of 1 to 2 minutes is necessary for most intracranial radiosurgery applications (15). If the target position is monitored less frequently, the margin must be increased to ensure the target receives the prescribed dose (14–17).

## Improvements in Beam-Delivery Technique
### Flattening Filter–*Free Delivery*

One shortcoming of the use of small radiosurgery fields is the reduction of the effective dose rate. Treatments can therefore be lengthy, and the resulting discomfort for the patient can result in an increased risk of motion. Flattening filter–free (FFF) beams, now entering widespread clinical use, have dose rates up to 2.4 times higher than conventional flattened beams and can significantly mitigate these risks. Removing the flattening filter increases the dose rate near the central axis by a factor of two to four, depending on the beam energy, which can lead to significantly shorter delivery times for hypofractionated treatment regimens. C-arm LINACs without a flattening filter became commercially available in 2010, and early clinical experience demonstrated treatment times for central nervous system (CNS) radiosurgery approaching those of conventional fractionation. Concerns regarding the use of FFF include an increased surface dose and the radiobiological effect relative to conventional flattened beams. For the dose range typical of hypofractionated radiation therapy, the radiobiological effect is expected to increase when treatment time is reduced. Ling et al showed that late-responding normal tissues have a larger increase than tumor and early-responding normal tissues, suggesting caution when implementing any technology that significantly shortens overall treatment time (18). Early reports on FFF beams have shown low rates of acute toxicity (19–23). Long-term experience with FFF beams is limited; however, preliminary results have not demonstrated unexpected toxicity.

## Intensity-Modulated Radiation Therapy and Volumetric Modulated Arc Therapy

Multileaf collimators (MLCs) coupled with computer-optimized planning have made intensity-modulated radiation therapy (IMRT) and volumetric-modulated arc therapy (VMAT) possible. IMRT and VMAT can generate highly conformal dose distributions that have rapid dose falloff, even for complex target shapes. IMRT and VMAT are more efficient to deliver than shot-based techniques, reducing treatment times. VMAT is a rotational technique in which the MLC aperture shape varies with the gantry angle. In most modern applications, the dose rate and the gantry speed also vary. VMAT differs from conformal arc therapy because the aperture shapes and weights are inverse planned to meet dosimetric objectives, rather than conforming to the target shape at all gantry angles. Conformal arc therapy has been widely used for LINAC intracranial radiosurgery (24–27), so it was a natural extension to use VMAT for stereotactic applications. VMAT's primary advantage over nonmodulated techniques is its ability to improve conformity and/or the sparing of critical structures.

## Dose Falloff

Recent discussions in the literature have focused on whether any particular system (Gamma Knife, Cyberknife, LINAC) confers a dosimetric advantage in terms of dose falloff. In other words, is dosimetric precision greater for any given platform compared to another? This is a clinically relevant question because any advantage in healthy tissue sparing will increase a given system's capacity to safely treat multiple targets or recurrent disease.

For single targets, dose falloff characteristics of three modalities—Perfexion, Cyberknife, and Novalis—were examined (28). Almost identical dose falloff was seen despite the large differences in delivery methods and treatment-planning strategies. This shows that when prescribing the same biologic effective dose (BED) to the target periphery, the radiobiologic effective dose as measured by the equivalent uniform biologic effective dose (EUBED) produced similar normal tissue–sparing properties among these modalities. This suggests that the dependence of normal brain toxicity on the Gamma Knife's 10-Gy or 12-Gy volumes (29–31) is most likely transferable from one modality to another. In particular, the EUBED for the surrounding normal brain tissue decreases with increasing numbers of fractions for target a/b, ranging from 10 to 20. In contrast, it clearly increases with increasing numbers of fractions for targets with a/b ratios close to that of the normal brain, such as a/b = 2. In the former case, the decrease in EUBED to the normal tissue is most significant within the first few fractions of treatments; for example, as with 10 fractions.

For multiple targets, the integral dose to the normal brain tissue was found to be apparatus-dependent (32). A comparison of Perfexion, CyberKnife, and Novalis modalities for up to 12 targets showed that Gamma Knife Perfexion plans resulted in much smaller normal brain volumes receiving any particular dose. The difference favored the Gamma Knife Perfexion on the order of two to three times. The Paddick conformity indices were also better for Perfexion, and no degradation in dose conformity was seen with increasing numbers of targets. To ensure consistent comparisons, the normal brain volume was normalized to the total target volume obtained with each modality. This avoided the rounding or scaling errors associated with different dose grid resolutions from computations at each treatment-planning system. This effect is almost insignificant for large target volumes but can be important for small target volumes.

The dose distribution for multiple targets exhibits complex beam interplay effects and requires a relatively large number of dose-volume constraints in the planning process. For multiple-lesion treatment plans, the total number of beams plus the number of constraints approximately scale proportionally with the total number of targets. Differences in dose calculation algorithms may also partially explain the apparatus-dependent effect. It is known that CyberKnife's low-isodose lines (eg, 10%–20%) often show islands of dose in nontarget regions that are not observed in the Novalis or Perfexion plans. These islands are basically associated with CyberKnife's nonisocentric planning algorithm rather than with its hardware design. However, these factors are unlikely to explain the large differences observed, because the calculations in the brain are in a relatively homogeneous space, and all systems have been well validated (33–35).

The hypothesis of improved sparing of normal brain tissue with Gamma Knife SRS when treating multiple targets has been challenged by other studies, which have shown that "for multiple target SRS, 4-arc VMAT produced clinically equivalent conformity, dose fall-off, 12 Gy isodose volume, and low isodose spill, and reduced treatment time compared to [the Gamma Knife]" (36). A discussion in the literature was sparked: some argued that although VMAT delivers faster treatment it significantly increases the normal tissue dose (37), while others argued that VMAT confers improved conformity and plan quality due to the high resolution 2.5-mm MLC leaves and an optimal four-arc technique with advanced inverse planning (38). The results of yet another recent study (39) have indicated that the most optimal VMAT plans yield normal brain isodose lines that are 100% to 200% higher than those with the Gamma Knife. The same study indicated that even for a single brain metastasis the peripheral dose falloff was lower for Gamma Knife surgery compared to VMAT by approximately a factor of two (39).

Current studies on dose falloff are problematic because they are all retrospective in nature and suffer from the issues of bias and a lack of proper control. Multiple studies have demonstrated that the dose falloff for a given system is most affected by the total target volume being treated, as well as the number of targets, including the dose interplay between them (40,41). After accounting for target size, further differences in dose falloff can be realized through differences in clinical practice and technique. For example, allowing multiple noncoplanar arcs, with heavy beam modulation and a willingness to allow target hot spots in excess of 150% of the prescription, will assuredly produce more rapid dose falloff than a single arc with limited modulation and a target hot spot of less than 120%. Furthermore, the Gamma Knife procedure is planned and prescribed fundamentally differently than VMAT, and it is not surprising that conflicts exist in the literature regarding dose falloff due to variability in plan quality, especially when forward planning. In Figure 3.4 a sample slice of a radiation dose distribution is shown for a single brain metastasis planned with a LINAC-based VMAT approach (one arc and four arcs) and with the Gamma Knife Perfexion. At first glance, one would conclude that the Gamma Knife distribution is the most precise since the isodose lines are the most tightly packed. However, other aspects must be considered: dose heterogeneity in the target, time required for planning, time required for performing quality assurance, beam deliverability, et cetera. Additionally, when performing hypofractionation and using a PTV margin to account for daily setup variation, the heterogeneous dose distribution of the Gamma Knife may be detrimental because a larger dose will be deposited in the normal brain tissue within the PTV but outside the gross tumor volume (GTV). In such cases where a PTV margin is

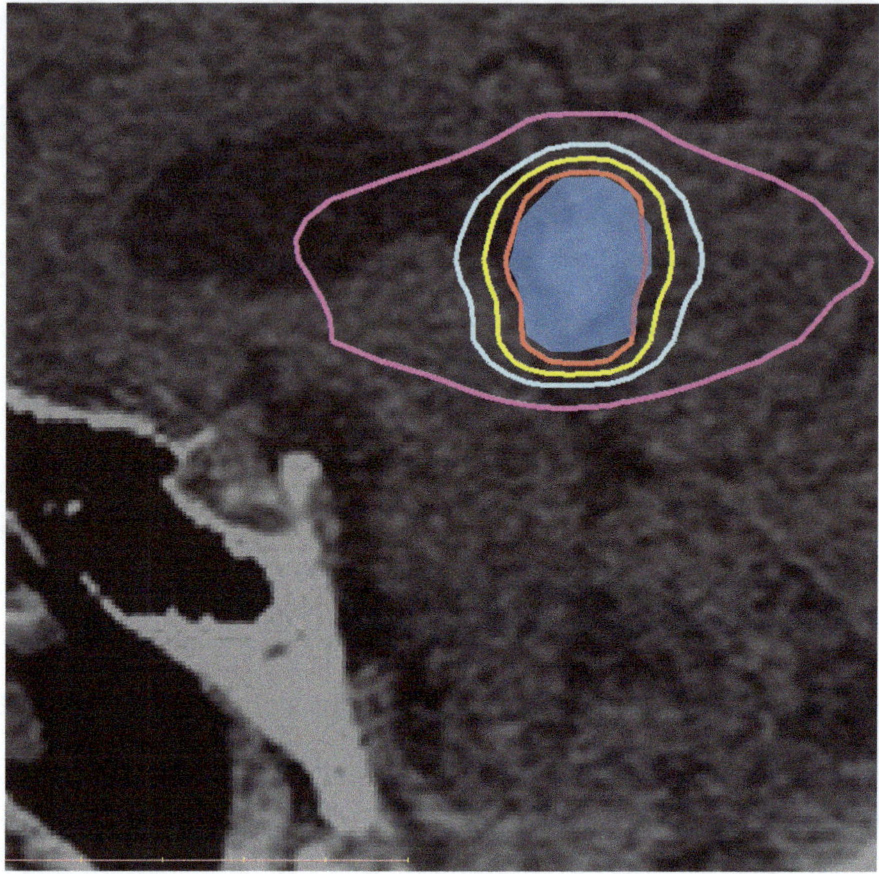

**FIGURE 3.4** Typical dose distribution and the resulting statistics for a single target shown in sagittal view

*Note:* Blue color wash = target volume. Isodose lines: gray = 30 Gy; red = 20 Gy (prescribed dose); yellow = 16 Gy; light blue = 12 Gy; pink = 5 Gy. VMAT (volumetric modulated arc therapy) was planned using a 4 mm MLC (multileaf collimator) Elekta beam modulator. Plans were all generated so that the target volume receiving 20 Gy was 98%.

needed, a more homogeneous dose distribution, as shown in Figure 3.4, may be the safest approach.

An unbiased, prospective, and high-powered multi-institutional study is required to answer whether a given technology truly confers a dosimetric advantage over the others. Due to differences in prescription and planning practices, this will be a challenging study to design, but if it can be done, it will hopefully resolve the current debate.

## Improvements in Small-Field Dosimetry

An MV photon field is traditionally defined as "small" when one or both of the following conditions are satisfied: (a) lateral charge particle equilibrium (CPE) is lost (ie, field dimensions are comparable to or smaller than the range of lateral secondary electrons); and (b) the collimator setting obstructs the source size.

Given the previous definition, with either cobalt 60 or LINAC-produced 6-MV photon beams, the fields become small below around 10 mm (42). In 2007 Doblado et al showed the importance of selecting a detector in small-field dosimetry (43). They observed that especially for field sizes less than 3.0 cm, results from different detectors start deviating. Such deviations exceed 50% at field sizes less than 10 mm if inappropriate detectors (eg, large-volume ionization chambers) are used. The results of these and similar studies indicate a strong need for international guidelines and recommendations for best practices in small-field dosimetry to maintain a consistent level of accuracy across all sites practicing SRS.

## Dose Calibration

National and international societies are currently developing a number of reports on small-field dosimetry. Most notably, these include: the American Association of Physicists in Medicine (AAPM) Task Group 155 report on small-field photon beam dosimetry, as well as the Task Group 178 report on Gamma Knife dosimetry; the joint report of the International Atomic Energy Agency (IAEA) and the AAPM on the dosimetry of small static fields used in external beam radiotherapy; the International Commission on Radiation Units and Measurements (ICRU) report on the prescription, recording, and reporting of stereotactic radiosurgery using small fields; and report 103 of the Institute of Physics and Engineering in Medicine (IPEM) on small-field MV photon dosimetry.

At the time of this book's publication, some of the small-field dosimetry protocols and reports previously noted were not yet available. However, given that most of the dosimetry protocols addressing small fields rely on the formalism outlined by Alfonso et al (44), a short summary of it will be provided to highlight some of the challenges in SRS and small-field dosimetry.

*Reference Dosimetry.* Currently, the AAPM Task Group 51 protocol (45) and its update (46), as well as the IAEA TRS-398 (47), form the basic formalism for clinical reference dosimetry. These protocols require reference conditions ($10 \times 10$ cm$^2$ field size, 100-cm source-to-axis or source-to-surface distance, etc) and rely on the use of an ionization chamber in a large water phantom under reference conditions that ensure the existence of electronic charged particle equilibrium. The problem arises that with the exception of LINAC-based SRS, all other specialized SRS delivery units (Gamma Knife, CyberKnife, and Tomotherapy) cannot meet the reference conditions outlined by protocols. The proposed remedy in the absence of an available $10 \times 10$ cm$^2$ field size has been to use the intermediate field size and measurement condition that most closely resembles the reference condition. The *machine-specific reference* (MSR) field is the technical terminology used to describe such a stationary intermediate field. The larger the differences between the MSR field and the reference field and the reference conditions (ie, the calibration conditions of the detector), the larger the potential differences in the beam quality and the variations in detector response. Only a handful of national laboratories have begun providing calibrations under specific MSR fields for a few models of SRS delivery equipment. More commonly, calibrations are provided under broad beam reference conditions. The physicist must first be sure to use an appropriate reference-caliber detector for the given MSR field and second, make sure to apply appropriate beam quality correction factors to account for differences between the MSR and the reference field/conditions.

The reference conditions for common SRS radiotherapy units are noted below:

- For LINAC-based SRS programs in which a conventional LINAC is fitted with either SRS cones or micro-MLC add-ons, the reference conditions should be taken as the conventional $10 \times 10$ cm$^2$ reference field at 100 cm from the source (or a field as close to this as possible; eg, a $9.8 \times 10.2$ cm$^2$ field if the MLC does not allow for an exact $10 \times 10$ cm$^2$ setting). All other collimator settings and field sizes are calibrated through relative dosimetry.
- For CyberKnife, the 60-mm diameter fixed collimator (80 cm from the source) provides a relatively flat and uniform field that normally is recommended as the MSR field.
- If tomotherapy is used for small-target therapy, the $5 \times 10$ cm$^2$ field size (85 cm from the source) is the recommended MSR field.
- Gamma Knife perhaps poses the largest challenge for dosimetry. Since the calibration of each individual source is impractical and of limited use, an appropriate MSR field would be the largest diameter collimator helmet (16 mm or 18 mm, depending on the model) with all sources out.

*Relative Dosimetry.* As previously mentioned, relative dosimetry is concerned with the measurement of output factors, or the ratio of absorbed dose to water at a point in any nonreference field to that determined under the reference conditions. It is noteworthy here to stress that the ratio is that of absorbed dose to water and not detector reading. It has been common practice in radiotherapy to interchange the two, and although the implications may be insignificant in relative ion chamber dosimetry in broad beams, they can be devastatingly large in small-field dosimetry. Indeed, detector responses can vary significantly over a wide range of field sizes, and they especially change as we move toward smaller field sizes. As a general practice, the difference between detector response in the MSR field relative to that in the reference field must be taken into account; for example, by using Monte Carlo calculated corrections (48,49).

The choice of a detector and understanding the response behavior of those choices in small-field dosimetry is of the utmost importance. Indeed, in SRS the size of the fields of interest often approaches the size of the detector. This may have consequences, such as volume averaging, perturbations, and more. Some of these will be briefly discussed next.

## Dosimeters in Small Fields
The choice of a dosimeter in small fields is contingent on its application and whether reference or relative dosimetry is the main focus.

*Reference Dosimetry.* Small-volume ionization chambers that satisfy the dosimetric requirements of stability, reproducibility, linearity, energy, dose and dose-rate independence, and more in small field sizes are obvious choices for reference dosimetry. Although high–spatial resolution detectors can minimize the volume-averaging effect, care should also be taken to select detectors that have minimal beam perturbation. As an example, some microchambers may cause large perturbations due to the nonwater equivalence of some of their components (50). The previously noted IAEA-AAPM report on small-field dosimetry will have a specific list of recommended reference class detectors for use with the various MSR fields and radiotherapy delivery units.

In relative dosimetry the detector choices are much wider, and selecting an ideal detector is perhaps more difficult. Since relative dose measurements need to be made at the smallest of SRS field sizes and the volume-averaging effect can be large even during beam profile measurements, it is important to select a detector whose sensitive volume is smaller than the field sizes of interest. A number of dosimeters have been used in radiosurgical fields: small-volume ionization chambers (51,52), microionization chambers (50,52), liquid ionization chambers (53,54), diamond detectors (55–58), silicon diodes (55,56,59), plastic and organic scintillators (57,60), radiochromic and radiographic films (60,61), metal oxide semiconductor filed effect transistors (MOSFET) (61,62), thermoluminescent dosimeters (TLD) (59,61), optically stimulated luminescence (OSL) detectors (63), alanine detectors (57), and polymer gels (64).

## OVERVIEW OF MAJOR STEREOTACTIC RADIOSURGERY TECHNOLOGIES AND HOW THEY INTEGRATE TO MANAGE RADIOSURGERY UNCERTAINTY

The three most advanced systems for delivering SRS to treat brain metastases are:

1. Leksell Gamma Knife (LGK)
2. CyberKnife
3. LINAC-based systems (IMRT/VMAT/cones)

Each system has its own unique set of features, which confer various advantages and disadvantages over the other. We will provide a brief overview of each system and its capabilities.

### Leksell Gamma Knife Perfexion and Icon™

The LGK system (Elekta Instruments AB, Stockholm, Sweden) delivers high-dose radiotherapy in a single fraction. All models of the Gamma Knife employ many (201 or 192) small beamlets that enter through the brain from different directions and converge to a point within the lesion to deliver an ablative dose of radiation with a steep dose gradient. Traditionally, LGK systems use a rigid head frame that immobilizes the patient's head and defines a stereotactic coordinate system with a direct mechanical linkage between the patient's head and the isocenter of the Gamma Knife suitable for localization and targeting (65,66). Stereotactic definition is based on up-front imaging of the patient using fiducial systems mounted to the patient's head frame to localize anatomy relative to the stereotactic frame of reference.

The clinical success of single-fraction Gamma Knife–based SRS for controlling disease of limited size has been well studied and published. For treating larger or recurrent disease, or for treating tumors close to critical organs at risk (OAR), the emerging treatment of hypofractionated SRS has recently shown favorable local control and normal tissue sparing compared to single-fraction SRS. This has pushed research toward making the Gamma Knife system more flexible and capable of delivering hypofractionated treatments while ensuring accurate and reproducible patient localization without the use of an invasive head frame.

Elekta designed a relocatable frame system called Extend that employed a suctioned dental mold of the hard palate and maxillary teeth. The system removed the requirement for surgical intervention needed for frame placement and was evaluated for safety, comfort, and accuracy prior to commercial release (6). The mean setup uncertainty of the Gamma Knife Extend system has been shown to be approximately 0.4 mm to 1.3 mm (6,7,67,68), which is comparable to other relocatable frame systems on the market.

But the Extend system had many limitations, including a complicated workflow (mouthpiece creation, application, and reposition check tool [RCT] measurement system) and the use of vacuum as a proxy of motion. The system relied on the assumption that any change in the vacuum pressure of greater than 10% equated to a displaced target. Also, the system required a high level of patient compliance, which limited its use to patients with good performance status and good dentition and without a sensitive gag reflex.

However, the development of onboard image-guidance technologies for LINACs led to new ideas to remedy the shortcomings of the Extend system. A group in the Department of Radiation Oncology at the University of Toronto developed a kV-CBCT system that they successfully integrated with the Gamma Knife Perfexion (69). The initial prototype allowed the system to translate from a parked position above the shield doors of the Perfexion to an imaging position between the patient and the shield doors. A rotational axis enabled the system to rotate 210° for imaging. With this prototype Ruschin et al demonstrated sufficient image quality for image-guided radiosurgery with down to 0.5 mm isotropic voxel resolution and a reconstruction field of view of $25.6 \times 25.6 \times 19.3$ cm (70).

Elekta built on the work of Ruschin et al and created an integrated CBCT system of sufficient quality to provide onboard verification of patient position and correction. They also integrated an optical tracking system intended to monitor intrafraction patient position and gate the treatment delivery during positional excursions from the planned treatment position. In 2015 Elekta branded the new treatment device as the Gamma Knife Icon (at the European Society for Radiotherapy and Oncology 3rd Forum), which as of the date of this publication is Food and Drug Administration (FDA) cleared in the United States and "CE" marked in the European Union. (Figure 3.5)

The Icon CBCT system currently includes two preset imaging modes—a high-dose and low-dose mode. Each has a 200° rotation and results in reconstructed voxels of 0.5 mm. Published proceedings by the vendor report a high-contrast resolution of eight line pairs per centimeter using 332 projections at 90 kVp. The high-dose mode has a CT dose index (CTDI) of approximately 7.0 mGy and has a higher signal-to-noise ratio compared to the low-dose mode, which has a CTDI of 2.8 mGy. Preliminary tests on localization uncertainty using a phantom suggest a mean positional uncertainty of less than 0.2 mm

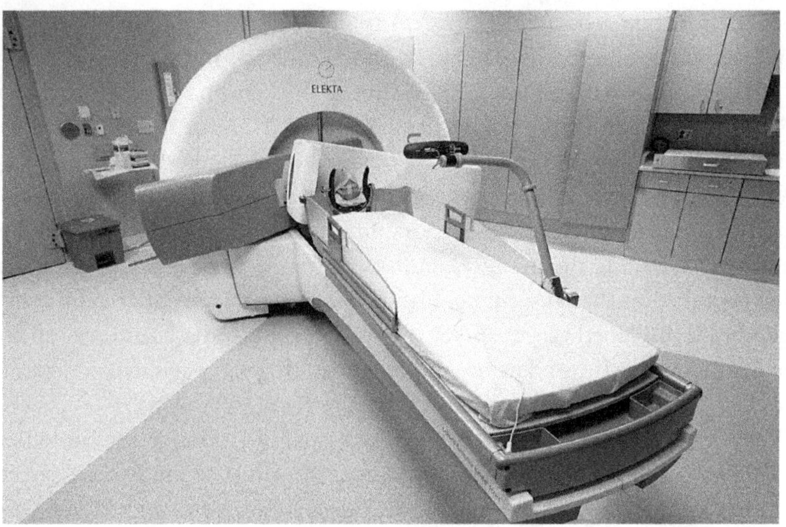

**FIGURE 3.5** Illustration of the Gamma Knife Icon system

(71,72). The results of a preliminary assessment of the Icon's thermoplastic mask system in conjunction with a LINAC system have indicated that sub-millimeter immobilization accuracy is attainable, and in conjunction with real-time optical tracking, it can match the precision of treatment using invasive frames (73).

## Linear Accelerator–Based Stereotactic Radiosurgery

Historically, LINAC-based SRS units were built upon standard LINACs with add-on collimation systems and couch stabilization devices. The majority of these SRS units employed tertiary cones to yield small circular beams with a minimum diameter of 0.5 cm to 1 cm or add-on micro- or mini-MLCs to deliver noncoplanar converging arc beams to the isocenter. The arrangement of these noncoplanar arc beams aimed to deliver an elliptical dose distribution similar to that of a single isocenter in Gamma Knife delivery. In general, the tertiary cones were made from high-Z materials and were intended to extend the source to diaphragm distance to sharpen the beam penumbra at the isocenter. Modifications to the treatment couch and the in-room laser system were also required to ensure submillimeter precision in delivery. Similar to Gamma Knife–based SRS, an invasive head frame was required for both immobilization and stereotaxy.

**TABLE 3.2** Comparison of dosimetric indices across treatment techniques

|  | VMAT-1 arc | VMAT-4 arcs (noncoplanar) | Gamma Knife Perfexion |
|---|---|---|---|
| PIV | 4.56 cm³ | 4.40 cm³ | 3.97 cm³ |
| CI Paddick | 0.75 | 0.77 | 0.84 |
| GI Paddick | 4.6 | 3.6 | 2.7 |
| V12Gy | 15.0 cm³ | 12.3 cm³ | 8.5 cm³ |
| Dmax | 23.3 Gy | 25.5 Gy | 39.1 Gy |
| Beamontime | ~7 min | ~ 10 min | ~ 40 min (at 3 Gy/min) |

*Note:* CI, conformity index; GI, gradient index; PIV, prescription isodose volume; VMAT, volumetric modulated arc therapy.

As shown in Figure 3.2, standard modern-day LINACs are equipped with online image-guidance systems in the form of CBCT. Furthermore, 6DOF robotic couches have paved the way for frameless systems, relying on imaging rather than the mechanical coupling of lasers to the stereotactic system to provide the required accuracy. The decision of whether to use tertiary cones (see Figure 3.1) or MLC-based delivery involves a discussion and balance around dose falloff, small-field dose calibration, treatment time, and the integration of other novel features, such as FFF mode. Table 3.2 shows a comparison of dosimetric indices across treatment techniques.

## CyberKnife

The CyberKnife (Accuray, Sunnyvale, CA, United States) (74), developed by the neurosurgeon John Adler in the late 1990s, is an alternative to the Gamma Knife to deliver frameless SRS (11,75). The CyberKnife system is a LINAC mounted on a robotic arm specifically designed for stereotactic treatments. Highly conformal dose distributions are achieved by using hundreds of noncoplanar, nonisocentric beams around the patient. Stereotactic targeting accuracy is achieved by combining near-real-time stereoscopic orthogonal x-ray images with advanced image recognition software, without the need for rigid fixation devices.

The CyberKnife consists of an X-band cavity magnetron and a side-coupled standing wave LINAC mounted on a robotic manipulator (Kuka Roboter GmbH, Augsburg, Germany). The LINAC produces an unflattened 6 MV-photon beam with a dose rate up to 1000 cGy/min. Treatment is delivered from hundreds of beams arranged around the target. Each beam is defined by a source point (called a *node*), a direction, and a field size. The complete set of nodes, called the *path set*, can range from 23 to 133 depending on the site and patient position. The image-guided system consists of two diagnostic x-ray sources mounted in the ceiling and two amorphous silicon flat-panel detectors embedded in the floor, imaging the patient from two orthogonal views at plus or minus 45° oblique angles. Images can be taken every 15 to 150 seconds (the typical imaging frequency is 30–60 seconds, depending on the treatment site). For organs such as the liver and the prostate, fiducials are implanted and tracked; for intracranial cases, six-dimensional skull tracking is used; and for spine cases, the Xsight spine-tracking algorithm is used, and its accuracy is 0.61 mm (76).

The CyberKnife M6 system has the option to use 1 of 12 fixed circular tungsten cones (with diameters ranging from 5 mm to 60 mm), an Iris collimator, or a recently developed micro–MLC. The Iris collimation system consists of two hexagonal banks of tungsten, producing a 12-sided aperture. The mechanical uncertainty of the Iris field sizes is 0.2 mm, which affects the output factor for the smallest field size (5 mm, 7.5 mm, and 10 mm). The uncertainty in output factor for the 5-mm aperture can be up to 10%, and thus the manufacturer restricts the use of this aperture. The micro–MLC consists of 41 pairs of fully interdigitated tungsten leaves 2.5 mm thick and 100 mm wide at 80 cm source-to-axis distance (SAD), allowing a maximum field size of 120 mm (leaf motion direction) by 100 mm. The vendor specification for interleaf leakage is a maximum of less than 0.5% (Accuray Inc) (74). The addition of the micro–MLC is expected to expand the clinical applications of the CyberKnife, allowing the treatment of large lesions (>6 cm) and the use of conventionally fractionated dose regimens. Early investigations have shown that plans generated with the micro–MLC result in a more homogeneous dose distribution, a lower number of monitoring units (Mu), and a significantly shorter treatment time (77,78).

Target localization during patient setup and treatment delivery is achieved by comparing the live camera images with a library of DRRs generated from the planning CT at 45° angles through the imaging center. Based on this comparison, the tracking software calculates the differences in the three translational and three rotational directions between simulation and treatment positions. The targeting accuracy of the CyberKnife system has been reported in the literature to be submillimeter and subdegree for both static and dynamic tracking methods (16,79). In 2014 a micro–MLC was added to the collimator system, which significantly reduces treatment time while maintaining or improving treatment quality. This system was branded as the CyberKnife M6 series.

## THE IMPACT OF TECHNOLOGY ON CLINICAL DEVELOPMENTS IN STEREOTACTIC RADIOSURGERY: MULTIPLE METASTASES AND HYPOFRACTIONATION

So far in this chapter, we have discussed the technical aspects, precision, and accuracy of the radiation platforms for SRS. In this part we focus on the impact of this technology on the clinical application of SRS. In the 1980s and 1990s, SRS was used in big academic centers and mainly for a single brain metastasis. With recent current technical developments such as IGRT, 6DOF robotic couches, optical systems, fine MLCs, IMRT/VMAT, et cetera, SRS platforms are now available in a large number of radiation therapy facilities, which has expanded the utilization of intracranial SRS. Furthermore, the clinical data support a major role for SRS for patients with brain metastases.

In the beginning, SRS was used as an adjunct to WBRT for patients with up to four metastases. The data concluded that there were significant improvements in local control and survival (80,81). Then, three randomized controlled trials compared SRS alone to WBRT plus SRS for patients with one to four brain metastases. Although they showed no overall survival (OS) benefit, they did show improved distant brain control and local control with additional WBRT (82–84). However, given the lack of survival advantage, SRS alone has been concluded to be the routine treatment option due to favorable neurocognitive outcomes, less risk of late side effects, and no adverse effects on a patient's performance status (85). Recently, an individual patient data meta-analysis of the same three trials challenged this impact on survival by showing a survival benefit for patients under 50 years of age who were treated with SRS alone (86). At this time several professional societies endorse SRS alone for patients with limited brain metastases.

Recent and ongoing trials are investigating the benefit of SRS alone in patients with 5 to 10 brain metastases. The first major prospective study evaluating SRS alone for multiple brain metastases was reported in 2014 (87). Patients with 1 to 10 brain metastases were treated with SRS alone using the Gamma Knife and stratified to 1, 2 to 4, and 5 to 10 metastases. Survival, distant brain relapse, and local control rates were not significantly different in patients with 5 to 10 metastases versus 2 to 4 metastases. These results are of major significance because they challenge the dogma that patients with more than four metastases will not benefit from SRS alone due to shortened survival and inevitable failure elsewhere in the brain. Therefore, this trial supplies evidence to support SRS alone in good Karnofsky performance status (KPS) patients with up to 10 metastases, provided the individual tumor volume is no more than 10 mL and less than 3 cm in the largest diameter, and the total cumulative volume of all tumors in the brain is less than or equal to 15 mL. Several ongoing randomized trials are evaluating WBRT alone versus SRS alone in similar patients, and a trial is being designed to evaluate SRS alone versus WBRT plus SRS boost in patients with 10 to 20 metastases (88).

One of the limitations of single-fraction SRS is its inverse relationship with the dose prescribed to the tumor diameter. As a result the upper limit of SRS eligibility is generally a maximum diameter of 3 cm to 4 cm. Furthermore, metastases within, or proximal to, critical structures would inadvertently be underdosed or untreated with SRS due to fear of causing necrosis and major clinical functional impairments. With the new advances in SRS technology and the advent of frameless and image-guided treatments, hypofractionated SRS has appeared to be a reasonable solution for those tumors, ensuring a higher BED is delivered while improving the safety profile on the normal tissue by exploiting the benefits of fractionation. Many centers are currently adopting hypofractionated SRS as a standard practice for tumors greater than 2 cm or near or within critical structures, and they report better local control than single-fraction SRS with similar or better radionecrosis rates (89,90).

Our approach at the Department of Radiation Oncology at the University of Toronto has been to favor single-fraction SRS for targets less than 1.5 cm and hypofractionated radiotherapy for targets greater than 2 cm in diameter. For targets 1.5 cm to 2 cm, either technique can be used while considering other factors as well, such as patient preference, et cetera. The preferred technique for hyperfractionated radiotherapy (HFRT) is a single-arc VMAT, reserving multiple arcs/beams for complex cases involving close proximity to OAR. For multiple targets spaced less than 8 cm apart, one isocenter is considered, thereby limiting the susceptibility of plan deliverability to off-axis image matching, leaf speed accuracy, and off-axis small-field beam modeling. For single-fraction SRS, we use a tertiary mounted cones system.

The GTV, in the case of intact metastases; the clinical target volume (CTV), in the case of surgical cavities; and the OAR, consisting of the brainstem, globes, lens, optic nerves, and chiasm are contoured on volumetric T1 postgadolinium MRI fused to the treatment-planning CT. For intact metastases, no additional expansion to the GTV is applied for microscopic spread; therefore, the CTV is equal to the GTV. For surgical cavities the CTV is contoured as the postoperative bed, and the meningeal margin is scrutinized for dural-based lesions. For single-fraction SRS, with the patient immobilized in an invasive head frame, no margin for PTV is applied. However, with the frameless PinPoint system, we apply a 1-mm PTV margin in all directions except craniocaudally, where the margin is grown to 1.5 mm based on our internal study. For hypofractionated SRS we immobilize in a simple thermoplastic mask and apply a uniform PTV margin of 2 mm. The target objective is to cover greater than 98% of the PTV (V100>98%) with the prescribed dose while limiting the maximum dose to less than 130% of the prescribed dose. For hypofractionated SRS the prescription dose ranges from 20 Gy to 35 Gy in five fractions or 24 Gy in three fractions and depends on tumor volume.

## CONCLUSIONS

Both accuracy and precision are important to the clinical success of SRS. In recent years technology and technologic publications have focused on comparing the precision of various systems, with arguments made in favor of certain systems under specific conditions. However, each institution must carefully measure the accuracy of the entire system, including dose calculation and calibration at small field, prior to embarking on an SRS program. The trade-offs that exist between various techniques, in particular hypofractionated treatments, may eventually translate to clinical benefits. It is imperative that the reporting of outcomes is accompanied by dosimetric data in order to generate guidelines for safe practice. There is no doubt that technology is driving advances in SRS applications. It behooves us to ensure that we practice safely and evaluate technologies prior to routine application.

## References


1. Li G, Ballangrud A, Kuo LC, et al. Motion monitoring for cranial frameless stereotactic radiosurgery using video-based three-dimensional optical surface imaging. *Med Phys.* 2011;38: 3981–3994.
2. Ramakrishna N, Rosca F, Friesen S, et al. A clinical comparison of patient setup and intra-fraction motion using frame-based radiosurgery versus a frameless image-guided radiosurgery system for intracranial lesions. *Radiother Oncol.* 2010;95:109–115.
3. Gill SS, Thomas DG, Warrington AP, et al. Relocatable frame for stereotactic external beam radiotherapy. *Int J Radiat Oncol Biol Phys.* 1991;20:599–603.
4. Graham JD, Warrington AP, Gill SS, et al. A non-invasive, relocatable stereotactic frame for fractionated radiotherapy and multiple imaging. *Radiother Oncol.* 1991;21:60–62.
5. Das S, Isiah R, Rajesh B, et al. Accuracy of relocation, evaluation of geometric uncertainties and clinical target volume (CTV) to planning target volume (PTV) margin in fractionated stereotactic radiotherapy for intracranial tumors using relocatable Gill-Thomas-Cosman (GTC) frame. *J Appl Clin Med Phys.* 2011;12:3260.
6. Ruschin M, Nayebi N, Carlsson P, et al. Performance of a novel repositioning head frame for gamma knife perfexion and image-guided linac-based intracranial stereotactic radiotherapy. *Int J Radiat Oncol Biol Phys.* 2010;78:306–313.
7. Sayer FT, Sherman JH, Yen CP, et al. Initial experience with the eXtend system: a relocatable frame system for multiple-session gamma knife radiosurgery. *World Neurosurg.* 2011;75:665–672.

8. Gevaert T, Verellen D, Tournel K, et al. Setup accuracy of the Novalis ExacTrac 6DOF system for frameless radiosurgery. *Int J Radiat Oncol Biol Phys*. 2012;82:1627–1635.

9. Gevaert T, Verellen D, Engels B, et al. Clinical evaluation of a robotic 6-degree of freedom treatment couch for frameless radiosurgery. *Int J Radiat Oncol Biol Phys*. 2012;83: 467–474.

10. Verellen D, Soete G, Linthout N, et al. Quality assurance of a system for improved target localization and patient set-up that combines real-time infrared tracking and stereoscopic X-ray imaging. *Radiother Oncol*. 2003;67:129–141.

11. Sahgal A, Ma L, Chang E, et al. Advances in technology for intracranial stereotactic radiosurgery. *Technol Cancer Res Treat*. 2009;271–280.

12. De Los Santos J, Popple R, Agazaryan N, et al. Image guided radiation therapy (IGRT) technologies for radiation therapy localization and delivery. *Int J Radiat Oncol Biol Phys*. 2013;87:33–45.

13. Jaffray DA, Siewerdsen JH, Wong JW, et al. Flat-panel cone-beam computed tomography for image-guided radiation therapy. *Int J Radiat Oncol Biol Phys*. 2002;53:1337–1349.

14. Hoogeman MS, Nuyttens JJ, Levendag PC, et al. Time dependence of intrafraction patient motion assessed by repeat stereoscopic imaging. *Int J Radiat Oncol Biol Phys*. 2008;70:609–618.

15. Murphy MJ, Chang SD, Gibbs IC, et al. Patterns of patient movement during frameless image-guided radiosurgery. *Int J Radiat Oncol Biol Phys*. 2003;55:1400–1408.

16. Murphy MJ. Intrafraction geometric uncertainties in frameless image-guided radiosurgery. *Int J Radiat Oncol Biol Phys*. 2009;73:1364–1368.

17. Kang KM, Chai GY, Jeong BK, et al. Estimation of optimal margin for intrafraction movements during frameless brain radiosurgery. *Med Phys*. 2013;40:051716.

18. Ling CC, Gerweck LE, Zaider M, et al. Dose-rate effects in external beam radiotherapy redux. *Radiother Oncol*. 2010;95:261–268.

19. Alongi F, Fogliata A, Clerici E, et al. Volumetric modulated arc therapy with flattening filter free beams for isolated abdominal/pelvic lymph nodes: report of dosimetric and early clinical results in oligometastatic patients. *Radiat Oncol*. 2012;7:204.

20. Alongi F, Cozzi L, Arcangeli S, et al. Linac based SBRT for prostate cancer in 5 fractions with VMAT and flattening filter free beams: preliminary report of a phase II study. *Radiat Oncol*. 2013;8:171.

21. Scorsetti M, Alongi F, Castiglioni S, et al. Feasibility and early clinical assessment of flattening filter free (FFF) based stereotactic body radiotherapy (SBRT) treatments. *Radiat Oncol*. 2011;6:113.

22. Wang PM, Hsu WC, Chung NN, et al. Feasibility of stereotactic body radiation therapy with volumetric modulated arc therapy and high intensity photon beams for hepatocellular carcinoma patients. *Radiat Oncol*. 2014;9:18.

23. Prendergast BM, Dobelbower MC, Bonner JA, et al. Stereotactic body radiation therapy (SBRT) for lung malignancies: preliminary toxicity results using a flattening filter-free linear accelerator operating at 2400 monitor units per minute. *Radiat Oncol*. 2013;8:273.

24. Cardinale RM, Benedict SH, Wu Q, et al. A comparison of three stereotactic radiotherapy techniques: ARCS vs. noncoplanar fixed fields vs. intensity modulation. *Int J Radiat Oncol Biol Phys*. 1998;42:431–436.

25. Leavitt DD. Beam shaping for SRT/SRS. *Med Dosim*. 1998;23:229–236.

26. Shiu AS, Kooy HM, Ewton JR, et al. Comparison of miniature multileaf collimation (MMLC) with circular collimation for stereotactic treatment. *Int J Radiat Oncol Biol Phys*. 1997;37:679–688.

27. Solberg TD, Boedeker KL, Fogg R, et al. Dynamic arc radiosurgery field shaping: a comparison with static field conformal and noncoplanar circular arcs. *Int J Radiat Oncol Biol Phys*. 2001;49:1481–1491.

28. Ma L, Sahgal A, Descovich M, et al. Equivalence in dose fall-off for isocentric and non-isocentric intracranial treatment modalities and its impact on dose fractionation schemes. *Int J Radiat Oncol Biol Phys*. 2010;76:943–948.

29. Chin LS, Ma L, DiBiase S. Radiation necrosis following gamma knife surgery: a case-controlled comparison of treatment parameters and long-term clinical follow up. *J Neurosurg*. 2001;94:899–904.

30. Flickinger JC, Kondziolka D, Maitz AH, et al. An analysis of the dose-response for arteriovenous malformation radiosurgery and other factors affecting obliteration. *Radiother Oncol*. 2002;63:347–354.

31. Korytko T, Radivoyevitch T, Colussi V, et al. 12 Gy gamma knife radiosurgical volume is a predictor for radiation necrosis in non-AVM intracranial tumors. *Int J Radiat Oncol Biol Phys*. 2006;64:419–424.

32. Ma L, Petti P, Wang B, et al. Apparatus dependence of normal brain tissue dose in stereotactic radiosurgery for multiple brain metastases. *J Neurosurg*. 2011;114:1580–1584.

33. Yin FF, Zhu J, Yan H, et al. Dosimetric characteristics of Novalis shaped beam surgery unit. *Med Phys*. 2002;29:1729–1738.

34. Chang SD, Main W, Martin DP, et al. An analysis of the accuracy of the CyberKnife: a robotic frameless stereotactic radiosurgical system. *Neurosurgery*. 2003;52:140–146, discussion 6–7.

35. Ma L, Chuang C, Descovich M, et al. Whole-procedure clinical accuracy of gamma knife treatments of large lesions. *Med Phys*. 2008;35:5110–5114.

36. Thomas EM, Popple RA, Wu X, et al. Comparison of plan quality and delivery time between volumetric arc therapy (RapidArc) and Gamma Knife radiosurgery for multiple cranial metastases. *Neurosurgery*. 2014;75:409–417, discussion 17–18.

37. Ma L, Sahgal A, Larson DA. Letter: volumetric arc therapy (RapidArc) vs Gamma Knife radiosurgery for multiple brain metastases. *Neurosurgery*. 2015;76:E353.

38. Thomas EM, Popple RA, Markert JM, et al. In reply: volumetric arc therapy (RapidArc) vs Gamma Knife radiosurgery for multiple brain metastases. *Neurosurgery*. 2015;76:e353–e354.

39. Hossain S, Keeling V, Hildebrand K, et al. Normal brain sparing with increasing number of beams and isocenters in volumetric-modulated arc beam radiosurgery of multiple brain metastases. *Technol Cancer Res Treat*. 2015; 15:766–771.

40. Ruschin M, Lee Y, Beachey D, et al. Investigation of dose falloff for intact brain metastases and surgical cavities using hypofractionated volumetric modulated arc radiotherapy. *Technol Cancer Res Treat*. 2015; 15:130–138.

41. Bohoudi O, Bruynzeel AM, Lagerwaard FJ, et al. Isotoxic radiosurgery planning for brain metastases. *Radiother Oncol*. 2016;120:253–257.

42. Bjärngard BE, Tsai JS, Rice RK, et al. Doses on the central axes of narrow 6-MV x-ray beams. *Med Phys*. 1990;17:794–799.

43. Sánchez-Doblado F, Hartmann GH, Pena J, et al. A new method for output factor determination in MLC shaped narrow beams. *Phys Med*. 2007;23:58–66.

44. Alfonso R, Andreo P, Capote R, et al. A new formalism for reference dosimetry of small and nonstandard fields. *Med Phys*. 2008;35:5179–5186.

45. Almond PR, Biggs PJ, Coursey BM, et al. AAPM's TG-51 protocol for clinical reference dosimetry of high-energy photon and electron beams. *Med Phys*. 1999;26:1847–1870.

46. McEwen M, DeWerd L, Ibbott G, et al. Addendum to the AAPM's TG-51 protocol for clinical reference dosimetry of high-energy photon beams. *Med Phys.* 2014;41: 041501.

47. Andreo P, Huq MS, Westermark M, et al. Protocols for the dosimetry of high-energy photon and electron beams: a comparison of the IAEA TRS-398 and previous international codes of practice. *Phys Med Biol.* 2002;47:3033–3053.

48. Dieterich S, Cavedon C, Wilcox EE. *Clinical Dosimetry Measurements in Radiotherapy.* Madison, WI: Medical Physics; 2009.

49. Bouchard H, Seuntjens J. Ionization chamber-based reference dosimetry of intensity modulated radiation beams. *Med Phys.* 2004;31:2454–2465.

50. Capote R, Sánchez-Doblado F, Leal A, et al. An EGSnrc Monte Carlo study of the microionization chamber for reference dosimetry of narrow irregular IMRT beamlets. *Med Phys.* 2004;31:2416–2422.

51. Agostinelli S, Garelli S, Piergentili M, et al. Response to high-energy photons of PTW31014 PinPoint ion chamber with a central aluminum electrode. *Med Phys.* 2008;35:3293–3301.

52. Laub WU, Wong T. The volume effect of detectors in the dosimetry of small fields used in IMRT. *Med Phys.* 2003;30:341–347.

53. Le Roy M, de Carlan L, Delaunay F, et al. Assessment of small volume ionization chambers as reference dosimeters in high-energy photon beams. *Phys Med Biol.* 2011;56: 5637–5650.

54. Andersson J, Kaiser FJ, Gómez F, et al. A comparison of different experimental methods for general recombination correction for liquid ionization chambers. *Phys Med Biol.* 2012;57:7161–7175.

55. Chung E, Davis S, Seuntjens J. Experimental analysis of general ion recombination in a liquid-filled ionization chamber in high-energy photon beams. *Med Phys.* 2013;40:062104.

56. Heydarian M, Hoban PW, Beddoe AH. A comparison of dosimetry techniques in stereotactic radiosurgery. *Phys Med Biol.* 1996;41:93–110.

57. Mack A, Scheib SG, Major J, et al. Precision dosimetry for narrow photon beams used in radiosurgery-determination of Gamma Knife output factors. *Med Phys.* 2002;29: 2080–2089.

58. Ralston A, Tyler M, Liu P, et al. Over-response of synthetic microDiamond detectors in small radiation fields. *Phys Med Biol.* 2014;59:5873–5881.

59. Westermark M, Arndt J, Nilsson B, et al. Comparative dosimetry in narrow high-energy photon beams. *Phys Med Biol.* 2000;45:685–702.

60. Zhu XR, Allen JJ, Shi J, et al. Total scatter factors and tissue maximum ratios for small radiosurgery fields: comparison of diode detectors, a parallel-plate ion chamber, and radiographic film. *Med Phys.* 2000;27:472–477.

61. Duggan DM, Coffey CW. Small photon field dosimetry for stereotactic radiosurgery. *Med Dosim.* 1998;23:153–159.

62. Francescon P, Cora S, Cavedon C, et al. Use of a new type of radiochromic film, a new parallel-plate micro-chamber, MOSFETs, and TLD 800 microcubes in the dosimetry of small beams. *Med Phys.* 1998;25:503–511.

63. Aguirre JF, Alvarez P, Ibbott GG, et al. *Standards, Applications and Quality Assurance in Medical Radiation Dosimetry (IDOS).* Vienna: International Atomic Energy Agency; 2010. Series 1:411–421.

64. Pantelis E, Antypas C, Petrokokkinos L, et al. Dosimetric characterization of CyberKnife radiosurgical photon beams using polymer gels. *Med Phys.* 2008;35:2312–2320.

65. Lunsford LD, Flickinger JC, Steiner L. The gamma knife. *JAMA.* 1988;259:2544.

66. Lindquist C, Paddick I. The Leksell Gamma Knife Perfexion and comparisons with its predecessors. *Neurosurgery.* 2007;61:130–140, discussion 40–41.

67. Schlesinger D, Xu Z, Taylor F, et al. Interfraction and intrafraction performance of the Gamma Knife Extend system for patient positioning and immobilization. *J Neurosurg.* 2012;117(suppl):217–224.

68. Ma L, Pinnaduwage D, McDermotee M, et al. Whole-procedural radiological accuracy for delivering multisession gamma knife radiosurgery with a relocatable frame system. *Technol Cancer Res Treat.* 2014;13:403–408.

69. Ruschin M, Komljenovic PT, Ansell S, et al. Cone beam computed tomography image guidance system for a dedicated intracranial radiosurgery treatment unit. *Int J Radiat Oncol Biol Phys.* 2013;85:243–250.

70. Cohen RA, Amrani O, Ruschin S. Linearized electro-optic racetrack modulator based on double injection method in silicon. *Opt Express.* 2015;23:2252–2261.

71. Eriksson M., Paper presented at: 17th International Leksell Gamma Knife Society Meeting; 2014; New York, NY.

72. Eriksson M, Nutti B, Hennix M, et al. Paper presented at: 17th International Leksell Gamma Knife Society Meeting; 2014; New York, NY.

73. Li W, Bootsma G, Von Schultz O, et al. Preliminary evaluation of a novel thermoplastic mask system with intra-fraction motion monitoring for future use with image-guided Gamma Knife. *Cureus.* 2016;8:e531.

74. Accuray Inc CyberKnife M6 Series [technical specifications].Sunnydale, CA, 2017.

75. Dieterich S, Gibbs IC. The CyberKnife in clinical use: current roles, future expectations. *Front Radiat Ther Oncol.* 2011;43:181–194.

76. Ho AK, Fu D, Cotrutz C, et al. A study of the accuracy of cyberknife spinal radiosurgery using skeletal structure tracking. *Neurosurgery.* 2007;60:ONS147-ONS156, discussion ONS56.

77. van de Water S, Hoogeman MS, Breedveld S, et al. Variable circular collimator in robotic radiosurgery: a time-efficient alternative to a mini-multileaf collimator? *Int J Radiat Oncol Biol Phys.* 2011;81:863–870.

78. McGuinness CM, Gottschalk AR, Lessard E, et al. Investigating the clinical advantages of a robotic linac equipped with a multileaf collimator in the treatment of brain and prostate cancer patients. *J Appl Clin Med Phys.* 2015;16:5502.

79. Kilby W, Dooley JR, Kuduvalli G, et al. The CyberKnife Robotic Radiosurgery System in 2010. *Technol Cancer Res Treat.* 2010;9:433–452.

80. Kondziolka D, Patel A, Lunsford LD, et al. Stereotactic radiosurgery plus whole brain radiotherapy versus radiotherapy alone for patients with multiple brain metastases. *Int J Radiat Oncol Biol Phys.* 1999;45:427–434.

81. Andrews DW, Scott CB, Sperduto PW, et al. Whole brain radiation therapy with or without stereotactic radiosurgery boost for patients with one to three brain metastases: phase III results of the RTOG 9508 randomised trial. *Lancet.* 2004;363:1665–1672.

82. Aoyama H, Shirato H, Tago M, et al. Stereotactic radiosurgery plus whole-brain radiation therapy vs stereotactic radiosurgery alone for treatment of brain metastases: a randomized controlled trial. *JAMA.* 2006;295:2483–2491.

83. Chang EL, Wefel JS, Hess KR, et al. Neurocognition in patients with brain metastases treated with radiosurgery or radiosurgery plus whole-brain irradiation: a randomised controlled trial. *Lancet Oncol.* 2009;10:1037–1044.

84. Kocher M, Soffietti R, Abacioglu U, et al. Adjuvant whole-brain radiotherapy versus observation after radiosurgery or surgical resection of one to three cerebral metastases: results of the EORTC 22952–26001 study. *J Clin Oncol.* 2011;29:134–141.

85. Tsao M, Xu W, Sahgal A. A meta-analysis evaluating stereotactic radiosurgery, whole-brain radiotherapy, or both for patients presenting with a limited number of brain metastases. *Cancer.* 2012;118:2486–2493.

86. Sahgal A, Aoyama H, Kocher M, et al. Phase 3 trials of stereotactic radiosurgery with or without whole-brain radiation therapy for 1 to 4 brain metastases: individual patient data meta-analysis. *Int J Radiat Oncol Biol Phys.* 2015;91:710–717.

87. Yamamoto M, Serizawa T, Shuto T, et al. Stereotactic radiosurgery for patients with multiple brain metastases (JLGK0901): a multi-institutional prospective observational study. *Lancet Oncol.* 2014;15:387–395.

88. Soliman H, Das S, Larson DA, et al. Stereotactic radiosurgery (SRS) in the modern management of patients with brain metastases. *Oncotarget.* 2016;7:12318–12330.

89. Minniti G, D'Angelillo RM, Scaringi C, et al. Fractionated stereotactic radiosurgery for patients with brain metastases. *J Neurooncol.* 2014;117:295–301.

90. Minniti G, Scaringi C, Paolini S, et al. Single-fraction versus multifraction (3×9 Gy) stereotactic radiosurgery for large (>2 cm) brain metastases: a comparative analysis of local control and risk of radiation-induced brain necrosis. *Int J Radiat Oncol Biol Phys.* 2016;95:1142–1148.

# Spine Radiosurgery in the Management of Spine Metastasis

4

*Neil K. Taunk and Sharad Goyal*

## SPINAL METASTASIS

Estimates show that approximately one-quarter million adults are living with a diagnosis of metastatic bone disease in the United States (1). Nearly 40% of patients with metastatic cancer will have disease in the spine at the time of death, making the spine the most common site of osseous metastatic disease (2). Of all cancer patients, an estimated 10% will develop symptomatic spinal metastases with some type of epidural cord compression (3). If undetected or left untreated, metastatic spine disease can lead to severe pain secondary to pathologic fracture or even catastrophic neurologic compromise if epidural spinal cord compression is present. More than 90% of metastatic lesions involving the spine are extradural. Intradural and intramedullary lesions are much less common and represent less than 5% and 1% of lesions, respectively. Nearly half of metastatic lesions originate from breast, lung, or prostate cancers—both because of total cancer incidence and their propensity to spread to bone. With improvements in systemic treatment and survival times, it is expected that patients with other tumor histologies will develop secondary lesions (4).

It is critically important to diagnosis spinal metastatic disease early. This is largely due to the understanding that functional outcomes depend on the neurologic condition at the time of presentation (eg, patients without ambulatory difficulty are more likely to retain the ability to ambulate). Tumor-related pain, or biologic pain, tends to appear early in the morning or at night, generally improves with physical activity, and often precedes the development of other neurological symptoms by weeks or months. This is likely due to the decreased production of endogenous steroids in the evening. Uncontrolled spinal tumors tend to produce pain and to diminish ambulatory ability and performance status secondary to malignant cord compression. The goal of local treatment is generally palliative, as the competing risks of systemic disease and mortality are often significant. In selected cases chemotherapy, targeted therapy, or initial surgery may pose as alternatives. The proper management of patients with spinal metastasis demands multidisciplinary treatment from spine surgeons, radiation oncologists, neuroradiologists, medical oncologists, and pain management specialists (5,6).

Even with advances in systemic treatment, radiation therapy (RT) plays a critical role in managing patients with spine metastasis. RT is used for the palliation of painful bone metastases and the relief of symptoms related to malignant spinal cord compression. Significant technological advances in RT have occurred beyond the traditional two-dimensional treatment. Newer modalities instrumental in modernizing treatment to the spine include intensity-modulated RT (IMRT), image-guided treatment (IGRT), stereotactic body RT (SBRT), and stereotactic radiosurgery (SRS). These treatments, specifically SBRT and SRS, allow radiation oncologists to deliver high-dose radiation with an accuracy within millimeters. Durable local control of spine metastasis may exceed 90% with SRS to the spine. This local control benefit is independent of histology, providing select patients with excellent palliation and long disease-free intervals (7).

Spine radiosurgery (SR) has emerged in the last several years as an excellent treatment option for patients with spine metastasis (see Figures 4.1 and 4.2).

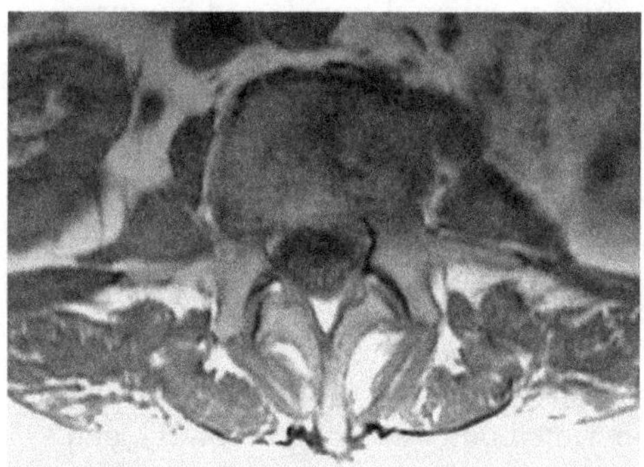

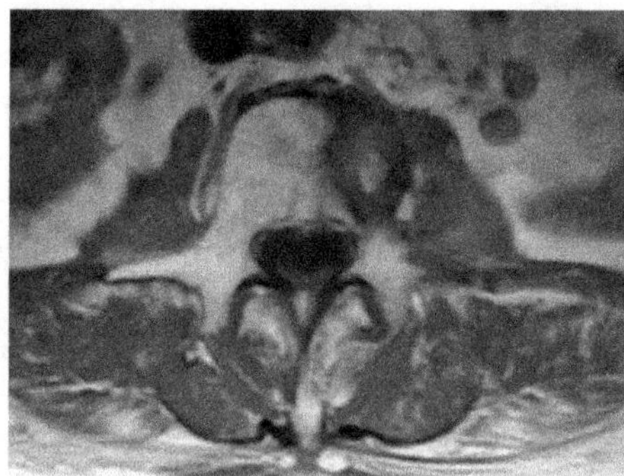

**FIGURE. 4.1** Woman aged 74 years with L3 body and pedicle disease with paraspinal extension (T1 weighted axial MRI): before treatment

**FIGURE 4.2** Woman aged 74 years from Figure 4.1 with 24 Gy in a single fraction, showing stable treated disease (T1 weighted axial MRI): eight months after treatment

This treatment allows the delivery of ultra-high, dose-targeted radiation to spine disease with relative sparing of adjacent healthy tissues and generally low toxicity when using sound technique. This technique is a high-technology approach to a long-standing problem in managing these patients. SR requires high-quality imaging with MRI, strict immobilization of the patient, modern radiation treatment planning, and IGRT for the delivery of therapy.

## Relative Radioresistance and the Case for Dose Escalation

Radiation is the principle local treatment for intra- and extracranial metastases. Conventionally fractionated RT may be ablative with definitive doses, but normal tissue tolerance limits the use of high-dose conventionally fractionated RT. A typical palliative schedule in conventional radiation includes 8 Gy×1, 4 Gy×5, or 3 Gy×10 fractions, which is suboptimal for some tumor histologies, such as melanoma, renal cell carcinoma (RCC), or sarcoma (8). SR provides ablative doses of highly conformal radiation to tumor targets in one to five treatments. In the era of targeted therapy and improved survival, SR offers durable local control for patients with metastatic radioresistant histologies.

Conventionally fractionated RT (eg, 1.8–2 Gy per fraction during the course of radiotherapy) mediates DNA damage in cancer cells, ultimately leading to mitotic catastrophe. Single-fraction RT and high-dose hypofractionated RT are thought to act upon a different mechanism. High-dose RT is expected to cause rapid endothelial cell apoptosis and subsequent microvascular damage, which ultimately leads to tumor killing (9). An additional mechanism indicates that immediately after high-dose RT, ceramide-mediated signaling of tumor necrosis factor-alpha and Fas ligand (FasL)-mediated apoptosis of cells occurs (10). This continues to be an active area of study, but SR is likely tumoricidal due to the ablation of both microvasculature and disease.

Tumor histologies are presumed to have an inherent radiosensitivity or relative radioresistance. For example, tumors of the lymphoid system, breast, and small cell lung cancer are relatively radiosensitive. Other diseases, such as melanoma, non–small cell lung cancer, or RCC are thought to be relatively radioresistant to RT (11).

Dose escalation using high biologically effective dose (BED) radiation may overcome the presumed radioresistance from conventionally fractionated RT. Based upon the linear- quadratic model of cell response, the BED is commonly used to calculate isoeffective RT schedules. The model accounts for *early effect* (tumor tissue), *late effect* (normal tissue), and inherent differences in the radiosensitivity of the tumor and the normal tissue. Studies using this model to determine BED have indicated that higher equivalent doses may yield improved outcomes. An early study showed that higher BED (as a continuous variable) independently predicted the overall response to palliative radiotherapy in patients with RCC (12). This study assumed an alpha to beta ratio of 10 Gy for tumor tissue, compared to data reported previously that empirically showed a lower alpha to beta ratio. Although the linear–quadratic model is reasonable to use with high-dose RT (even potentially up to 18 Gy per fraction), further refinements in the model are necessary, and it may better predict the effects of high-dose radiation or SR (13,14). An alternative model, the universal survival curve, incorporates the linear–quadratic and the multitarget models to account for both vascular and stromal damage caused by ablative radiotherapy (15).

Compared to conventionally fractionated regimens, SR often results in very high BED radiation in only one to five fractions. This high-dose treatment may overcome the presumed radioresistance of several solid tumor histologies. Only with advanced radiation techniques can this high-dose treatment be delivered safely without exceeding the tolerance of adjacent normal tissues.

## PATIENT ASSESSMENT AND SELECTION

Potentially any patient with spine metastasis is a candidate for SR, but indications are currently being both expanded and refined. These indications may include pain related to an involved vertebral body, radiographic tumor progression, lesions associated with progressive neurologic deficits, adjuvant therapy after surgical interventions for radioresistant histology metastasis, and reirradiation therapy (16).

It is optimal to use a multidisciplinary approach to identify and treat those patients who would most benefit from SR. A comprehensive algorithm, NOMS, has been developed that incorporates four fundamental assessments in guiding optimal treatment paths for patients with spine metastasis: (N)eurologic, (O)ncologic, (M)echanical instability, and (S)ystemic disease (11). The goal of this decision framework is to provide a reliable assessment incorporating key factors such as histology, grade of compression, and the presence of mechanical symptoms.

Several examples show how this framework would work in clinical practice. A patient with an NSCLC metastasis (radioresistant histology) who presents with high-grade cord compression and a mechanically unstable spine would first go for posterior decompression (eg, *separation surgery*) and hardware stabilization, followed by SR for local control. A patient with breast cancer, low-grade or absent compression, and a mechanically stable spine would go directly to conventionally fractionated radiation.

## TECHNIQUE

Conventional RT with various treatment schedules utilizes generous margins around the gross tumor volume, indiscriminately irradiating normal tissue, including the spinal cord. In conventional spine treatment planning, the involved vertebral bodies are covered, as well as an immediately superior and inferior body. Margins are typically 2 cm lateral to the vertebral body edge. However, immediate and durable palliation is often limited to radiosensitive tumors, such as breast and prostate cancers (8).

SR requires a number of special techniques to deliver ablative RT safely and effectively. This includes custom and strict immobilization, the use of multiple beams to create conformal dose distribution, image guidance during each treatment with cone-beam CT, and accuracy within millimeters. Multiple beams allow for the shaping of a highly conformal dose, sparing the spinal cord in particular, which is usually within millimeters of the target volume (17).

Custom immobilization requires reproducible patient positioning while securely immobilizing the shoulders, neck, abdomen, or pelvis, as appropriate (18). For SR, patients are held in an immobilization cradle or a rigid stereotactic body frame, of which there are several commercially available. Often, multiple methods are combined, such as using an immobilization cradle combined with an alpha cradle or a five-point mask for upper cervical lesions. Although these immobilization modalities are noninvasive and cannot guarantee perfect positioning (such as with a rigid head frame), they are suitably comfortable and accurate. An immobilization accuracy rate of approximately 95%, based on pre- and posttreatment onboard-imaging findings, is reported for the noninvasive cradles currently in use (19).

Image guidance uses daily onboard imaging, ideally with pretreatment cone-beam CT, with or without additional tracking, such as intrafraction motion tracking (20). An orthogonal pair is generally not sufficient to account for movement in all planes. Further advancements include using a 6-degrees-of-freedom treatment couch or surface-based imaging, which allows for the correction of positioning errors in any plane and the potential interruption of treatment if the patient is outside tolerances on positioning.

Spinal cord identification is of the utmost importance to allow for an accurate estimation of cord dose and protection of the cord. This is exceptionally important in the reirradiation setting, when the cord has already received a significant dose, and errors in estimating the cord dose can be catastrophic (21). Most institutions use fusion of T2 weighted spine imaging with CT simulation. This is easy to practice and with fusion limited to the area of interest can often provide high-quality cord localization. In addition, this is a noninvasive approach. The preferred approach at the Memorial Sloan Kettering Cancer Center (MSKCC) is to use a presimulation CT myelogram, unless contraindicated, and simulate the patient before losing the contrast. MSKCC found this method superior to image fusion with MRI because MRI is prone to artifacts from implanted hardware; imperfect image fusion of MRI with the CT-simulation scan may also occur. Filling defects can identify epidural disease, as well. However, this is an invasive approach not feasible at all institutions.

The International Spine Radiosurgery Consortium uses the Spratt six-segmentation method to delineate the treatment volume, which treats the gross tumor, an abnormal marrow signal, and an adjacent normal bony segment to account for subclinical tumor spread to create the clinical target volume (CTV) (22). For example, if the body contains the gross tumor volume (GTV), then the pedicles would be included to account for subclinical tumor spread. Some practitioners treat the GTV only, but the consortium method accounts for the failures that most commonly occur outside the GTV. A margin of 2 mm to 3 mm is added from the CTV to create the planning target volume (PTV).

Controversy remains regarding the effective dose required for tumor eradication. The dose prescribed typically ranges from 16 Gy to 24 Gy in a single fraction or a number of hypofractionated regimens. Although some groups practice up to 24 Gy in a single fraction, other groups indicate that 16 Gy to 18 Gy may be sufficient for a tumoricidal dose. In addition, the reduced dose may be associated with improved toxicity, such as a reduced incidence of vertebral compression fracture or myelopathy (23–25).

## CLINICAL EFFECTIVENESS

SR is understood to provide very high rates of local control, based on pain response and radiographic response.

Schipani et al reported on 165 spine metastases in 124 patients. These patients were treated with 18 Gy in a single fraction, prescribed to the 90% isodose line. With a median follow-up of 7 months, 92% of patients achieved local control. There were no Radiation Therapy Oncology Group (RTOG) grade 2 through 4 acute or late complications. A constraint of 10 Gy to 10% of the spinal cord was utilized. The maximum dose ($D_{max}$) of the spinal cord after organ-at-risk analysis was 13.8 Gy (range: 5.4 Gy–21 Gy), indicating that a cord $D_{max}$ of 14 Gy was a reasonable and safe constraint (25).

The Cleveland Clinic reported a series of single-fraction treatments with 88 lesions in 57 patients. The median dose was 15 Gy in a single fraction. Nearly

20% of the lesions had received prior in-field radiation. At a median follow-up of 5.4 months, actuarial radiographic progression-free survival was 92.3% and 71.2% at 3 months and 12 months, respectively. Adjusted pain-free survival was 84.9% and 67.7% at 3 months and 12 months, respectively (26).

Gerszten et al evaluated 500 lesions in 393 patients using radiosurgery. These patients ranged in age from 18 to 85 years and had lesions in all segments of the spine; 344 lesions had been previously radiated. All patients were treated with the CyberKnife (Accuray, Sunnyvale, CA) system with a mean dose of 20 Gy (range: 12.5–25 Gy) in one fraction. The mean tumor volume was 46 mL (range: 0.2–264 mL). At a median follow-up at 21 months, long-term pain had improved by 86%. Long-term tumor control was demonstrated in 90% of lesions treated with SR. There was no acute or subacute myelopathy (27).

MSKCC treated 105 RCC metastases with single-dose SR or hypofractionated SR. It found 3-year actuarial local progression-free survival to be 44% (Table 4.1). In patients with disease treated in a single fraction with a dose greater than or equal to 24 Gy, 3-year local progression-free survival was 88%. However, patients receiving hypofractionated treatment in three to five fractions had significantly reduced 3-year local control, at 17%. In a multivariate analysis, single- fraction treatment and treatment with a total dose greater than or equal to 24 Gy was predictive of improved local control (28). The group treated 88 patients with 120 sarcoma metastases with the same treatment approach. Patients were treated with a single-fraction dose at a median of 24 Gy or hypofractionated treatment in three to six fractions at a median total dose of 28.5 Gy. Actuarial local control for all patients was 88% at 12 months. Single-fraction treatment showed superior local control compared to hypofractionated regimens (91% vs. 84%, $P = .007$) (29). Based on this data, several institutions generally prefer to treat patients with single-fraction treatment when feasible (eg, single-level disease or never-irradiated disease).

SR has significant durability with respect to local control as measured by either pain control or with radiographic progression. In several series, 3-year local control exceeded 90% (7,28). Other series have consistently reported local control to be over 80% for 12 to 36 months after completing therapy. In one series of 278 patients, approximately 11% (with 36 involved segments) lived for at least 5 years after completing SR, with a median follow-up of 6.1 years. This cohort experienced three treatment failures approximately 49 months after completing therapy: two were in field, and the final was at the treatment margins (30). The importance of this durable local control is tremendous given that improvements in systemic therapy may allow patients to live much longer than previously expected.

**TABLE 4.1**  Selected series for spine SRS in RCC and mixed histologies

| Name | Patients | Lesions | Histology | Dose (Gy) | Treatment fractions | Local control | Follow-up (actuarial) |
|---|---|---|---|---|---|---|---|
| Balagamwala EH, et al (2012) (26) | 57 | 88 | RCC | 15 | 1 | 71.2% | 12 months |
| Gerszten PC, et al (2005) (43) | 48 | 60 | RCC | 20 (mean) | 1 | 89% | 37 months (median) |
| Gerszten PC, et al (2007) (27) | 393 | 500 | Mixed | 20 (mean) | 1 | 88% | 21 months (median) |
| Sohn S, et al (2014) (58) | 13 | 13 | RCC | 38 (marginal dose) | 1–5 | 85.7% | 12 months |
| Thibault I, et al (2014) (59) | 37 | 71 | RCC | 24 | 2 | 83% | 12 months |
| Wang XS, et al (2012) (55) | 149 | 166 | Mixed | 27–30 | 3 | 80.5% | 12 months |
| Yamada Y et al (2008) (7) | 93 | 103 | Mixed | 24 | 1 | 90% | 15 months |
| Zelefsky MJ, et al (2012) (28) | 45 | 45 | RCC | 24 | 1 | 88% | 36 months |

*Source:* Adapted from References 7, 26, 27, 28, 43, 55, 58, 59.

## POSTOPERATIVE SPINE RADIOSURGERY

There is little doubt that patients with metastatic disease to the spine can achieve durable local control with SR. However, it may not always be used independently of other modalities. Patients with mechanically unstable spines may benefit from initial stabilization or, for those with high-grade compression, immediate surgery for neurologic preservation. Anterior decompression is associated with higher rates of mean neurologic improvement; however, posterior decompression may be associated with improved perioperative mortality. Combined modality therapy, such as the addition of laminectomy and stabilization to radiation, can improve neurologic function (31). The debate regarding the criteria for surgery in metastatic cord compression is ongoing. The following are usually necessary for improved outcomes: favorable performance status and expected overall survival, a relatively radioresistant tumor type, and cord compression accompanied by mechanical instability (11,32,33).

Epidural disease is one of the important factors limiting the efficacy of SR. In order to administer an ablative radiation dose more safely, it is now possible to create a gap between the metastatic lesion and the thecal sac or cord. This often involves a laminectomy and the removal of the posterior elements—not necessarily with gross resection of all disease—as well as posterior spine stabilization with hardware. The goal of this manner of surgery is not gross total resection, or even significant tumor debulking. It is to administer a full dose of SR to the entire tumor volume while minimizing the radiation dose to the spinal cord (31).

Series regarding the combined modality treatment of separation surgery followed by SR show the effectiveness of this approach. MSKCC reported on patients treated from 2002 to 2011 who received separation surgery followed by single-fraction or hypofractionated SR (34,35). Of these patients, 136 exhibited high-grade cord compression. The full cohort received posterior decompression and stabilization, followed by SR. Postoperative SR provided durable local control, with a cumulative incidence of progression at 1 year of 16.4%. This finding is in line with patients who do not necessarily require separation surgery.

## Complications

Early reports demonstrate the relative safety of SR with respect to the bone and spinal cord, even with previous in-field RT. Other side effects of treatment are largely site-specific, such as esophagitis during cervical spine treatment or myositis in lumbosacral lesions.

A vertebral compression fracture (VCF) is reported relatively frequently after SR, although a symptomatic VCF is less often encountered. VCFs have been reported with approximately 20% incidence. They are associated with a higher dose per fraction ($\geq$20 Gy) and when three out of the six original Spinal Instability Neoplastic Score (SINS) components are met: a baseline VCF, a lytic tumor, and a pre-existing spinal deformity (36).

Practitioners must note high-risk patients who would initially benefit from some type of intervention, such as kyphoplasty, percutaneous screws, or hardware stabilization. Sahgal et al reported a cumulative incidence of VCFs at 13.49% at 2 years in a cohort of 410 lesions in 252 patients. The greatest risk factors for VCFs in a multivariate analysis were treatments of a high dose per fraction ($\geq$24 Gy and 20–23 Gy, compared to lower doses), a pretreatment VCF, lytic spine disease, and spinal deformity. Kyphoplasty, percutaneous screws, surgery, or another intervention were required in 43% of these lesions (37). Other series report similar rates of compression fractures, from 11% to 39% (38,39). Although some series indicate a significant incidence of VCFs, it is important to note that they are less often symptomatic or in need of an intervention. Symptomatic disease primarily revolves around patients who may require increased pain medication, or later surgical intervention. Although most VCFs can be conservatively managed, further characterization of the fracture is certainly warranted given the heterogeneity in reporting, symptomatology, and interventions (37).

A pain flare or an acute worsening of pain due to the index lesion can occur in nearly 20% of cases after SR. The flare may occur within 24 hours of a single dose or a few days after hypofractioned schemes (40). Some patients may also experience myositis due to having a high volume of usually lumbar musculature exposed to high-dose RT. Both the pain flare and the myositis are usually temporary and can be remedied by nonsteroidal anti-inflammatory drugs (NSAIDs) or steroids if needed.

Myelopathy is the most concerning toxicity of SR. This is usually due to physicians exceeding the presumed cord tolerance or errors in positioning during treatment. Fortunately, myelopathy is uncommon, and many series report minimal to no incidence of it. The best way to prevent myelopathy is to avoid any unnecessary dose to the spinal cord and respect the planning dose constraints. The Gerszten series and multiple MSKCC series indicated no acute myelopathy, regardless of the dose used. The Cleveland Clinic series reported a nearly 5% rate of grade 1 and 2 motor neuropathy. A Stanford series using a CyberKnife-based SR reported 3 out of 62 (approximately 5%) patients experiencing severe myelopathy after treatment. Interestingly, all of these complications in this series occurred in patients who were treated for thoracic spine lesions. Two of the three patients had received prior treatment with anti–vascular endothelial growth factor (VEGF) targeted therapies (41). We have an incomplete understanding of the spinal cord's true tolerance and how either prior or current systemic therapy can affect this tolerance. Given this fact, it is generally recommended that patients not be treated concurrently with systemic therapy while receiving SR (7,17,26,42,43).

Other events are associated with SR, such as the risk of mucositis, skin dermatitis, and esophageal toxicity, and many factors may influence additional SR toxicity. These factors include the proximity and the extension of the tumor to adjacent normal tissues, the receipt of concurrent systemic therapy and targeted therapies, and the presence of comorbidities (acute infection, prior surgery, diabetes, collagen vascular disease, or any genetic predisposition).

## REPORTING CRITERIA AND ASSESSING LOCAL CONTROL WITH IMAGING

Local control is the most meaningful outcome, but it can be reported in a number of ways, including radiographic response or physician- or patient-reported pain response. Serial total spine MRI is the current standard of care modality to assess the response to treatment and to conduct a long-term follow-up.

MRI is the cornerstone of spine imaging, allowing for the assessment of both the bony anatomy and the cord. After radiation treatment, there are characteristic T1 and T2 weighted changes in the tumor and the bone marrow (44). MRI is the best imaging modality for spine metastases and offers exquisite sensitivity in detecting lesions (45–47). T1 weighted images allow both the size and the volume of individual lesions to be assessed. After treatment, T1 weighted images can also provide anatomic information regarding the treatment response. Functional MRI techniques, including diffusion-weighted MRI imaging (DW-MRI) and dynamic contrast–enhanced MRI (DCE-MRI), can significantly augment the information gained beyond anatomic details. DW-MRI accounts for tumor-specific changes in water diffusion due to the changes in cellular density that may occur after radiation treatment (48). DCE-MRI, also known as *perfusion MRI*, offers additional data regarding tumor vascularity and can outperform simple diagnostic MRI. However, significant limitations exist in its initial diagnostic utility, given the limited field of view attained (it is recommended that the entire spinal axis be imaged during diagnosis and to monitor the treatment response). In addition, there is little interinstitutional agreement on acquiring images, making it difficult to compare images between institutions (49,50).

CT primarily provides information on bony anatomy and the mineralization status. It offers cortical and trabecular bone assessment with high spatial resolution and anatomical detail. It is best at evaluating bony structures and can readily reveal reossification after a successful tumor treatment. However, CT offers incomplete information on the response of epidural disease (51–53). Unfortunately, CT is also highly susceptible to artifacts from implanted metal hardware, even when orthopedic metal artifact reduction (O-MAR) is used. Molecular imaging techniques may also be used to image both a patient's spine and total systemic disease burden. However, common tracers such as $^{99m}$Tc and $^{18}$F-NaF are unable to accurately detect visceral metastasis. Furthermore, these agents are largely imaging the secondary bone matrix response to lytic and blastic tumor changes. This matrix response often clouds the assessment after treatment, as opposed to tumor-directed agents that may reflect the actual tumor burden.

Given the revolution and the expansion in the multidisciplinary treatment of spine disease, the SPine response assessment in Neuro-Oncology (SPINO) group issued guidelines for disease monitoring after SBRT (54). The group formed with the goals of surveying and standardizing the methods of reporting local disease control and pain with imaging after treatment with spine SBRT. Local control is largely defined as no tumor progression in the SBRT-treated volume or no progression of any treated epidural extension. Few centers strictly used the Response Evaluation Criteria in Solid Tumors (RECIST) to determine treatment response. Nearly all centers imaged patients with MRI for 2 to 3 months after treatment and then every 2 to 6 months thereafter. No institution surveyed used fluorodeoxyglucose PET (FDG-PET) alone routinely to follow patients, although some used the modality as an adjunct to ambiguities in MRI response. The authors acknowledge that future issues to resolve in response assessment include the utility of functional imaging techniques, such as PET and MRI; the criteria for assessing epidural disease; the use of the RECIST criteria versus developing an independent spine criteria; and the difficulties in assessing response in the setting of a VCF. The SPINO group ultimately recommends MRI for disease monitoring, performed 2 to 3 months after initial treatment for the first year and then every 3 to 6 months thereafter, and defines local control as the absence of any progression in the treated region.

The SPINO group's recommendations include MRI for baseline assessment, as well as a 2-to-3 month posttreatment MRI to determine the initial response. Most centers, including our own, define local control as the absence of progressive disease in the SBRT-treated volume. Further consensus is pending regarding integrating multiparametric MRI and molecular imaging to assess the treatment response. Spine SBRT has offered remarkably high rates of local control with limited toxicity to patients with even potentially catastrophic spine disease; however, much is required to best determine how to assess treatment responses in patients and predict who will benefit the most from spine SBRT. Patients should be followed with MRI but offered nonstandard imaging techniques in trials when available to further advance our understanding of image-based assessment after SBRT.

## FUTURE CONCERNS AND CONCLUSIONS

A preponderance of low-level evidence indicates that SR is a very effective tool in managing patients with spine metastasis. However, significant issues remain in further validating this treatment modality and refining its applications.

Early series, which are primarily retrospective, report on a heterogeneous case mix. In addition, significant heterogeneity exists with regard to prior therapy, such as previous radiation, mechanical symptoms and stabilization, systemic therapy, and separation surgery. There is a further lack of clarity with respect to toxicity reporting and the time frame in which to report. The expectation is that as prospective data continue to emerge, there will be more homogeneous groups of patients reported upon, and the reporting on toxicity will be more uniform and stringent.

Prospective evaluation has largely been limited to single-institution experiences (55). A phase II/III study (RTOG-0631) of spine SRS has already established the feasibility of studying this technique in a multi-institutional cooperative group setting (56). Patients with one to three lesions and a numerical pain scale score greater than or equal to 5 were treated; 44 patients received 16 to 18 Gy of single-fraction SR. Grade 1/2 and grade 3 SBRT-related adverse events were observed in 7 and 0 patients, respectively. These cooperative groups will further standardize technique, outcome, and toxicity reporting in future trials.

In addition, consensus groups have formed to standardize reporting. We also expect standards to form in terms of treatment. This will primarily revolve around prescribed doses, where the current dose ranges from 16 to 24 Gy in a single fraction; normal tissue constraints, particularly with the cord; and further implementation of the International Spine Radiosurgery consortium guidelines (22,57).

Spine radiosurgery is an effective tool in managing patients with spine metastasis, particularly those with prior RT or instrumentation. We know from multiple series that spine SRS has extremely high rates of durable local control and palliation. However, it demands high quality control, precision guidance, and careful patient selection to be safely and effectively implemented.

## References


1. Li S, et al. Estimated number of prevalent cases of metastatic bone disease in the US adult population. *Clin Epidemiol.* 2012;4:87–93.
2. Wong DA, Fornasier VL, MacNab I. Spinal metastases: the obvious, the occult, and the impostors. *Spine (Phila Pa 1976).* 1990;15(1):1–4.
3. Perrin RG, Laxton AW. Metastatic spine disease: epidemiology, pathophysiology, and evaluation of patients. *Neurosurg Clin N Am.* 2004;15(4):365–373.
4. Bohm P, Huber J. The surgical treatment of bony metastases of the spine and limbs. *J Bone Joint Surg Br.* 2002;84(4):521–529.
5. Bilsky MH, et al. The diagnosis and treatment of metastatic spinal tumor. *Oncologist.* 1999;4(6):459–469.
6. Gokaslan ZL, et al. Transthoracic vertebrectomy for metastatic spinal tumors. *J Neurosurg.* 1998;89(4):599–609.
7. Yamada Y, et al. High-dose, single-fraction image-guided intensity-modulated radiotherapy for metastatic spinal lesions. *Int J Radiat Oncol Biol Phys.* 2008;71(2):484–490.
8. Hartsell WF, et al. Randomized trial of short- versus long-course radiotherapy for palliation of painful bone metastases. *J Natl Cancer Inst.* 2005;97(11):798–804.
9. Haimovitz-Friedman A, et al. Ionizing radiation acts on cellular membranes to generate ceramide and initiate apoptosis. *J Exp Med.* 1994;180(2):525–535.
10. Garcia-Barros M, et al. Tumor response to radiotherapy regulated by endothelial cell apoptosis. *Science.* 2003;300(5622):1155–1159.
11. Laufer I, et al. The NOMS framework: approach to the treatment of spinal metastatic tumors. *Oncologist.* 2013;18(6):744–751.
12. DiBiase SJ, et al. Palliative irradiation for focally symptomatic metastatic renal cell carcinoma: support for dose escalation based on a biological model. *J Urol.* 1997;158(3):746–749.

13. Brenner DJ. The linear-quadratic model is an appropriate methodology for determining isoeffective doses at large doses per fraction. *Semin Radiat Oncol.* 2008;18(4):234–239.

14. Kirkpatrick JP, Meyer JJ, Marks LB. The linear-quadratic model is inappropriate to model high dose per fraction effects in radiosurgery. *Semin Radiat Oncol.* 2008;18(4):240–243.

15. Park C, et al. Universal survival curve and single fraction equivalent dose: useful tools in understanding potency of ablative radiotherapy. *Int J Radiat Oncol Biol Phys.* 2008;70(3):847–852.

16. Harel R, Zach L. Spine radiosurgery for spinal metastases: indications, technique and outcome. *Neurol Res.* 2014;36(6):550–556.

17. Yamada Y, et al. Multifractionated image-guided and stereotactic intensity-modulated radiotherapy of paraspinal tumors: a preliminary report. *Int J Radiat Oncol Biol Phys.* 2005;62(1):53–61.

18. Chang EL, et al. Phase I/II study of stereotactic body radiotherapy for spinal metastasis and its pattern of failure. *J Neurosurg Spine.* 2007;7(2):151–160.

19. Benedict SH, et al. Stereotactic body radiation therapy: the report of AAPM Task Group 101. *Med Phys.* 2010;37(8):4078–4101.

20. Wen N, et al. Clinical use of dual image-guided localization system for spine radiosurgery. *Technol Cancer Res Treat.* 2012;11(2):123–131.

21. Chow E, et al. Palliation of bone metastases: a survey of patterns of practice among Canadian radiation oncologists. *Radiother Oncol.* 2000;56(3):305–314.

22. Cox BW, et al. International spine radiosurgery consortium consensus guidelines for target volume definition in spinal stereotactic radiosurgery. *Int J Radiat Oncol Biol Phys.* 2012;83(5):e597-e605.

23. Sahgal A, et al. Probabilities of radiation myelopathy specific to stereotactic body radiation therapy to guide safe practice. *Int J Radiat Oncol Biol Phys.* 2013;85(2):341–347.

24. Chang JH, et al. Stereotactic body radiotherapy for spinal metastases: what are the risks and how do we minimize them? *Spine.* 2016;41(Suppl. 20):S238-S245.

25. Schipani S, et al. Spine radiosurgery: a dosimetric analysis in 124 patients who received 18 Gy. *Int J Radiat Oncol Biol Phys.* 2012;84(5):e571-e576.

26. Balagamwala EH, et al. Single-fraction stereotactic body radiotherapy for spinal metastases from renal cell carcinoma. *J Neurosurg Spine.* 2012;17(6):556–564.

27. Gerszten PC, et al. Radiosurgery for spinal metastases: clinical experience in 500 cases from a single institution. *Spine (Phila Pa 1976).* 2007;32(2):193–199.

28. Zelefsky MJ, et al. Tumor control outcomes after hypofractionated and single-dose stereotactic image-guided intensity-modulated radiotherapy for extracranial metastases from renal cell carcinoma. *Int J Radiat Oncol Biol Phys.* 2012;82(5):1744–1748.

29. Folkert MR, et al. Outcomes and toxicity for hypofractionated and single-fraction image-guided stereotactic radiosurgery for sarcomas metastasizing to the spine. *Int J Radiat Oncol Biol Phys.* 2014;88(5):1085–1091.

30. Moussazadeh N, et al. Five-year outcomes of high-dose single-fraction spinal stereotactic radiosurgery. *Int J Radiat Oncol Biol Phys.* 2015;93(2):361–367.

31. Moussazadeh N, et al. Separation surgery for spinal metastases: effect of spinal radiosurgery on surgical treatment goals. *Cancer Control.* 2014;21(2):168–174.

32. Bilsky MH, et al. Reliability analysis of the epidural spinal cord compression scale. *J Neurosurg Spine.* 2010;13(3):324–328.

33. Loblaw DA, et al. Systematic review of the diagnosis and management of malignant extradural spinal cord compression: the Cancer Care Ontario Practice Guidelines Initiative's Neuro-Oncology Disease Site Group. *J Clin Oncol.* 2005;23(9):2028–2037.

34. Moulding HD, et al. Local disease control after decompressive surgery and adjuvant high-dose single-fraction radiosurgery for spine metastases. *J Neurosurg Spine.* 2010;13(1): 87–93.

35. Laufer I, et al. Local disease control for spinal metastases following "separation surgery" and adjuvant hypofractionated or high-dose single-fraction stereotactic radiosurgery: outcome analysis in 186 patients. *J Neurosurg Spine.* 2013;18(3):207–214.

36. Fisher CG, et al. A novel classification system for spinal instability in neoplastic disease: an evidence-based approach and expert consensus from the Spine Oncology Study Group. *Spine (Phila Pa 1976).* 2010;35(22):E1221-E1229.

37. Sahgal A, et al. Vertebral compression fracture after stereotactic body radiotherapy for spinal metastases. *Lancet Oncol.* 2013;14(8):e310–e320.

38. Boehling NS, et al. Vertebral compression fracture risk after stereotactic body radiotherapy for spinal metastases. *J Neurosurg Spine.* 2012;16(4):379–386.

39. Cunha MVR, et al. Vertebral compression fracture (VCF) after spine stereotactic body radiation therapy (SBRT): analysis of predictive factors. *Int J Radiat Oncol Biol Phys.* 2012;84(3):e343–e349.

40. Pan HY, et al. Incidence and predictive factors of pain flare after spine stereotactic body radiation therapy: secondary analysis of phase 1/2 trials. *Int J Radiat Oncol Biol Phys.* 2014;90(4):870–876.

41. Gibbs IC, et al. Image-guided robotic radiosurgery for spinal metastases. *Radiother Oncol.* 2007;82(2):185–190.

42. Nguyen Q.-N, et al. Management of spinal metastases from renal cell carcinoma using stereotactic body radiotherapy. *Int J Radiat Oncol Biol Phys.* 2010;76(4):1185–1192.

43. Gerszten, PC, et al. Stereotactic radiosurgery for spinal metastases from renal cell carcinoma. *J Neurosurg Spine.* 2005;3(4):288–295.

44. Ramsey RG, Zacharias CE. MR imaging of the spine after radiation therapy: easily recognizable effects. *Am J Roentgenol.* 1985;144(6):1131–1135.

45. Lecouvet FE, et al. MRI for response assessment in metastatic bone disease. *Eur Radiol.* 2013;23(7):1986–1997.

46. Costelloe CM, et al. Fast dixon whole-body MRI for detecting distant cancer metastasis: a preliminary clinical study. *J Magn Reson Imaging.* 2012;35(2):399–408.

47. Tombal B, et al. Magnetic resonance imaging of the axial skeleton enables objective measurement of tumor response on prostate cancer bone metastases. *Prostate.* 2005;65(2): 178–187.

48. Cappabianca S, et al. Assessing response to radiation therapy treatment of bone metastases: short-term followup of radiation therapy treatment of bone metastases with diffusion-weighted magnetic resonance imaging. *J Radiother.* 2014;2014:8.

49. Padhani AR, Miles KA. Multiparametric imaging of tumor response to therapy. *Radiology.* 2010;256(2):348–364.

50. Spratt DE, et al. Early magnetic resonance imaging biomarkers to predict local control after high dose stereotactic body radiotherapy for patients with sarcoma spine metastases. *Spine J.* 2016;16(3):291–298.

51. Vassiliou V, et al. Combination ibandronate and radiotherapy for the treatment of bone metastases: clinical evaluation and radiologic assessment. *Int J Radiat Oncol Biol Phys.* 2007;67(1):264–272.

52. Vassiliou V, et al. A novel study investigating the therapeutic outcome of patients with lytic, mixed and sclerotic bone metastases treated with combined radiotherapy and ibandronate. *Clin Exp Metastasis.* 2007;24(3):169–178.

53. Chiu N, et al. Radiological changes on CT after stereotactic body radiation therapy to non-spine bone metastases: a descriptive series. *Ann Palliat Med.* 2016;5(2):116–124.

54. Thibault I, et al. Response assessment after stereotactic body radiotherapy for spinal metastasis: a report from the SPIne response assessment in Neuro-Oncology (SPINO) group. *Lancet Oncol.* 2015;16(16):e595-e603.

55. Wang XS, et al. A prospective analysis of the clinical effects of stereotactic body radiation therapy in cancer patients with spinal metastases without spinal cord compression. *Lancet Oncol.* 2012;13(4):395–402.

56. Ryu S, et al. RTOG 0631 phase 2/3 study of image guided stereotactic radiosurgery for localized (1–3) spine metastases: phase 2 results. *Pract Radiat Oncol.* 2014;4(2):76–81.

57. Sahgal A, Larson DA, Chang EL. Stereotactic body radiosurgery for spinal metastases: a critical review. *Int J Radiat Oncol Biol Phys.* 2008;71(3):652–665.

58. Sohn S, et al. Stereotactic radiosurgery compared with external radiation therapy as a primary treatment in spine metastasis from renal cell carcinoma: a multicenter, matched-pair study. *J Neurooncol.* 2014;119(1):121–128.

59. Thibault I, et al. Spine stereotactic body radiotherapy for renal cell cancer spinal metastases: analysis of outcomes and risk of vertebral compression fracture. *J Neurosurg Spine.* 2014;21(5):711–718.

# Body Radiosurgery 5

*Jordan A. Torok, Manisha Palta,*
*and Joseph K. Salama*

## INTRODUCTION

Stereotactic body radiation therapy (SBRT), also referred to as stereotactic ablative body radiotherapy (SABR), is a treatment coupling precise and reproducible anatomic targeting accuracy with high doses of externally generated ionizing radiation, with the goal of maximizing target cell kill while minimizing radiation-related injury to adjacent normal tissues. SBRT uses multiple coplanar and non-coplanar beams that converge on a target area, resulting in complete coverage of tumors and subsequent steep dose gradients with relatively low doses of radiation to uninvolved tissue. Although early versions of SBRT employed the use of an external coordinate reference system to localize extracranial targets (stereotaxis) (1), modern implementation now primarily relies on orthogonal kV images or volumetric image guidance using implanted fiducials, bony reference landmarks, and/or soft tissues for target localization. An alternative description that takes this modern practice into account is *hypofractionated image-guided radiation therapy* (HIGRT). Patient immobilization and respiratory motion management are key components in the precision and reproducibility of this technique. SBRT has proven successful for a variety of extracranial tumors and is now considered a standard treatment approach for primary malignancies in the lung, liver, prostate, and pancreas, in addition to multiple metastatic sites.

## LUNG RADIOSURGERY

Surgery has long been the treatment modality of choice for medically operable patients with early-stage (stage I/II) lung cancer. For inoperable patients, conventional radiation therapy has been the only potentially curative treatment. In nonselected patients with non–small cell lung cancer (NSCLC), locoregional failure rates approached 50% at 2 years with conventional radiotherapy (2). For early-stage NSCLC (stage I/II), efforts to improve local control culminated in the use of SBRT. Extrapolating from the success and techniques of intracranial radiosurgery, the first reports of SBRT for primary and metastatic lung cancer used a stereotactic frame with external fiducial markers for target localization and patient setup (1). As opposed to applying relatively large population-based margins for respiration, respiratory motion was individually assessed using fluoroscopy with or without a device to apply pressure to the abdomen to limit diaphragmatic motion. An initial phase I dose escalation trial of SBRT from the University of Indiana used these techniques to treat patients with cT1-2 N0 NSCLC. After delineating the gross tumor volume (GTV) on CT, the planning target volume (PTV) was enlarged by 0.5 cm in the axial plane and 1.0 cm in the cranial-caudal plane. The dose escalation was stopped at 20 Gy per fraction in three fractions for T1 ($\leq$3 cm) lesions without reaching the dose-limiting toxicity (3). For T2 (>3 but $\leq$7 cm) lesions, the maximum tolerated dose was 22 Gy per fraction. The 20 Gy$\times$3 dosing regimen was then evaluated prospectively in a single institution phase II study demonstrating a 95% control rate at 2 years (4). This trial noted the importance of tumor location in the development of treatment-related toxicity and death, with a grade 3+ toxicity of 46% versus 17% for perihilar/central and peripherally located tumors, respectively. Tumor size was also predictive of toxicity, with GTVs greater than 10 cc associated with an eightfold risk of high-grade toxicity compared to smaller tumors. Some of the more common high-grade toxicities included pneumonias, pleural or pericardial effusions, a decline in pulmonary function tests, and skin reactions. Most treatment-related deaths were related to pneumonia.

These initial promising results prompted the multicenter Radiation Therapy Oncology Group (RTOG) 0236 trial to determine if acceptable local control could be obtained for early- stage NSCLC in the cooperative group setting. Based on the initial experience with SBRT, patient eligibility was restricted to tumors 5 cm or less that were not within or touching the zone of the proximal bronchial tree (2 cm expanded volume from the carina, main stem, and secondary lobar bronchi). The prescription dose was 60 Gy in three fractions (20 Gy/fraction) without heterogeneity correction and approximately 54 Gy (18 Gy/fraction) when taking this into account. The patient immobilization and treatment techniques were similar to those used in the initial University of Indiana reports. The three-year results confirmed excellent primary tumor control of 98% (5). Consistent results were also noted in Asian and European trials of SBRT using different dosing regimens, with 3-yr tumor control rates of 92% to 98% (6,7).

In parallel with the development of SBRT in Europe and North America, a frameless system emphasizing image guidance was pioneered in Japan (8). This system utilized an in-room CT and fluoroscopy unit that shared the same axis as the treatment unit, allowing precise translation from simulation to treatment. Modern treatment machines equipped with cone-beam CT (CBCT) similarly are able to match patients on the treatment couch without the use of a body frame. The routine incorporation of tumor motion assessment, often with four-dimensional CT, further advanced the treatment planning. Four-dimensional CT generates volumetric data sets from different phases of the respiratory cycle (9). A custom assessment of respiratory motion for the GTV can then be made to define an internal target volume (ITV). This volume can be constructed by contouring the GTV on each individual CT data set or more efficiently, by contouring on a maximum intensity projection (MIP) image set that represents the highest pixel intensity in a given voxel over the entire respiratory cycle (10). Alternatives to four-dimensional CT motion assessment include fluoroscopy tracking of tumors or implanted fiducial markers. These methods allow for the personalized assessment of motion and reduce further expansion of the PTV to set up the margin alone.

Multiple dose fractionation regimens have been utilized for SBRT, and the optimal treatment remains unknown. To date only one randomized trial has compared different SBRT regimens (34 Gy×1 vs. 12 Gy×4), and no significant differences were noted (11). For many of these treatment schemes, the biologically equivalent dose (BED) has been calculated using the linear quadratic equation and correlated with clinical outcomes. Investigators from Japan determined that treatments achieving a BED of 100 Gy or greater for the tumor ($\alpha/\beta = 10$) had improved local control and survival (12). Of note, the RTOG 0236 regimen (18 Gy×3) has a $BED_{10}$ of 150 Gy, which is the highest among commonly used regimens. This dose has the potential to cause significant normal tissue injury and is therefore only recommended for peripherally located lesions. An additional consideration for peripheral lesions is the proximity of the target to the chest wall. When utilizing the RTOG 0236 regimen, several studies found a correlation between chest wall toxicity (rib fracture and/or severe pain) and the volume of the chest wall receiving 30 Gy and above (13,14). If the absolute volume of the chest wall receiving this dose can be kept below 30 cc, the risk of significant toxicity is relatively low. When this is not possible, an alternative dosing scheme associated with lower rates of chest wall toxicity should be considered, such as 10 Gy×5 ($BED_{10}$ = 100) (15). This risk-adapted approach based on chest wall dosimetry has been shown to decrease the incidence of toxicity while maintaining high rates of control (16,17).

For centrally located lesions, an increase in fractionation is warranted given the toxicity noted in the early phase I/II trials of SBRT. Experience from the Netherlands utilizing an eight-fraction regimen of 7.5 Gy ($BED_{10}$ = 105) in 63 patients demonstrated minimal grade 3 and no grade 4/5 toxicity (18). When compared to a similar cohort with peripheral lesions, local control and survival were equivalent. A variety of other dosing schemes have been described, including 48 Gy to 50 Gy in four fractions, 50 Gy to 60 Gy in five fractions, and 70 Gy in ten fractions. Different SBRT regimens for central lesions have also been analyzed to correlate BED with tumor control and toxicity outcomes. Similar to the findings with peripheral tumors, a $BED_{10}$ greater than or equal to 100 Gy results in high rates of tumor control (19). Treatment-related mortality appears to be limited when the BED for normal tissue injury ($\alpha/\beta$ = 3; $BED_3$) was kept at or below 210 Gy. RTOG 0813, a phase I/II dose escalation study looking at the tolerability and efficacy of a variety of five-fraction dose levels, has completed accrual, and the results are awaiting publication. This information will assist in identifying doses that can maximize tumor control while limiting normal tissue toxicity. Figure 5.1 shows a representative treatment plan for a patient with a central lung tumor.

Although many single-arm SBRT experiences have been promising, until recently, comparisons with standard radiation were lacking. The Stereotactic Precision and Conventional Radiotherapy Evaluation (SPACE) study comparing SBRT (66 Gy in three fractions over 1 week) to three-dimensional CRT (70 Gy in 35 fractions over 7 weeks) did not show a difference in overall survival (OS) or progression-free survival, but SBRT was associated with less toxicity and an improved quality of life (20). Large data sets demonstrate what appears to be an improvement in OS among medically inoperable patients receiving SBRT compared to those receiving conventionally fractionated RT (21). The ongoing Trans Tasman Radiation Oncology Group (TROG) Hypofractionated Radiotherapy (Stereotactic) Versus Conventional Radiotherapy for Inoperable Early Stage I Non-small Cell Lung Cancer (NSCLC) study will contribute additional prospective evidence when completed. Long-term follow-ups after SBRT have shown the potential for late relapses, with 5-year local control approaching 80% in one study (22). Nevertheless, local control rates are high, and the predominant mode of failure is now distant (23). Higher rates of regional and distant failure and poorer survival are seen with larger tumor sizes,

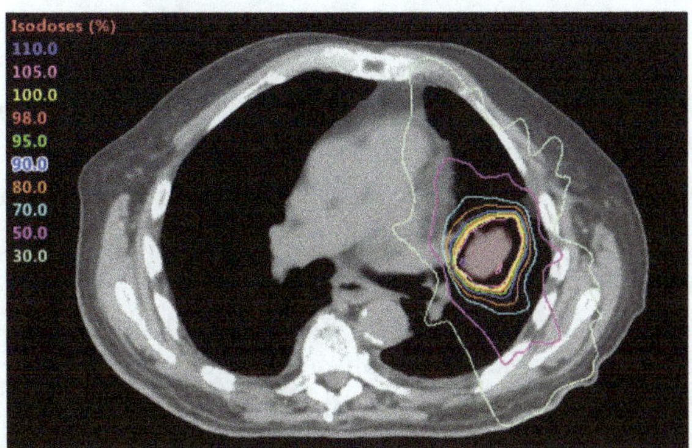


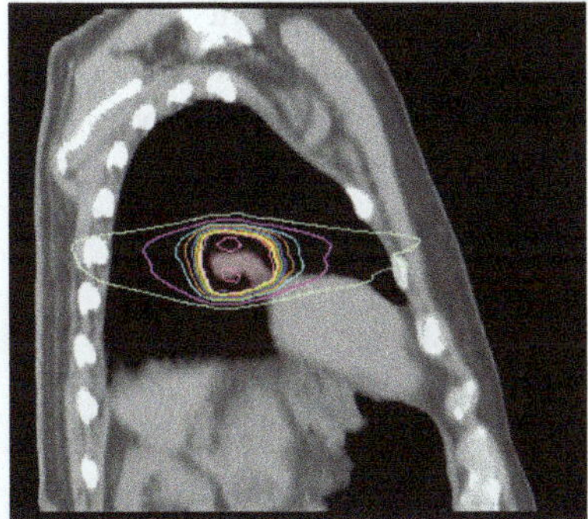

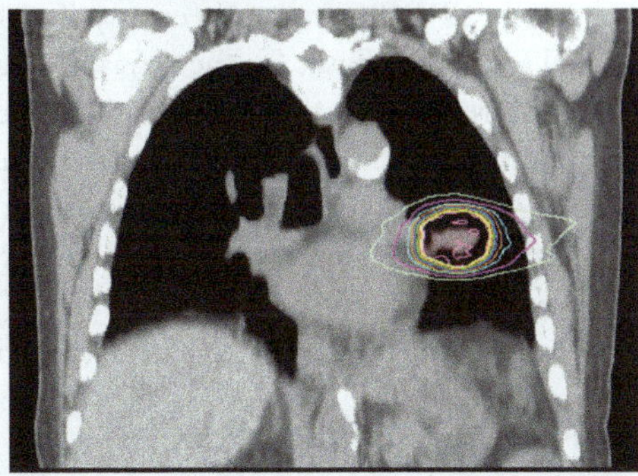

**FIGURE 5.1** Man aged 84 years with a central left lower lobe NSCLC treated with 7.5 Gy fractions × 8 (60 Gy total)

(Top) Isodose lines in the axial; (Left) coronal; and (Right) sagittal planes.

*Note:* NSCLC, non–small cell lung cancer.

suggesting the need for improved staging and/or the consideration of adjuvant therapy in select patients (24).

In modern practice, patients being considered for SBRT are often staged clinically with an integrated PET/CT and an endobronchial ultrasound (EBUS) with transbronchial needle aspiration (TBNA). In a randomized trial of surgical patients treated with a mediastinal lymph node dissection, EBUS-TBNA had a sensitivity, specificity, negative predictive value, and diagnostic accuracy of 81%, 100%, 91%, and 93%, respectively, which were similar to the results obtained with mediastinoscopy (25). Unlike surgical patients who have a comprehensive mediastinal evaluation at the time of surgery, mediastinal assessment prior to SBRT relies on imaging. The estimated sensitivity, specificity, and negative and positive predictive value for PET when identifying mediastinal metastases is 91%, 86%, 95%, and 74%, respectively (26). The high negative predictive value is particularly useful in excluding mediastinal disease for SBRT candidates. Particular patient populations at greater risk for occult nodal metastases despite a negative PET include adenocarcinoma histology, large or centrally located primary tumors, and those with a high standardized uptake value (SUV) in the primary tumor (27). Patients with a PET-positive mediastinal node should have it biopsied due to the potential for a false-positive result, particularly in those with underlying inflammatory conditions. Prospective experience of PET utilization for radiation planning has shown low rates of failure in PET-negative lymph nodes (28). Collectively, these results indicate that PET is critical in the workflow of SBRT planning.

The success of SBRT in primarily inoperable patients has led to multiple trials comparing SBRT versus lobectomy in medically operable patients. Although accrual proved difficult for these trials, a pooled analysis of two trials that closed early was recently reported. In this combined analysis, 58 patients with primary peripheral or central NSCLC less than 4 cm were randomly allocated to SBRT (risk-adapted based on location) or an anatomic lobectomy with hilar/mediastinal lymph node dissection. After a median follow-up of 40 months, recurrence-free survival was equivalent (29). Interestingly, an improved survival rate was found in patients treated with SBRT, with a 3-year OS of 95% compared to 79% in patients treated with surgery. Although surgery continues to be the standard of care for now, these provocative results provide equipoise for ongoing trials that will further define the role of SBRT in the medically operable population.

## LIVER RADIOSURGERY

Body radiosurgery has several applications in the liver, including for primary malignancies such as hepatocellular carcinoma (HCC) and cholangiocarcinoma, as well as for the treatment of liver metastases. SBRT for primary liver tumors is primarily based on the treatment of HCC, the most common primary liver tumor. The majority of patients diagnosed with HCC have varying degrees of liver cirrhosis. The Child–Turcotte–Pugh (CTP) classification is a tool used to estimate liver function, taking into account the presence of encephalopathy and ascites and albumin and bilirubin levels as well as the prothrombin time/international normalized ratio (PT/INR) (30). Patients with the best liver function are classified as CTP A, while classes B and C denote progressive liver decompensation. Treatment selection for HCC is best made in the multidisciplinary setting with the consideration of patient comorbidity and performance status, tumor extent (size and multifocality), and liver function. The Barcelona Clinic Liver Cancer (BCLC) classification incorporates these factors into a staging system with an associated treatment algorithm (31). For patients who are awaiting or are ineligible for resection or transplantation, multiple ablative approaches can be used, either as bridging or primary therapy, respectively. These ablative techniques include radiofrequency ablation (RFA), percutaneous ethanol/acetic acid injection (PEI), transarterial chemoembolization (TACE), and radioembolization (eg, Y-90 microspheres). More recently, SBRT has been utilized as an alternative ablative modality. Although not mentioned in the BCLC treatment algorithm, SBRT can be considered for the primary therapy of early-stage HCC unsuitable for surgery, as a bridge to transplant, and for advanced cases that are either refractory or unsuitable for other techniques (32).

Investigators at Princess Margaret Hospital have recently described the prospective experience for locally advanced HCC. This sequential phase I/II trial included patients with CTP class A liver disease who were felt to be unsuitable for resection, transplantation, or RFA. Up to five tumors were allowed, with a maximum dimension of 15 cm. Other permissible unfavorable findings included the presence of extrahepatic disease, tumor vascular thrombosis, and prior liver-directed therapy. Patients were simulated using active breathing control or abdominal compression in end-expiration breath-holding. The GTV was contoured with the use of triphasic CT and/or MRI (tumor vascular thrombosis included) and expanded at least 5 mm based on the motion management strategy. The radiation dose was delivered in six fractions, with the total dose contingent on a normal tissue complication probability model based on the effective volume of liver receiving the prescription dose (range: 30 Gy to 54 Gy). After a median follow-up of 31 months, 1-year local control and OS were 87% and 55%, respectively, with 30% of patients experiencing a deterioration of CTP class at 3 months (33). RTOG 1112 is currently assessing the efficacy of sorafenib in combination with SBRT for locally advanced disease, where doses of 27.5 Gy to 50 Gy in five fractions are allowed depending on the mean liver dose. The effectiveness of SBRT as a bridging therapy was demonstrated in a study in which patients safely received 50 Gy in 10 fractions with the majority going on to transplantation (34). Few reports exist that guide SBRT over other treatment modalities for HCC. Researchers conducting a recent retrospective study compared their institution's experience with both RFA and SBRT for inoperable HCC. Despite worse adverse prognostic findings in the SBRT arm, freedom from local progression at 2 years was similar between the two modalities (80% RFA, 84% SBRT) (35). The authors noted that local control decreased with increasing lesion size with RFA but not SBRT, whereas local progression was significantly higher for RFA in lesions greater than 2 cm. Ongoing clinical trials will further define SBRT utilization.

The majority of liver SBRT experience comes from the treatment of liver metastases. Compared to primary liver cancer patients, those with liver metastases tend to have better liver function, potentially increasing their tolerance of SBRT. The rationale for using local therapy to treat liver metastases is mostly based on the long-term survival of select patients treated with local therapy for limited colorectal metastases (36,37). In a multicenter phase I/II trial of patients with liver metastases from a variety of histologies (the majority colorectal), the SBRT dose was escalated safely to a total of 60 Gy in three fractions (38). Local control was 92% at 2 years with only one grade 3 toxicity (skin ulcer/pain) in 63 treated lesions. In this study at least 700 cc of liver was kept below a dose of 15 Gy. A second phase II trial also evaluated the safety and efficacy of a higher dose regimen, treating to 75 Gy in three fractions (39). Like the earlier trial, the most common histology was colorectal, but a variety of primary sites were included. After a median of 12 months, the in-field local response was 94%, and only one patient experienced grade 3 toxicity (chest wall pain) out of 73 treated lesions (61 patients). Together, these studies demonstrate high rates of local control with minimal toxicity.

From a technical standpoint, a variety of immobilization devices are available to create a custom mold of the patient for abdominal radiosurgery. These may be combined with a vacuum system to further enhance immobilization. The liver is highly subject to respiratory motion, as in the treatment of lung tumors, and this motion can be evaluated using four-dimensional CT. Abdominal compressive devices reduce this motion further by blunting the diaphragmatic excursion. Other techniques for respiratory motion management include treatment in a voluntary breath hold, using an active breathing control (ABC) system that further controls a static respiratory phase. Implanted fiducial markers can also be used—but cautiously, as patients with decompensated liver function may be unable to synthesize coagulation factors. Figure 5.2 shows a representative liver SBRT plan for a patient with intrahepatic cholangiocarcinoma.


## PANCREAS

The management of resectable pancreatic cancer has traditionally been based on surgery followed by adjuvant therapy. Despite this approach, the prognosis remains poor even for the favorable subset amenable to a potentially curative resection and treated with modern systemic therapy and often adjuvant radiotherapy (40). Patients with locally advanced or borderline resectable disease make up a larger proportion of those with pancreatic cancer whose treatment

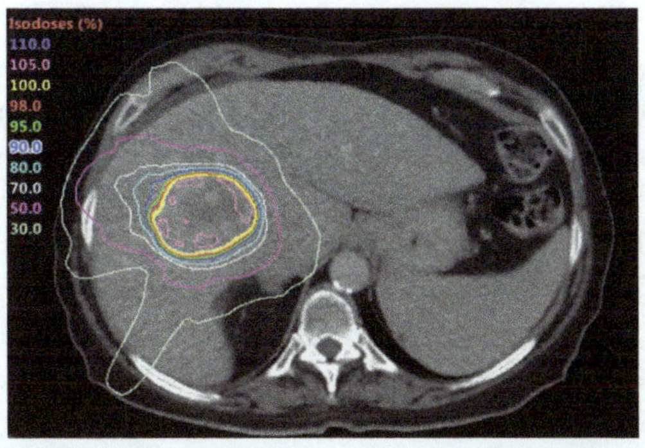

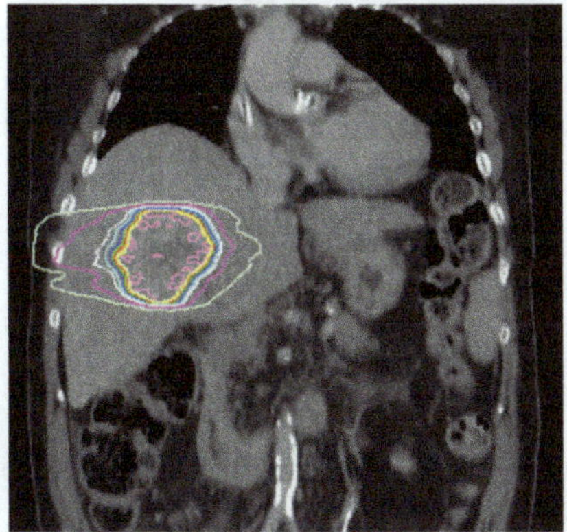

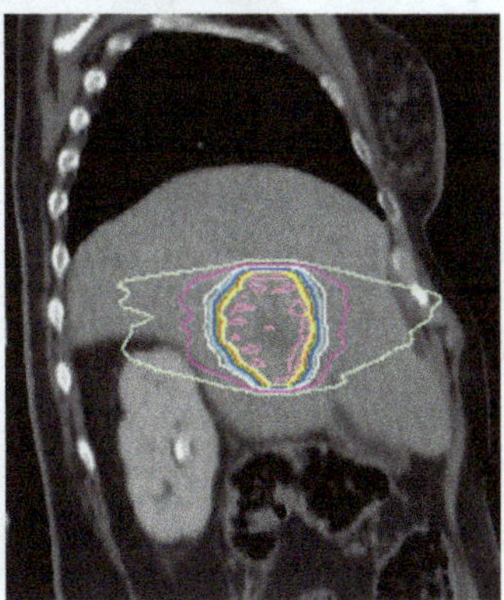

**FIGURE 5.2**  Woman aged 64 years with unresectable intrahepatic cholangiocarcinoma treated with 10 Gy fractions × 5 (50 Gy total)
   (Top) Isodose lines in the axial; (Left) coronal; and (Right) sagittal planes.

options are limited. Efforts to intensify neoadjuvant therapy for borderline and some locally advanced patients, to facilitate resection, are being studied, while durable local control and symptom palliation is the goal for the remaining patients with locally advanced disease. Local progression remains a critical issue in pancreatic cancer, with one autopsy series showing that approximately 30% of patients die with only local disease (41). Even among patients without disease progression during induction chemotherapy and who receive consolidation chemoradiation, the rates of isolated and any local progression are approximately 30% and 50%, respectively (42). This serves as a potential rationale for dose escalation utilizing SBRT.

Early experience with SBRT for locally advanced pancreatic cancer comes from Stanford, where a robotic radiosurgery system was used to treat 15 patients in a phase I dose escalation trial, ultimately reaching 25 Gy without dose-limiting toxicity (43). The same SBRT dosing regimen was then used as a boost after standard chemoradiation in a phase II study, confirming excellent local control (only 1:15 patients experienced local progression). However, despite these gains, there was no apparent improvement in survival compared to previous studies with high distant progression rates (44). In an attempt to improve distant control, SBRT was integrated into a gemcitabine regimen without prior chemoradiation. This platform highlighted the potential toxicity of single-fraction SBRT. Of the 16 treated patients, 5 developed duodenal ulcers, one developed duodenal stenosis, and one patient had a duodenal perforation (44% grade 2 or higher toxicity) (45). An association between duodenal volume and toxicity was noted. The largest phase II study using this platform consisted mostly of patients with locally advanced disease but also those with medically inoperable, locally recurrent, and metastatic disease who had received gemcitabine-based therapy. A total of 77 patients were treated, and the freedom from local progression and isolated local recurrence rates at a median follow-up of 6 months were 91% and 5%, respectively (46). Despite the promising local control, 1-yr OS was 21%, and the majority of patients progressed distantly. In addition, toxicity was not trivial, with 25% of patients experiencing grade 2 or higher late toxicity at 1 year.

Fractionated pancreatic SBRT has also been investigated in Denmark, with one trial treating a cohort of 22 patients to a total dose of 45 Gy in three fractions. Local control was notably worse in this study (57% at 1 year) compared to the Stanford series, with a high rate of grade 2 or higher toxicity (79%). Lower total doses of 30 Gy in three fractions appeared to be better tolerated in another trial, with no grade 2 toxicity observed and local control of 83% at a follow-up of 6 months (47). These studies ultimately culminated in a multi-institutional phase II trial of locally advanced pancreatic cancer patients in which 49 patients received SBRT to a total dose of 33 Gy in five fractions integrated into a systemically dosed gemcitabine backbone. After a median follow-up of 14 months, the local disease progression at 1 year was 78%, and median OS was only 14 months (48). Of particular interest was that 8% of patients went on to have no residual tumor (R0) resections, suggesting the potential for down-staging. Late grade 2 or greater toxicity was 11%, comparing favorably to previously described regimens. Proximal duodenum, stomach, and small bowel were limited such that 9 cc received less than 15 Gy, 3 cc received less than 20 Gy, and 1 cc received less than 33 Gy, respectively. In addition to the favorable local control and toxicity profile, significant pain improvement was documented, highlighting an important but often overlooked palliative benefit to this treatment.

In patients who have borderline resectable disease, a window of opportunity exists to use aggressive neoadjuvant therapy to possibly convert a subset to resection and offer the only chance for long-term survival. Although intensive systemic therapy combinations and standard chemoradiation are being investigated for this purpose, SBRT may also play a role. Investigators at the Moffitt Cancer Center utilized a 7 to 10 Gy/fx dosing scheme after induction chemotherapy, delivering 25 Gy to the whole tumor and 35 Gy to the region of vessel involvement in patients with borderline or unresectable tumors (49). Of 73 patients treated in this manner, 31 underwent an R0 resection. After a median follow-up of 10 months, 1-yr local control in nonoperative patients was 80%, and late grade 3 or higher toxicity was 5%. Neoadjuvant hypofractionated proton therapy has been investigated in resectable pancreatic cancer patients, which may guide further SBRT trials. A phase I dose escalation trial of 15 resectable patients demonstrated the feasibility of 5 Gy×5 given daily and concurrently with capecitabine followed by adjuvant gemcitabine (50). The phase II portion of the trial, which included an additional 35 patients, showed a locoregional recurrence rate of 16%, a median survival of 17 months, and a grade 3+toxicity of 4% (51). Similar to other approaches with SBRT, distant failure was the predominant mode of recurrence. The role of SBRT is being investigated in Alliance A021501, in which patients with borderline resectable disease will be randomized to induction folinic acid, fluorouracil, and oxaliplatin (FOLFOX) alone or FOLFOX followed by SBRT prior to surgery.

Practically speaking, SBRT to the pancreas is augmented with the placement of fiducial markers, typically via endoscopic ultrasound, to assist in target localization given the difficulty in visualizing the primary tumor on CBCT. Customized immobilization is routinely used, as are both intravenous (IV) and oral contrast, so that careful delineation of the target, duodenum, stomach, and bowel may be accomplished. Additionally, improved delineation of the primary pancreatic tumor can be seen with triphasic, bolus-tracked IV contrast administration (Figure 5.3) (52). Four-dimensional CT performed at the time of simulation can be used to assess motion, with further management depending on the degree of pancreas movement. Free- breathing treatments can be delivered to patients with less than 3 mm motion; otherwise, previously mentioned techniques such as breath-holding, phase-based gating, or ABC can be utilized. Abdominal compression should be used cautiously given the potential to push proximal bowel structures closer to the target (53). For planning following the generation of an ITV based on four-dimensional CT information, typical expansions for the PTV used in the literature range from 2 mm to 3 mm with the use of daily on-board imaging (matching to fiducials) and CBCT (primarily

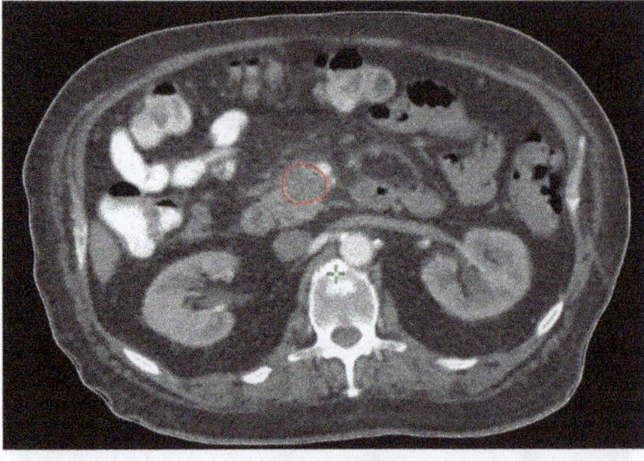

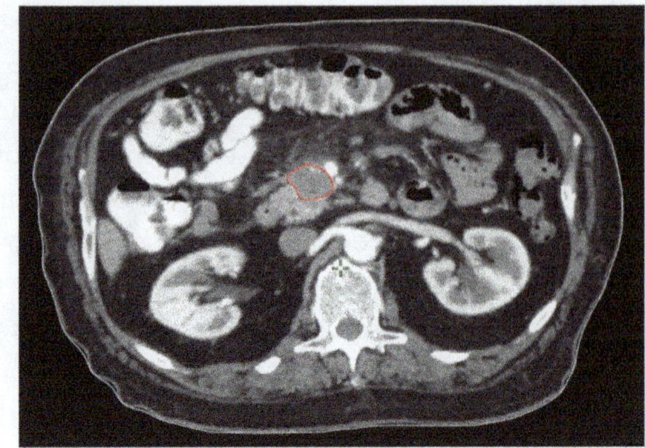

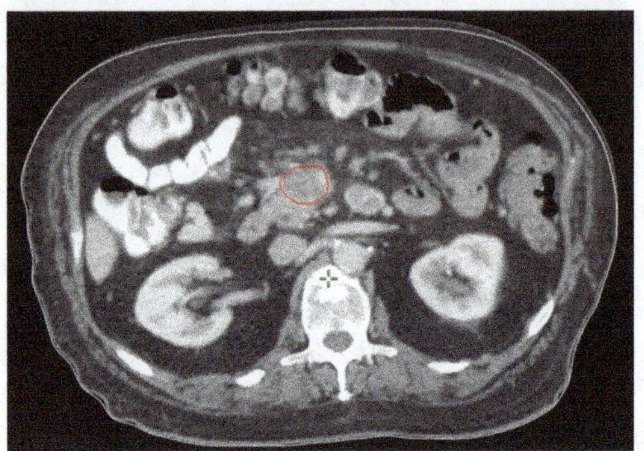

**FIGURE 5.3** Woman aged 67 years with locally advanced pancreatic cancer

Triphasic CT simulation images with intravenous and oral contrast demonstrate the gross tumor volume (*outlined in red*) in each phase.

for verification of adjacent organs at risk). Figure 5.4 provides an example of SBRT for a patient with locally advanced pancreatic cancer.

## OLIGOMETASTASES

*Oligometastases* refers to a distinct clinical state in which patients with a presumably unique tumor biology have distant metastases limited in number and destination organ, rendering the potential for a cure with metastasis-directed therapy (54). The state of oligometastases is more prevalent than one might expect. In breast cancer, for example, a pooled analysis of patients enrolled in first-line metastatic breast cancer trials found that approximately half of patients had fewer than or equal to 2 metastatic sites (55). In lung cancer, oligometastatic presentation may be less frequent in those with de novo metastatic disease (56) but is closer to 50% in those with recurrent disease after surgical resection (57). One trial of melanoma patients found that 78% developed a solitary metastasis (58). Patients with limited metastases, especially those with a single or solitary lesion, have an improved prognosis compared to those with a greater disease extent (59,60). Patterns of failure analyses show

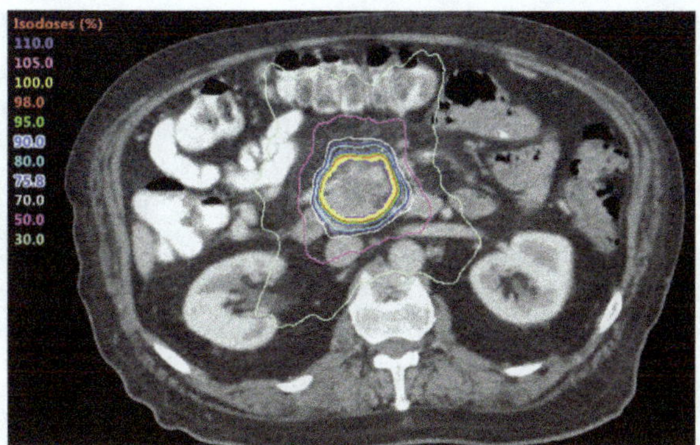

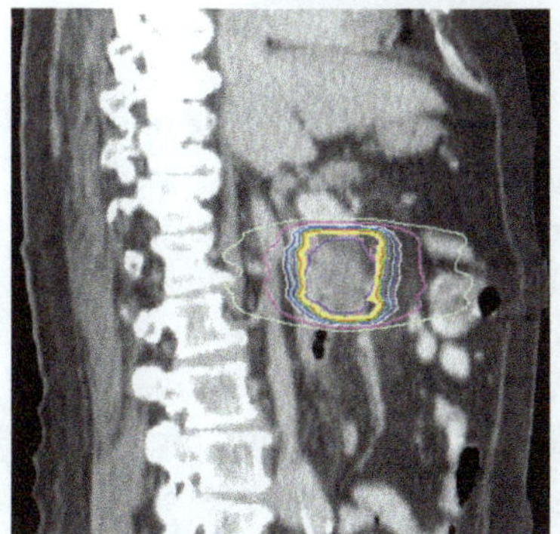
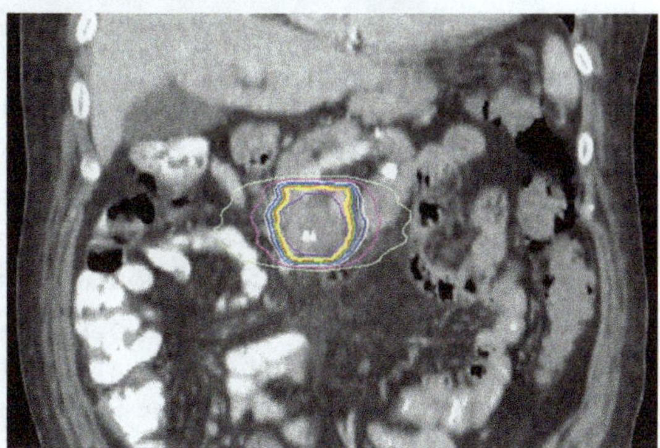

**FIGURE 5.4** Same patient in Figure 5.3 demonstrating a treatment plan of 6.6 Gy fractions × 5 (33 Gy total)
(Top) Isodose lines in the axial; (Left) coronal; and (Right) sagittal planes.

that the predominant mode of progression is at known sites of metastases (61), suggesting that local therapy may extend progression-free survival in select patients.

A surgical series of metastasectomy patients demonstrating the potential for curative treatment in select patients supports the rationale for SBRT. For lung metastases from a variety of histologies, pulmonary metastasectomy has been associated with long-term survival, particularly in patients with long disease-free intervals and a single metastasis (62). A large series of liver resections for metastatic colorectal cancer has also shown the potential for long-term survival in select patients (63). Adrenalectomy for predominantly NSCLC metastases has demonstrated similar findings (64). SBRT is uniquely suited for the treatment of oligometastases, particularly when surgery may not be feasible and when ablative doses can be delivered for local control with minimal morbidity. In some patients this can facilitate the initiation of a systemic therapy that may prove critical for disease control.

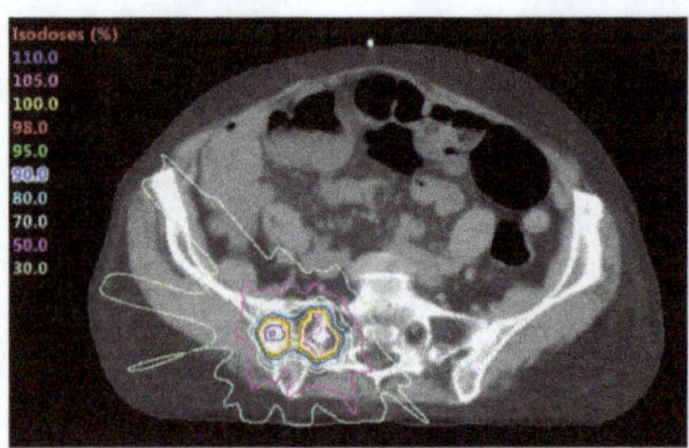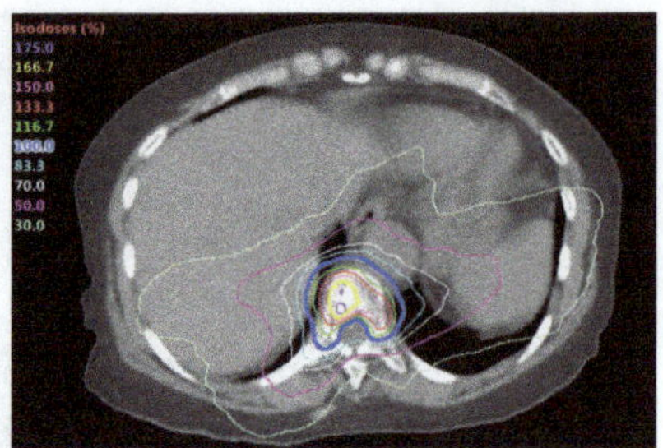

**FIGURE 5.5**  Woman aged 68 years with oligometastatic NSCLC

Axial isodose lines show treatment to the right ilium (Left; 5 Gy fractions × 10) and T10 vertebral body (Right; 3 Gy fractions × 10).

*Note:* NSCLC, non–small cell lung cancer.

A multi-institutional phase I/II trial that included patients with one to three metastases (cumulative maximum tumor diameter < 7 cm) demonstrated the efficacy and tolerability of SBRT for lung metastases. Utilizing a three-fraction regimen, the total dose was safely escalated to 60 Gy, which resulted in a 2-year local control of 96% (65). Simulation and planning techniques are essentially identical to those used for early-stage NSCLC. Additional studies have been published utilizing different dose fractionation schemes but similarly high rates of treated metastasis control in the 90% range (66). Numerous retrospective series show the feasibility and safety of SBRT for adrenal metastases, with one of the largest series utilizing 36 Gy in three fractions reporting a 2-year local control rate of 90% (67). The use of SBRT has been well described for vertebral body metastases (covered in a separate chapter), but a growing body of literature also suggests benefits in nonspine osseous locations. A recent series including patients with predominantly osseous pelvic metastases used SBRT dose regimens of 18 Gy to 24 Gy in a single fraction or 30 Gy in three fractions among several other less commonly used fractionations. Of 85 sites treated, the 1-year local control was 92%, with two asymptomatic pathologic fractures reported (68). The total dose is important because it is in primary sites; prescription doses of at least 48 Gy to 54 Gy are associated with optimal local control (69,70). Figure 5.5 demonstrates the treatment of two separate osseous sites in a patient with oligometastatic NSCLC.

SBRT has also been shown to safely and effectively treat multiple sites and organs in individual patients (70,71). NRG BR001 is the first National Cancer Institute (NCI)–sponsored multi-institutional prospective effort to assess the safety of SBRT for the treatment of multiple metastatic lesions in several anatomic sites (72). Eligible sites in this trial include the lungs (peripheral or central), the lymph nodes (mediastinal or cervical), the liver, spinal/paraspinal tissue, and osseous and abdominal/pelvic metastases (lymph node or adrenal gland). Initial starting doses for central lung and mediastinal lymph nodes are 50 Gy in 10 fractions, while liver, peripheral lung, and abdominal nodes/adrenal metastases will start at 45 Gy in 3 fractions. Spinal/paraspinal and other osseous sites will receive 30 Gy in 3 fractions. Treating multiple sites presents several challenges that include but are not limited to optimal immobilization (occasionally requiring two separate simulation scans depending on anatomic sites), the most appropriate motion-management strategy for all treated sites, image guidance and the use of multiple versus single isocenters, treatment using different fractionations, and the implications of organ dose constraints. The results from this trial will be critical to how SBRT becomes integrated into oligometastatic management.

It is important to recognize that prognostic and survival analyses have found that long-term survival in oligometastatic patients is most likely in those with very good performance status who have received previous chemotherapy and have small (≤3 cm) solitary metastases that are metachronous with their primary tumor (73). Beyond patient selection, a major challenge of SBRT for oligometastases is applying the general principles from mixed and heterogeneous studies to specific body sites where the optimal dose and fractionation are unknown. Fortunately, promising retrospective and single-institution outcomes have led to larger multicenter prospective trials, such as NRG BR001, that have outlined dosing parameters and toxicity limits for a variety of locations. As these trials mature, refinements in SBRT techniques will likely be made to optimize the therapeutic ratio for both individual sites and for those who require more complex planning for multiple-site disease.

## CONCLUSIONS

SBRT is an innovative approach that can reproducibly deliver ablative radiation doses to targets that previously required long courses of conventional radiation and were significantly limited by normal tissue tolerance. It has gained wide acceptance as a primary treatment modality in medically inoperable lung cancer and has found multiple indications in a variety of gastrointestinal malignancies, genitourinary cancers, and metastatic sites. Ongoing clinical trials will further define the role of SBRT, which will likely be a key component in the future of radiation therapy.

### References

1. Blomgren H, Lax I, Naslund I, et al. Stereotactic high dose fraction radiation therapy of extracranial tumors using an accelerator: clinical experience of the first thirty-one patients. *Acta Oncol.* 1995;34(6):861–870.

2. Mauguen A, Le Pechoux C, Saunders MI, et al. Hyperfractionated or accelerated radiotherapy in lung cancer: an individual patient data meta-analysis. *J Clin Oncol.* 2012; 30(22):2788–2797.

3. Timmerman R, Papiez L, McGarry R, et al. Extracranial stereotactic radioablation: results of a phase I study in medically inoperable stage I non-small cell lung cancer. *Chest.* 2003;124(5):1946–1955.

4. Timmerman R, McGarry R, Yiannoutsos C, et al. Excessive toxicity when treating central tumors in a phase II study of stereotactic body radiation therapy for medically inoperable early-stage lung cancer. *J Clin Oncol.* 2006;24(30):4833–4839.

5. Timmerman R, Paulus R, Galvin J, et al. Stereotactic body radiation therapy for inoperable early stage lung cancer. *JAMA.* 2010;303(11):1070–1076.

6. Baumann P, Nyman J, Hoyer M, et al. Outcome in a prospective phase II trial of medically inoperable stage I non-small-cell lung cancer patients treated with stereotactic body radiotherapy. *J Clin Oncol.* 2009;27(20):3290–3296.

7. Nagata Y, Takayama K, Matsuo Y, et al. Clinical outcomes of a phase I/II study of 48 Gy of stereotactic body radiotherapy in 4 fractions for primary lung cancer using a stereotactic body frame. *Int J Radiat Oncol Biol Phys.* 2005;63(5):1427–1431.

8. Uematsu M, Shioda A, Tahara K, et al. Focal, high dose, and fractionated modified stereotactic radiation therapy for lung carcinoma patients: a preliminary experience. *Cancer.* 1998;82(6):1062–1070.

9. Underberg RW, Lagerwaard FJ, Cuijpers JP, et al. Four-dimensional CT scans for treatment planning in stereotactic radiotherapy for stage I lung cancer. *Int J Radiat Oncol Biol Phys.* 2004;60(4):1283–1290.

10. Underberg RW, Lagerwaard FJ, Slotman BJ, et al. Use of maximum intensity projections (MIP) for target volume generation in 4DCT scans for lung cancer. *Int J Radiat Oncol Biol Phys.* 2005;63(1):253–260.

11. Videtic GM, Hu C, Singh AK, et al. A randomized phase 2 study comparing 2 stereotactic body radiation therapy schedules for medically inoperable patients with stage I peripheral non-small cell lung cancer: NRG Oncology RTOG 0915 (NCCTG N0927). *Int J Radiat Oncol Biol Phys.* 2015;93(4):757–764.

12. Onishi H, Araki T, Shirato H, et al. Stereotactic hypofractionated high-dose irradiation for stage I nonsmall cell lung carcinoma: clinical outcomes in 245 subjects in a Japanese multiinstitutional study. *Cancer.* 2004;101(7):1623–1631.

13. Dunlap NE, Cai J, Biedermann GB, et al. Chest wall volume receiving >30 Gy predicts risk of severe pain and/or rib fracture after lung stereotactic body radiotherapy. *Int J Radiat Oncol Biol Phys.* 2010;76(3):796–801.

14. Stephans KL, Djemil T, Tendulkar RD, et al. Prediction of chest wall toxicity from lung stereotactic body radiotherapy (SBRT). *Int J Radiat Oncol Biol Phys.* 2012;82(2):974–980.

15. Stephans KL, Djemil T, Reddy CA, et al. A comparison of two stereotactic body radiation fractionation schedules for medically inoperable stage I non-small cell lung cancer: the Cleveland Clinic experience. *J Thorac Oncol.* 2009;4(8):976–982.

16. Coroller TP, Mak RH, Lewis JH, et al. Low incidence of chest wall pain with a risk-adapted lung stereotactic body radiation therapy approach using three or five fractions based on chest wall dosimetry. *PLoS One.* 2014;9(4):e94859.

17. Bongers EM, Haasbeek CJ, Lagerwaard FJ, et al. Incidence and risk factors for chest wall toxicity after risk-adapted stereotactic radiotherapy for early-stage lung cancer. *J Thorac Oncol.* 2011;6(12):2052–2057.

18. Haasbeek CJ, Lagerwaard FJ, Slotman BJ, et al. Outcomes of stereotactic ablative radiotherapy for centrally located early-stage lung cancer. *J Thorac Oncol.* 2011;6(12):2036–2043.

19. Senthi S, Haasbeek CJ, Slotman BJ, et al. Outcomes of stereotactic ablative radiotherapy for central lung tumours: a systematic review. *Radiother Oncol.* 2013;106(3):276–282.

20. Nyman J, Hallqvist A, Lund JS, et al. SPACE—A randomized study of SBRT vs conventional fractionated radiotherapy in medically inoperable stage I NSCLC. *Radiother Oncol.* 2016;121(1):1–8.

21. Boyer MJ, Williams CD, Kelley MJ, et al. Improved survival with stereotactic body radiation therapy (SBRT) compared to conventional radiation in stage I NSCLC: A Veteran's Affairs Central Cancer Registry (VACCR) study. Paper presented at: American Society of Therapeutic Radiology and Oncology (ASTRO) Meeting; September 2016; Boston, MA.

22. Lindberg K, Nyman J, Riesenfeld Kallskog V, et al. Long-term results of a prospective phase II trial of medically inoperable stage I NSCLC treated with SBRT—the Nordic experience. *Acta Oncol.* 2015;54(8):1096–1104.

23. Senthi S, Lagerwaard FJ, Haasbeek CJ, et al. Patterns of disease recurrence after stereotactic ablative radiotherapy for early stage non-small-cell lung cancer: a retrospective analysis. *Lancet Oncol.* 2012;13(8):802–809.

24. Allibhai Z, Taremi M, Bezjak A, et al. The impact of tumor size on outcomes after stereotactic body radiation therapy for medically inoperable early-stage non-small cell lung cancer. *Int J Radiat Oncol Biol Phys.* 2013;87(5):1064–1070.

25. Yasufuku K, Pierre A, Darling G, et al. A prospective controlled trial of endobronchial ultrasound-guided transbronchial needle aspiration compared with mediastinoscopy for mediastinal lymph node staging of lung cancer. *J Thorac Cardiovasc Surg.* 2011;142(6):1393–1400, e1.

26. Pieterman RM, van Putten JW, Meuzelaar JJ, et al. Preoperative staging of non-small-cell lung cancer with positron-emission tomography. *N Engl J Med.* 2000;343(4):254–261.

27. Lee PC, Port JL, Korst RJ, et al. Risk factors for occult mediastinal metastases in clinical stage I non-small cell lung cancer. *Ann Thorac Surg.* 2007;84(1):177–181.

28. Bradley J, Bae K, Choi N, et al. A phase II comparative study of gross tumor volume definition with or without PET/CT fusion in dosimetric planning for non-small-cell lung cancer (NSCLC): primary analysis of Radiation Therapy Oncology Group (RTOG) 0515. *Int J Radiat Oncol Biol Phys.* 2012;82(1):435–441, e1.

29. Chang JY, Senan S, Paul MA, et al. Stereotactic ablative radiotherapy versus lobectomy for operable stage I non-small-cell lung cancer: a pooled analysis of two randomised trials. *Lancet Oncol.* 2015;16(6):630–637.

30. Child CGT, Turcotte JG. *Surgery and Portal Hypertension.* Child CG, ed. Philadelphia, PA: WB Saunders; 1964.

31. Forner A, Llovet JM, Bruix J. Hepatocellular carcinoma. *Lancet.* 2012;379(9822):1245–1255.

32. Klein J, Dawson LA. Hepatocellular carcinoma radiation therapy: review of evidence and future opportunities. *Int J Radiat Oncol Biol Phys.* 2013;87(1):22–32.

33. Bujold A, Massey CA, Kim JJ, et al. Sequential phase I and II trials of stereotactic body radiotherapy for locally advanced hepatocellular carcinoma. *J Clin Oncol.* 2013;31(13):1631–1639.

34. Katz AW, Chawla S, Qu Z, et al. Stereotactic hypofractionated radiation therapy as a bridge to transplantation for hepatocellular carcinoma: clinical outcome and pathologic correlation. *Int J Radiat Oncol Biol Phys.* 2012;83(3):895–900.

35. Wahl DR, Stenmark MH, Tao Y, et al. Outcomes after stereotactic body radiotherapy or radiofrequency ablation for hepatocellular carcinoma. *J Clin Oncol.* 2016;34(5):452–459.

36. Wong SL, Mangu PB, Choti MA, et al. American Society of Clinical Oncology 2009 clinical evidence review on radiofrequency ablation of hepatic metastases from colorectal cancer. *J Clin Oncol.* 2010;28(3):493–508.

37. Tomlinson JS, Jarnagin WR, DeMatteo RP, et al. Actual 10-year survival after resection of colorectal liver metastases defines cure. *J Clin Oncol.* 2007;25(29):4575–4780.

38. Rusthoven KE, Kavanagh BD, Cardenes H, et al. Multi-institutional phase I/II trial of stereotactic body radiation therapy for liver metastases. *J Clin Oncol.* 2009;27(10): 1572–1578.

39. Scorsetti M, Arcangeli S, Tozzi A, et al. Is stereotactic body radiation therapy an attractive option for unresectable liver metastases? a preliminary report from a phase 2 trial. *Int J Radiat Oncol Biol Phys.* 2013;86(2):336–342.

40. Neoptolemos JP, Stocken DD, Bassi C, et al. Adjuvant chemotherapy with fluorouracil plus folinic acid vs gemcitabine following pancreatic cancer resection: a randomized controlled trial. *JAMA.* 2010;304(10):1073–1081.

41. Iacobuzio-Donahue CA, Fu B, Yachida S, et al. DPC4 gene status of the primary carcinoma correlates with patterns of failure in patients with pancreatic cancer. *J Clin Oncol.* 2009;27(11):1806–1813.

42. Mukherjee S, Hurt CN, Bridgewater J, et al. Gemcitabine-based or capecitabine-based chemoradiotherapy for locally advanced pancreatic cancer (SCALOP): a multicentre, randomised, phase 2 trial. *Lancet Oncol.* 2013;14(4):317–326.

43. Koong AC, Le QT, Ho A, et al. Phase I study of stereotactic radiosurgery in patients with locally advanced pancreatic cancer. *Int J Radiat Oncol Biol Phys.* 2004;58(4): 1017–1021.

44. Koong AC, Christofferson E, Le QT, et al. Phase II study to assess the efficacy of conventionally fractionated radiotherapy followed by a stereotactic radiosurgery boost in patients with locally advanced pancreatic cancer. *Int J Radiat Oncol Biol Phys.* 2005; 63(2):320–323.

45. Schellenberg D, Goodman KA, Lee F, et al. Gemcitabine chemotherapy and single-fraction stereotactic body radiotherapy for locally advanced pancreatic cancer. *Int J Radiat Oncol Biol Phys.* 2008;72(3):678–686.

46. Chang DT, Schellenberg D, Shen J, et al. Stereotactic radiotherapy for unresectable adenocarcinoma of the pancreas. *Cancer.* 2009;115(3):665–672.

47. Polistina F, Costantin G, Casamassima F, et al. Unresectable locally advanced pancreatic cancer: a multimodal treatment using neoadjuvant chemoradiotherapy (gemcitabine plus stereotactic radiosurgery) and subsequent surgical exploration. *Ann Surg Oncol.* 2010; 17(8):2092–2101.

48. Herman JM, Chang DT, Goodman KA, et al. Phase 2 multi-institutional trial evaluating gemcitabine and stereotactic body radiotherapy for patients with locally advanced unresectable pancreatic adenocarcinoma. *Cancer.* 2015;121(7):1128–1137.

49. Chuong MD, Springett GM, Freilich JM, et al. Stereotactic body radiation therapy for locally advanced and borderline resectable pancreatic cancer is effective and well tolerated. *Int J Radiat Oncol Biol Phys.* 2013;86(3):516–522.

50. Hong TS, Ryan DP, Blaszkowsky LS, et al. Phase I study of preoperative short-course chemoradiation with proton beam therapy and capecitabine for resectable pancreatic ductal adenocarcinoma of the head. *Int J Radiat Oncol Biol Phys.* 2011;79(1):151–157.

51. Hong TS, Ryan DP, Borger DR, et al. A phase 1/2 and biomarker study of preoperative short course chemoradiation with proton beam therapy and capecitabine followed by early surgery for resectable pancreatic ductal adenocarcinoma. *Int J Radiat Oncol Biol Phys.* 2014;89(4):830–838.

52. Godfrey D, Patel B, Adamson J, et al. Triphasic bolus tracking CT simulation for SBRT of locoregionally advanced pancreatic cancer. Paper presented at: American Society of Therapeutic Radiology and Oncology (ASTRO) Meeting; September 2016; Boston, MA.

53. Taniguchi CM, Murphy JD, Eclov N, et al. Dosimetric analysis of organs at risk during expiratory gating in stereotactic body radiation therapy for pancreatic cancer. *Int J Radiat Oncol Biol Phys*. 2013;85(4):1090–1095.

54. Hellman S, Weichselbaum RR. Oligometastases. *J Clin Oncol*. 1995;13(1):8–10.

55. Salama JK, Chmura SJ. The role of surgery and ablative radiotherapy in oligometastatic breast cancer. *Semin Oncol*. 2014;41(6):790–797.

56. Parikh RB, Cronin AM, Kozono DE, et al. Definitive primary therapy in patients presenting with oligometastatic non-small cell lung cancer. *Int J Radiat Oncol Biol Phys*. 2014;89(4):880–887.

57. Yano T, Okamoto T, Haro A, et al. Local treatment of oligometastatic recurrence in patients with resected non-small cell lung cancer. *Lung Cancer*. 2013;82(3):431–435.

58. Howard JH, Thompson JF, Mozzillo N, et al. Metastasectomy for distant metastatic melanoma: analysis of data from the first Multicenter Selective Lymphadenectomy Trial (MSLT-I). *Ann Surg Oncol*. 2012;19(8):2547–2555.

59. Albain KS, Crowley JJ, LeBlanc M, et al. Survival determinants in extensive-stage non-small-cell lung cancer: the Southwest Oncology Group experience. *J Clin Oncol*. 1991;9(9):1618–1626.

60. Singh D, Yi WS, Brasacchio RA, et al. Is there a favorable subset of patients with prostate cancer who develop oligometastases? *Int J Radiat Oncol Biol Phys*. 2004;58(1):3–10.

61. Rusthoven KE, Hammerman SF, Kavanagh BD, et al. Is there a role for consolidative stereotactic body radiation therapy following first-line systemic therapy for metastatic lung cancer? a patterns-of-failure analysis. *Acta Oncol*. 2009;48(4):578–583.

62. Pastorino U, Buyse M, Friedel G, et al. Long-term results of lung metastasectomy: prognostic analyses based on 5206 cases. *J Thorac Cardiovasc Surg*. 1997;113(1):37–49.

63. Fong Y, Fortner J, Sun RL, et al. Clinical score for predicting recurrence after hepatic resection for metastatic colorectal cancer: analysis of 1001 consecutive cases. *Ann Surg*. 1999;230(3):309–318, discussion 18–21.

64. Tanvetyanon T, Robinson LA, Schell MJ, et al. Outcomes of adrenalectomy for isolated synchronous versus metachronous adrenal metastases in non-small-cell lung cancer: a systematic review and pooled analysis. *J Clin Oncol*. 2008;26(7):1142–1147.

65. Rusthoven KE, Kavanagh BD, Burri SH, et al. Multi-institutional phase I/II trial of stereotactic body radiation therapy for lung metastases. *J Clin Oncol*. 2009;27(10): 1579–1584.

66. Salama JK, Milano MT. Radical irradiation of extracranial oligometastases. *J Clin Oncol*. 2014;32(26):2902–2912.

67. Casamassima F, Livi L, Masciullo S, et al. Stereotactic radiotherapy for adrenal gland metastases: university of Florence experience. *Int J Radiat Oncol Biol Phys*. 2012;82(2): 919–923.

68. Owen D, Laack NN, Mayo CS, et al. Outcomes and toxicities of stereotactic body radiation therapy for non-spine bone oligometastases. *Pract Radiat Oncol*. 2014;4(2):e143–e149.

69. McCammon R, Schefter TE, Gaspar LE, et al. Observation of a dose-control relationship for lung and liver tumors after stereotactic body radiation therapy. *Int J Radiat Oncol Biol Phys*. 2009;73(1):112–118.

70. Salama JK, Hasselle MD, Chmura SJ, et al. Stereotactic body radiotherapy for multisite extracranial oligometastases: final report of a dose escalation trial in patients with 1 to 5 sites of metastatic disease. *Cancer*. 2012;118(11):2962–2970.

71. Milano MT, Katz AW, Zhang H, et al. Oligometastases treated with stereotactic body radiotherapy: long-term follow-up of prospective study. *Int J Radiat Oncol Biol Phys.* 2012;83(3):878–886.
72. Al-Hallaq HA, Chmura S, Salama JK, et al. Rationale of technical requirements for NRG-BR001: the first NCI-sponsored trial of SBRT for the treatment of multiple metastases. *Pract Radiat Oncol.* 2016;6(6):e291–e298.
73. Fode MM, Hoyer M. Survival and prognostic factors in 321 patients treated with stereotactic body radiotherapy for oligo-metastases. *Radiother Oncol.* 2015;114(2):155–160.

# Brachytherapy 6

*Dodul Mondal, Omar Mahmoud, and Atif J. Khan*

## INTRODUCTION

Since Finsen's invention of ultraviolet rays as a successful modality of therapy for lupus disorders, the history of radiation therapy has witnessed many advances and achievements. The discovery of x-rays in 1895 by Wilhelm Röntgen further paved the way. In 1896 Henri Becquerel discovered the radioactivity of uranium. It was soon succeeded by Marie Sklodowska Curie's identification of radium and polonium as radioactive elements in 1898. In 1896 Victor Despeignes attempted the first x-ray therapy for a stomach tumor (1).

The term *brachytherapy* is derived from a Greek word meaning "short," signifying a short distance between the source of radiation and the tumor. Dr. Gosta Forssell coined the word in 1931. French physician Henri-Alexandre Danlos performed the first brachytherapy procedure in 1901 by implanting a radium source within a tumor. Subsequently, on both sides of the Atlantic, brachytherapy started growing under the able leadership of Danlos at the Curie institute, Paris, and at St. Luke's and Memorial Hospitals in New York under Robert Abbe.

With passing time, the sources, techniques, indications, and outcomes of brachytherapy have changed dramatically. However, to date brachytherapy continues to be the most conformal of all radiation treatments simply by virtue of being delivered within the body ("inside out"). The initial enthusiasm and indications started mostly with skin, gynecologic, and head and neck cancers and gradually extended to almost every disease site. A detailed discussion, although desired, is beyond the scope of this chapter.

## BRACHYTHERAPY SOURCE TYPES

Brachytherapy sources are mostly sealed and encapsulated. They can be wires, needles, tubes, pellets, or seeds. Each has its own size, half-life, and activity and delivers a specific dose over a particular period of time. In modern-day practice with remote afterloader machines, a tiny source at the tip of a cable is most common. This type is called the *stepping source*, driven by a stepping motor.

### Different Types of Brachytherapy

Customarily, brachytherapy can be classified in the following different ways:

1. According to the method of placing the radioactive source:
   a. Interstitial brachytherapy (IBT): Brachytherapy radionuclides are placed directly into the tissue with a surgical procedure. The radionuclides can remain in place temporarily, for an indefinite period of time, or permanently.
   b. Intracavitary brachytherapy: The sources are housed inside an applicator, which is placed within a body cavity (such as the uterine cavity) for a defined time—usually a short duration.
   c. Intraluminal: Brachytherapy sources are placed in a natural luminal structure of the body, such as the esophagus or the bronchus. The source is located inside a catheter or an applicator, where it stays for a short period of time.
   d. Surface brachytherapy: Previously known as *plesiotherapy*, in this technique custom- made surface molds are made, along with catheters, to hold a radiation source. It is usually employed for very superficial and complex or irregular tumors, and treatment is usually conducted with high-dose rate (HDR) technique.
2. According to the method of loading the source:
   a. Manual afterloader: Initially, specific nonradioactive applicators or needles are placed. Radioactive sources are then manually loaded into these applicators or needles.
   b. Remote afterloader: A remote-controlled computer system mechanically loads the source, reducing the chance of radiation exposure to the staff and other medical personnel. The introduction of the remote-controlled afterloader has improved safety in the practice of brachytherapy.
3. According to dose rate. The International Commission on Radiation Unit and Measurements (ICRU) report 38 has provided following definitions:
   a. HDR: The rate of dose delivered is more than 12 Gy per hour. However, modern HDR brachytherapy units are capable of delivering a much higher dose than that.

b. Medium dose rate (MDR): The dose rate is 2 Gy to12 Gy per hour, an amount not routinely used for clinical practice.

c. Low dose rate (LDR): The dose rate is 0.4 Gy to 2 Gy per hour.

d. Ultra-low dose rate (ULDR): The delivered dose rate is 0.01 Gy to 0.3 Gy per hour.

e. Although not originally described in ICRU 38, pulsed dose rate (PDR) brachytherapy is important for permanent implants. PDR brachytherapy delivers a series of short (10-to-30 minute) pulses (short treatments) every hour. It essentially combines the technological advantages of afterloading HDR brachytherapy with the radiobiological advantage of LDR brachytherapy, allowing incomplete repair over the same treatment time. Unlike HDR techniques, it requires inpatient treatment.

4. Classification based on the duration of the implant:

a. Temporary: The radioactive material remains in place for a short duration of time and is removed from the body after the necessary dose is delivered.

b. Permanent: Once inserted in the body, the radioactive material remains there, delivering doses over the life of the isotope.

## THE ROLE OF BRACHYTHERAPY IN DIFFERENT MALIGNANCIES

Though historically, brachytherapy found its beginning with nonmalignant lupus, very rapidly its applicability extended to different malignant conditions, including skin cancers, gynecologic malignancies, and head and neck cancers. Today it is an integral part of the multimodality management of cancers of many sites. It can be used in radical treatment either as a primary modality or as part of a combined-modality approach. It can also be employed very effectively for the palliation of symptoms. Here we will discuss the applicability of brachytherapy to cancers of different systems.

### Brachytherapy in Gynecologic Malignancies

The historical importance of brachytherapy for gynecologic cancers can never be understated. Different schools of thought on brachytherapy techniques, dose rate systems, and dose calculation systems were developed in the early part of the twentieth century. Of note are the Paris system, the Manchester system, and the Stockholm system. Among these, the Manchester system was described for both intracavitary and interstitial implants. The large proportion of gynecologic cancers in which brachytherapy is applicable are comprised of cancers of the uterus, the uterine cervix, and the vagina. A few factors have made brachytherapy an essential component of treatment, including the presence of a hollow organ that can accommodate the brachytherapy applicator and the sources easily; the location of the genital tract and its anatomy, making implanting easy; the organ's high radiation tolerance, thus making the delivery of a high radiation dose possible; and of course the presence of OAR that can be easily separated from the target by manual techniques with easy maneuvers.

## Brachytherapy in Cervical Carcinoma

Brachytherapy is an integral part of cervical carcinoma treatment and can be employed at every stage of disease, starting from in situ tumors to invasive tumors of a very advanced stage. The dose is prescribed and reported at point A when the uterus and cervix are intact. For postoperative treatment the dose is prescribed at a depth of 5 mm from the vaginal surface mucosa. However, as more forms of image-guided brachytherapy become available, there is a steady and consistent change toward the adoption of volume-based dosimetry.

## Brachytherapy for Precancerous Lesions (Previous Stage 0, Tis)

Though the preferred treatment is either therapeutic conization or total abdominal hysterectomy (TAH) with or without a part of the vaginal cuff, radical brachytherapy can also be employed under the following circumstances:

1. Patients with contraindications to surgery or who do not consent to surgical resection
2. Multifocal disease either in the cervix or in the vagina
3. Disease extending to the vagina and requiring extended vaginal resection (2,3)

Treatment can be delivered either by tandem and ovoids or by vaginal cylinder and tandem with the LDR or the HDR technique. An LDR dose equivalent of 50 Gy to point A or 20 to 30 Gy by HDR therapy seems adequate for tumor control.

In a first-of-its-kind study from the Mallinckrodt Institute of Radiology, 21 patients with carcinoma in situ (CIS) and 34 patients with stage IA cancer were treated from January 1959 through December 1986 with LDR using an average dose of 4,612 cGy to point A (4). In 13 patients treated with ICRT alone, the average radiation dose was 5,571 cGy to point A. Other patients received combined external beam radiation therapy (EBRT) with ICRT with an average ICRT dose of 5,200 cGy to point A. Local, regional, and distant control were excellent, with 5.9% of patients developing severe toxicity. Only one patient with stage IA cancer developed a pelvic recurrence.

In a retrospective analysis from Japan, Ogino et al have shown excellent outcomes in 17 patients treated with HDR-ICRT alone (5). With a mean total dose of 26.1 Gy (range: 20–30) and 23.3 Gy (range: 15–30) for CIN-3 and VAIN-3, respectively, none of the patients showed any recurrence or died due to disease.

Kim et al have published their experiences from Korea in a recent study using HDR-ICRT and Co-60 or Ir-192 for 166 patients (6). The median radiation dose was 30 Gy/6 fractions (range: 30–52). After a median follow-up of 152 months, 2 patients developed recurrent disease, and 26 patients died from non-malignant intercurrent disease. Overall, the success rate with brachytherapy alone is nearly 100% in preinvasive disease, even in the presence of poor histological factors.

## Brachytherapy for Invasive Cervical Carcinoma Stage IA/IA2
### *Adjuvant Brachytherapy After Surgery*

- In many instances, microinvasive cervical carcinoma is an incidental finding after a TAH. Such patients, if found to have deep stromal invasion on the postoperative histopathology report, should receive adjuvant brachytherapy to a total dose of 65 Gy in an LDR-equivalent dose to the mucosa. This dose can be delivered in one or two divided treatment sessions. A HDR-ICRT with a dose of 7 Gy×6 fractions is also an acceptable and reasonable choice for a convenient outpatient procedure. The dose should be calculated at the vaginal mucosal surface.

- For patients having gross invasion or a postoperative residual tumor at the vault or parametrium after an inadvertent surgery, the situation becomes difficult, with poor outcomes in the absence of adjuvant treatment. A more extensive treatment using external beam radiation to the whole pelvis, concurrent platinum-based chemotherapy, and brachytherapy either by ICRT or by interstitial implant seems more appropriate. A whole pelvis dose from 40 Gy to 45 Gy and/or a parametrial boost of 10 Gy to 20 Gy is considered adequate with or without concurrent chemotherapy. Brachytherapy, when feasible, is performed via an intravaginal cylinder or ovoids, with the total vaginal mucosal dose reaching up to 60 Gy to 65 Gy. If ICRT is not possible, an interstitial implant should be considered. Survival with this approach after an inadvertent hysterectomy with poor clinicopathologic features often reaches 60% to 90%.

In their experience with 83 patients, Sharma et al (7) treated those who underwent inadvertent surgery with EBRT and brachytherapy. After an initial EBRT dose of 50 Gy to the pelvis, patients received a 30-Gy LDR equivalent dose to a 0.5-cm depth of the vaginal mucosa by ovoids or an 8 Gy×2 weekly HDR treatment with ovoids. Patients with gross residual disease were treated with interstitial implants. The cumulative 5-year overall survival (OS) was 62%. The results of this study, however, differed from a more historic study by Andras et al (8). In a similar clinical scenario, the 5-year OS was 89%. Intravaginal vault brachytherapy was combined with EBRT.

*Radical Brachytherapy Alone.* Radical brachytherapy alone can be delivered to patients with International Federation of Gynecology and Obstetrics (FIGO) stage IA1/IA2 malignancies who are not candidates for surgery or who are unwilling to undergo surgery. This can achieve excellent local control of disease, with a reported 10-year progression-free survival (PFS) of 98% to 100%. A total dose of 65 Gy to 75 Gy by LDR to point A is sufficient, keeping the vaginal mucosal surface dose 100 Gy to 120 Gy (9,10). An equivalent dose of HDR can also be employed. The American Brachytherapy Society (ABS) recommends an LDR dose equivalent of 50 Gy to 60 Gy to point A for clinical stage IA1 and IA2 (11).

## Brachytherapy in Combination With External Beam Radiation Therapy

ICRT in combination with EBRT is advocated for patients showing a lymphovascular space invasion (LVSI) in their conization specimen. A typical pelvic EBRT dose of 40 Gy to 45 Gy with or without midline shielding is delivered. This is followed by ICRT to a total dose of 70 Gy to 80 Gy to point A.

## Brachytherapy for Limited-Volume Invasive Cervical Carcinoma Stage IB1/IIA

These malignancies are a closely associated group characterized by the presence of a limited-volume disease within the cervix, upper vagina, or medial parametrium without a significant risk of pelvic lymph node involvement. Treatment modalities include radical surgery, radical radiotherapy, radical chemoradiation, postoperative radiotherapy, postoperative chemoradiation, and postoperative brachytherapy. The choice of any modality depends on several factors, including patient preference, the expertise available for any specific type of treatment, issues of fertility and ovarian function preservation, and the presence of high-risk features in biopsy specimens. Only a few randomized trials exist supporting the role of any modality with an equal cure rate. The prognosis is usually excellent, with 5-year survival reaching almost 90%.

*Brachytherapy Alone.* Brachytherapy alone is seldom a choice, except for a very rare group requiring vaginal brachytherapy alone after radical surgery with a risk of vaginal cuff recurrence. This may be justified for patients having close vaginal margins, without any other risk factors, in their pathology specimens after a successful radical surgery. However, this is controversial, and the ABS in its latest consensus statement declined to provide any specific guideline (12). An LDR-equivalent dose of 60 Gy to the vaginal mucosal surface should suffice in these patients. For limited-volume disease, brachytherapy is usually delivered in combination with adjuvant EBRT.

*Preoperative Brachytherapy.*  For tumors less than 4 cm (IB1), the Institut Gustave Roussy (IGR) technique uses a 60-Gy reference isodose to the volume encompassing the disease, the upper third of the vagina, the medial third of the parametrium, and the upper third of the uterus. Treatment is usually delivered in one to two sessions (13). For tumors more than 4 cm (IB2), a combination of brachytherapy of 40 Gy (reference isodose) and EBRT of 20 Gy is used.

Among 288 stage IB patients, this treatment provided excellent tumor control. The 5-year actuarial pelvic disease-free and disease-free survivals (DSF) were 92% and 89%, respectively. The 5-year OS among stage I patients was 92% (14).

*Postoperative Adjuvant Brachytherapy.*  Most patients require brachytherapy as part of adjuvant radiotherapy in combination with pelvic radiation such as those with high-risk features after a hysterectomy including deep stromal invasion, extensive lymphovascular invasion, parametrial or vaginal invasion, or the presence of positive or close margins.

The ABS recommends a total LDR-equivalent dose of 70 Gy to the vaginal mucosa. The treatment can be delivered either by HDR or LDR techniques. With HDR, the usual dose fraction is 6 Gy×3. The largest diameter vaginal cylinder suitable for a particular patient or vaginal ovoids can be used to deliver the treatment.

*Brachytherapy as Part of Radical Radiation.*  Brachytherapy in combination with external radiation, with or without chemotherapy, is an alternative approach. In a landmark study, Landoni et al have established radical radiotherapy as a comparable modality to surgery for patients with stage IB2 through IIA disease (15). Multiple randomized trials in patients with stage IB2 through IVA have utilized brachytherapy as an essential component of treatment (16–20).

The dose of brachytherapy depends on the dose rate of treatment. With HDR brachytherapy, a 5-week or 3-week intracavitary application 1 week apart and 7 Gy per fraction to point A is the standard, with various combinations of EBRT protocols, including midline shielding. Two LDR applications at 1 week intervals, each delivering 30 Gy to point A, is another alternative approach.

## Brachytherapy for Advanced Invasive Carcinoma Cervix Stage IB2, IIB–IVA

Brachytherapy is an essential component of a chemoradiation protocol. A total dose of 90 Gy to point A should be the target. EBRT delivers 45 Gy to 50 Gy; the HDR technique can deliver 7 Gy × 3 fractions at 1-week intervals or 9 Gy × 2 fractions for adequate tumor control. A single LDR application of 30 Gy to point A is adequate.

It would be wise to discuss modern image-guided brachytherapy at this point. CT- or MRI-based planning provides the opportunity to see the dose coverage and the actual location of organs at risk (OAR) and their dose-volume characteristics. The European Epidemiological Study of Familial Breast Cancer (EMBRACE) is a multi-institutional MRI-based brachytherapy protocol that takes the volume of disease as seen on MRI into account. The dose prescription is volume-based without compromising the point A dose. Different target volumes are described in this protocol, including the gross tumor volume at diagnosis ($GTV_D$), the gross tumor volume at brachytherapy ($GTV_B$), the high-risk clinical target volume (HR- CTV), and the intermediate-risk CTV (IR-CTV) (21). Interested readers can follow different Groupe Européen de Curiethérapie and the European Society for Radiotherapy and Oncology (GEC-ESTRO) definitions and brachytherapy applicator details.

It is important to keep in mind that patients who are not suitable for intracavitary insertion due to local anatomical distortion, or who have a small central recurrence, can be considered for interstitial brachytherapy. The dose and the fractionation are variable and depend on individual institutional preferences (22,23).

## Brachytherapy for Hemostatic and Palliative Purposes

In a series from the Mallinckrodt Institute of Radiology, patients with cervical cancer experiencing acute, severe vaginal bleeding were treated with vaginal brachytherapy to provide good bleeding control. A total dose of 10 Gy, in two weekly fractions of 5 Gy, was delivered to the surface of the cervix with a ring applicator (24).

## Brachytherapy for Uterine Cancer

*As Part of Definitive Management.* As with cervical cancer, brachytherapy is an integral component of endometrial cancer management. However, unlike the former, radical brachytherapy is not an option, and surgery remains the mainstay of treatment with or without various combinations of radiotherapy and chemotherapy. The brachytherapy in question is usually intravaginal, with a vaginal cylinder applicator of the maximum diameter that can snugly fit into the vagina.

The dose is prescribed at a depth of 5 mm from the applicator surface. The target volume for brachytherapy is usually the upper third of the vagina. IBT has a role in recurrent disease.

Largely, vaginal brachytherapy is limited to early-stage (stage I and stage II) endometrial cancer after a standard TAH plus a bilateral salpingo-oopherectomy (BSO). Patients over the age of 60 years who have a grade 3 tumor, deep stromal invasion, and/or LVSI have a 13% to 27% risk of local failure in the absence of adjuvant treatment (25,26).

A dose of 18 Gy to 21 Gy delivered in three weekly fractions of 6 Gy to 7 Gy at a depth of 5 mm from the applicator surface is adequate, depending on risk category. The benefits of vaginal brachytherapy include reduced local failure rates and avoidance of the side effects of EBRT.

In the combined National Cancer Institute of Canada (NCIC) and Efficacy of Systematic Pelvic Lymphadenectomy in Endometrial Cancer (MRC ASTEC) trial, the 5-year local or pelvic failure rate was significantly lower in patients undergoing adjuvant radiation; 52% of these patients received combined EBRT and intravaginal brachytherapy (IVBT) (27). In a randomized study of observation versus IVBT, Sorbe et al reported no significant differences between the two arms in terms of local or pelvic failures (28). The Post Operative Radiation Therapy in Endometrial Carcinoma (PORTEC-2) trial randomized 427 patients to pelvic EBRT or IVBT; they received a 7 Gy×3 weekly dose by HDR or a 30-Gy dose by LDR. The DFS and the OS did not differ significantly, demonstrating the adequacy of IVBT for this patient population (29).

Multiple studies have documented the benefit of a vaginal cuff brachytherapy boost after a dose of 45 Gy to 50.4 Gy EBRT to the pelvis. A dose of 6 Gy×3 or 6 Gy×2 by HDR brachytherapy is adequate. However, the role of EBRT remains controversial in this early-stage disease category.

Surgically staged II or III disease is managed by adjuvant radiotherapy with EBRT and brachytherapy. The previous stage IIA does not exist in the current FIGO staging and is currently not being discussed, but the treatment is the same as that for stage I. Table 6.1 summarizes the roles of brachytherapy.

***Concurrent Brachytherapy and Chemotherapy.***  In recent years, adjuvant and concurrent chemotherapy with intravaginal brachytherapy have proven they are not inferior to standard treatment (30,31). However, this requires further confirmation.

### Brachytherapy for Recurrent Disease

Brachytherapy alone or in combination with EBRT can be used for the curative treatment of uterine cancer with a small central recurrence. An intracavitary

**TABLE 6.1**  Indications and doses of various brachytherapy combinations

| Surgical stage | Presence of risk factor | Grade 1 | Grade 2 | Grade 3 | Dose of IVBT alone | Dose of IVBT in combination with EBRT | |
|---|---|---|---|---|---|---|---|
| IA | − | Observation | Observation or IVBT | Observation or IVBT | 21 Gy HDR or 30 Gy LDR | 21 Gy or 18 Gy | A lower IVBT dose is recommended when pelvic EBRT dose is 50–50.4 Gy. A higher IVBT dose is delivered when pelvic EBRT dose is 45 Gy. |
| | + | Observation or IVBT | Observation or IVBT and/or EBRT | Observation or IVBT and/or EBRT | 21 Gy HDR or 30 Gy LDR | 21 Gy or 18 Gy | |
| IB | − | Observation or IVBT | Observation or IVBT | IVBT and/or EBRT | 21 Gy HDR or 30 Gy LDR | 21 Gy or 18 Gy | |
| | + | Observation or IVBT and/or EBRT | Observation or IVBT and/or EBRT | EBRT and/or IVBT | 21 Gy HDR or 30 Gy LDR | 21 Gy or 18 Gy | |
| II | | IVBT and/or EBRT | IVBT and/or EBRT | EBRT and/or IVBT | 21 Gy HDR or 30 Gy LDR | 21 Gy or 18 Gy | |
| IIIA, IIIB, IIIC | | EBRT + IVBT with various combinations of chemotherapy | | | 21 Gy HDR or 30 Gy LDR | 21 Gy or 18 Gy | |

*Note:* EBRT, external beam radiotherapy; IVBT, intravaginal brachytherapy; HDR, high dose rate; LDR, low dose rate.

*Source:* Partially modified from NCCN guideline, 2016.

or interstitial boost and/or EBRT should be the treatment of choice, and dose fractionation usually depends on the previous treatment and the radiation dose profile. Properly assessing the extent of the vaginal growth, including the submucosal spread of the disease, is important.

***Brachytherapy as a Part of Radical Radiation.*** For medically inoperable patients with very early-stage disease, radical radiation for curative treatment can be delivered, just as in the management of cervical cancer, with a target dose of 80 Gy to 85 Gy LDR equivalence to point A. Usually, a radical brachytherapy of 70 Gy to 75 Gy alone for low-risk disease and 30 Gy to 35 Gy in combination with EBRT (45–50 Gy) for high- to intermediate-risk disease is adequate.

## Brachytherapy for Vulvovaginal Disease

Primary vulvovaginal cancers are relatively less common. Brachytherapy plays a distinct role in the management of vulvovaginal cancers or endometrial cancers with vaginal recurrences.

The primary treatment for vulvar cancers is surgical resection. Patients unwilling or unable for medical reasons to undergo surgery who have a localized central tumor in proximity to the urethra can be treated with radical radiation, and brachytherapy can be used as a boost with EBRT. Brachytherapy alone with an interstitial implant can be considered for recurrent central tumors. When used as a boost, 18 Gy to 21 Gy in 6 to 7 fractions is adequate. As a radical treatment, 45 Gy to 50 Gy in 15 to 18 fractions is recommended.

Primary vaginal cancers constitute only 1% to 2% of all gynecological cancers. In 2012 the ABS recommended the use of IBT for vaginal cancers (32). Any lesion more than 5 mm thick should be treated with IBT, either alone or in combination with EBRT. The recommendations are summarized in Table 6.2.

IBT can also be used to treat recurrent tumors. No specific guidelines exist for this treatment, and the dose fractionation depends on the previous dose administered to the tumor and the OAR.

Intracavitary brachytherapy is used in combination with EBRT to treat stage I tumors that are well differentiated and less than 5 mm in thickness. Either LDR or HDR can be used, depending on the institutional expertise and the facilities available.

## Genitourinary Brachytherapy

Brachytherapy as part of a management protocol is used for a variety of genitourinary malignancies—most commonly for prostate cancer, less commonly for penile and urethral cancer, and rarely for bladder cancer. Only prostate cancer will be discussed here.

**TABLE 6.2**  ABS recommendation summary for vaginal interstitial implant

| Interstitial vaginal brachytherapy | |
| --- | --- |
| Indication | Stage I–IVA with residual lesion >5 mm thick |
| Technique | Perineal template with vaginal cylinder for upper-third lesion |
| | Freehand or template-based implant for mid or lower-third lesion |
| Needles | Titanium or plastic needles to reduce artifacts |
| Implant guidance | USG or CT or MRI for needle placement |
| Planning | Image-based, volumetric. CT- or MRI-based planning |
| Dose | Gross disease 70–80 Gy<br>Uninvolved vagina 60 Gy<br>Pelvis/inguinal 45–50 Gy<br>OAR D2cc < 70 Gy |

*Note:* OAR, organs at risk; USG, ultrasonography.

**TABLE 6.3**  Different radioisotopes for prostate brachytherapy

| Type of implant | Radioisotope | Half-life | Energy (MeV) | Dose as monotherapy (Gy) | Dose with EBRT (Gy) | |
| --- | --- | --- | --- | --- | --- | --- |
| Temporary | $^{192}$Ir | 73.8 days | 0.38 (average) | 38 | 45–0.4 | |
| | $^{137}$Cs | 30 years | 0.662 | 110–120 | | |
| Permanent | $^{125}$I | 59.4 days | 0.028 | 140–160 | 108–110 | EBRT dose |
| | $^{103}$Pd | 17 days | 0.021 | 110–125 | 90–100 | 41.4–50.4 Gy |

*Note:* EBRT, external beam radiotherapy.

## Brachytherapy in Prostate Cancer

Brachytherapy has long been a cornerstone of managing prostatic cancer. Used either as monotherapy or as a boost to pelvic EBRT, it has provided excellent long-term outcomes. Like cervical cancer, as discussed previously, brachytherapy to the prostate can also be delivered by the HDR or LDR technique. Essentially, the implants are temporary. Most prostate brachytherapy, however, is performed using a brachytherapy seed implant. Table 6.3 shows radioisotopes and their usage in prostate brachytherapy.

*Different Brachytherapy Techniques.*  The different brachytherapy techniques can be enumerated as follows: (a) preplanned transperineal template–based implants, and (b) image-guided intraoperative real-time implants. As a general rule, imaging should be mandatory during prostate implanting whether employing permanent seed or HDR needles. Trans-rectal ultrasound (TRUS) guidance is used most of the time. Real-time TRUS image-guided brachytherapy has the ability to modify the needle or seed position in real time.

*Indications.* An LDR permanent seed implant is indicated as a form of monotherapy under the following conditions:

1. Life expectancy of at least 10 years
2. Localized low-risk prostatic adenocarcinoma:
   a. T1c through T2a, and
   b. Prostate-specific antigen (PSA) less than or equal to 10 ng/mL, and
   c. Gleason score less than or equal to 6
3. Absence of extracapsular invasion
4. International patient symptom score (IPSS) of 0 through 8
5. Prostate volume less than 40 cc to 50 cc
6. Intermediate-risk group, albeit with caution:
   a. T2b through T2c, or
   b. PSA 10 ng/mL to 20 ng/mL, or
   c. Gleason score of 7 (3+4)

Different societies have different recommendations, as summarized in Table 6.4.

HDR brachytherapy is indicated as a form of monotherapy for both low- and intermediate-risk disease. The data supporting HDR monotherapy are scarce at present but promising (33,34). The prescribed dose is 38 Gy in four fractions; each fraction delivering a dose of 9.5 Gy. In their study Zamboglou et al (34) from Germany treated 718 patients with 8-year biochemical control and a metastasis-free survival rate of 90% and 97%, respectively, using HDR brachytherapy alone. Patients received 38 Gy in four fractions in either one or two implants or 34.5 Gy in three single-fraction implants.

*LDR/HDR as a Boost.* Both LDR and HDR brachytherapy can be used to boost the dose to the prostate after EBRT to the pelvis of 41.4 Gy to 50.4 Gy. Hormonal manipulation with recommended agents can also be employed when indicated. Primary EBRT or neoadjuvant hormone therapy helps to shrink a large prostate gland, making it more convenient to place an implant. Both intermediate- and high-risk patients can be treated with a brachytherapy boost. However, the involvement of the seminal vesicles should be judged cautiously. Seminal vesicles receiving an implant should be treated with EBRT and covered within the implant volume.

**TABLE 6.4** Indications for prostate permanent seed implant

| Criteria | Indicated | Relative |
| --- | --- | --- |
| Life expectancy (year) | 10 | — |
| Stage | T1c–T2a | |
| PSA (ng/mL) | <10 | 10–20 |
| GS | 3–6 | 7 (3 + 4) |
| Extracapsular spread | None | Minimum |
| Prostate volume | <40 | 40–60 |
| IPSS | 0–8 | 9–19 |

*Note:* GS, Gleason score; IPSS, International patient symptom score; PSA, prostate-specific antigen.

1. Intermediate-risk group:
   a. T2b through T2c, or
   b. PSA 10 ng/mL to 20 ng/mL, or
   c. Gleason score of 7 (3+4)
2. High-risk group:
   a. T3a, or
   b. Gleason score of 8 through 10, or
   c. PSA greater than 20 ng/mL

***Contraindications to Permanent Seed Implants.*** The absolute contraindications to permanent seed implants include the following:

1. Limited life expectancy
2. Metastatic disease
3. Pubic interference
4. Absence of the rectum
5. Large transurethral resection of prostate (TURP) defect

The relative contraindications include:

1. Recent TURP
2. Inflammatory bowel disease
3. Prior pelvic radiotherapy
4. Coagulation disorder
5. Large prostate greater than 60 cc
6. Large median lobe
7. IPSS greater than 20 (35,36)

**TABLE 6.5**  Reported outcomes with brachytherapy in selected series

| Author | Year | Patient number | Monotherapy or combination | Median follow-up (years) | Maximum follow-up (years) | Biochemical failure-free survival (%) | Overall survival (%) |
|---|---|---|---|---|---|---|---|
| Potters (37) | 2008 | 1449 | Both | 7 | 12 | 81 | 81 |
| Sylvester (38) | 2011 | 215 | Monotherapy | 11.7 | 18.4 | 80.4 | 37.1 |
| Zelefsky (39) | 2012 | 1466 | Both | 4 | 13 | 80–98 | — |
| Vargas (40) | 2013 | 304 | Both | 10.3 | 14 | 78–98 | 62–83 |
| Buckstein (41) | 2013 | 131 | Both | 11.5 | — | 90.1 | — |
| Morris (42) | 2013 | 1006 | Monotherapy | 7.5 | >10 | 94.1 | 83.5 |
| Morris (43) (ASCENDE-RT) | 2015 | 400 | Combination | 6.5 | >9 | 83 | — |

*Note:* ASCENDE-RT, Androgen Suppression Combined With Elective Nodal and Dose Escalated Radiation Therapy.

*Source:* Adapted from References 37, 38, 39, 40, 41, 42, 43.

***Postimplant Dosimetry.*** Postimplant dosimetry is as important as the implant itself and is vital to the quality assurance aspect of both HDR and LDR brachytherapy to the prostate. The availability of computer- based software and high-quality imaging has made this part of treatment easy. The following are the ABS recommendations, for dosimetric reporting purposes, for prostate implants (35):

- Prostate: D90 (Gy and percent)
- V100 and V150 (in percent)
- Urethra: UV150 (in volume)
- UV5, UV30 (in percent)
- Rectum: RV100 (in volume)

Results with prostate brachytherapy have been excellent at experienced centers over the years when treated alone or in combination with EBRT (Table 6.5) (37–43). The recently published early data of the Androgen Suppression Combined With Elective Nodal and Dose Escalated Radiation Therapy (ASCENDE-RT) trial look promising for intermediate- and high-risk patients treated with a brachytherapy boost after initial pelvic EBRT (43). The biochemical relapse-free survival after 9 years for the combined group was 83%, which is significantly better than the EBRT-boost arm (83% vs. 63%).

Overall, the results with brachytherapy for early-stage prostate cancer are excellent. However, even with such consistent results over a long period of time, the trend toward brachytherapy is decreasing, which is of concern (44).

## Brachytherapy for Breast Cancer

Needless to say, revolutionary changes in brachytherapy have occurred in breast cancer, with versatile applicators and treatment protocols. A full array of techniques, including interstitial implant, intracavitary application, intraoperative application, boost treatment, radical treatment, and different applicators, have made this an interesting domain for brachytherapy advocates.

## Types of Breast Brachytherapy

### Depending on Time of Application

1. Perioperative brachytherapy boost: Brachytherapy catheters are implanted during the surgical resection itself (45). Treatment is delivered within a few days.
2. Postoperative implant: Catheters or applicators are implanted after surgery, within weeks to months depending on the protocol.
3. Intraoperative radiotherapy (IORT): Brachytherapy applicator insertion and treatment are both done during the surgical resection itself while the wound is still open.

### Depending on Technique

1. Template-based IBT
2. Freehand IBT
3. Intracavitary balloon-based brachytherapy
4. Intraoperative applicator-based brachytherapy

### Depending on Fractionation and Schedule

1. Brachytherapy as a boost to the cavity
2. Accelerated partial breast irradiation (APBI)

### Brachytherapy Applicators

1. Interstitial needle and plastic catheters
2. Balloon-based applicators:
   a. Single lumen: MammoSite
   b. Multilumen: SAVI, Contura
3. Intraoperative applicators:
   a. Harrison-Anderson-Mick (HAM) applicator
   b. Modified HAM applicator
   c. CT-HDR multilumen balloon catheter

Special mention must be made that a majority of IORT techniques do not use brachytherapy sources. The sources of radiation in the ELIOT and the TARGIT studies were 6-MV linear accelerators for electron use and 50-kV

**TABLE 6.6**  Selected studies of brachytherapy boost

| Author | Year | Total number | Number of brachytherapy boosts | Other modality for boost | Median follow-up (years) | Cosmesis (good to excellent) % | Local recurrence |
|---|---|---|---|---|---|---|---|
| Perez (80) | 1996 | 701 | 129 | Electron | 5.6 | No difference | No difference |
| Resch (81) | 2002 | 410 | 410 | None | 8.7 (mean) | 38 | LR = 3.9% |
| Polgár (82) | 2002 | 207 | 52 | Electron | 5.3 | 88.5 | No difference |
| Budrukkar (83) | 2007 | 1022 | 536 (LDR + HDR) | Electron | 3.5 | Similar | Similar |
| Sharma (45) | 2013 | 100 | 100 | None | 4.5 | 87% | 100% |
| Gitt (84) | 2016 | 107 | 107 | None | 1.9 | | |
| Hennequin (85) | 1999 | 106 | 106 | None | 3.6 | 63 | 5.8 |
| Neumanova (86) | 2007 | 215 | 215 | None | 5.8 | 73 | 1.5 |

*Note:* HDR, high dose rate; LDR, low dose rate.

*Source:* Adapted from References 45, 80, 81, 82, 83, 84, 85, 86.

x-rays. For the same reason, electronic brachytherapy is not covered in this discussion.

## Indications for Breast Brachytherapy

Even before APBI came into vogue, breast brachytherapy was routinely performed to boost the tumor cavity after breast-conserving surgery (BCT) (Table 6.6). Traditionally, this was done in conjunction with EBRT to the whole breast. Presently, this can be divided into three major indications:

1. Boost to the tumor cavity as part of standard BCT
2. APBI as the sole modality of treatment
3. Recurrent tumor treatment

## What to Treat?

Both interstitial and intracavitary techniques usually treat the same target, the lumpectomy cavity. The ASTRO in 2009, in its recommendation related to APBI, advised targeting 1 cm and not more than 2 cm around the cavity for treatment (46). This is also true for brachytherapy when used as a boost. In 2001 the ABS recommended targeting a 2-cm margin around the cavity using at least two planes of catheter insertion, with the exception of a very small or large cavity, where a single plane or more than two planes can be used (47). Recently, the GEC-ESTRO has also published guidelines to treat lumpectomy cavities for boost and APBI purposes with multicatheter IBT after closed and open cavity resections (48,49). This is important, considering the adoption of more closed-cavity surgical techniques during BCS. As a standard, the resection cavity along with a 1-cm to 2-cm margin should be treated, keeping the skin dose within tolerance limits for adequate cosmesis and to avoid skin and fat necrosis. This applies to both the boost and the APBI techniques.

## Brachytherapy as a Boost to the Tumor Cavity

Patients who are young or have close, positive, or unknown cavity resection margins; a deep-seated tumor along with large breasts; an irregular cavity; or extensive intraductal components will benefit the most from a boost with a multicatheter brachytherapy implant.

A brachytherapy boost to the tumor cavity is performed prior to or 2 to 3 weeks after the completion of EBRT. Perioperatively implanting catheters and then delivering a boost dose before EBRT leads to a second surgical trauma to the patient (45). When such treatment is given after EBRT, the brachytherapy boost is usually delivered 2 to 3 weeks after EBRT is completed.

The boost dose is 10 Gy to 16 Gy in two to four fractions with the HDR technique. Usually, two fractions at 6-hour intervals are delivered per day. Good cosmetic outcomes and local control are reported in high-risk patients receiving PDR brachytherapy with 20-Gy doses to the cavity (50). This study documented an 87% rate of good-to-excellent cosmesis with only 1.5% local recurrence. However, the reported follow-up period was short.

Of 84 patients treated with a single-fraction HDR boost of 7 Gy in combination with EBRT, all showed excellent cosmetic outcomes, and only one showed local recurrence (51). In a large cohort of patients receiving brachytherapy as a boost after BCS, Budrukkar et al reported similar local control and cosmesis; 536 patients received brachytherapy with LDR or HDR, and 486 patients received an EBRT boost with electrons. However, the authors have reported more late sequelae with the HDR boost compared to other modalities. Overall, there is no difference in oncologic and cosmetic outcome after a brachytherapy boost.

## Brachytherapy in Accelerated Partial Breast Irradiation

The largest area of brachytherapy use for breast cancer has revolved around APBI for the last decade. Because the majority of tumor recurrences are seen within close proximity to the index tumor, the need for whole-breast irradiation has been questioned (52,53). Multiple large controlled studies have effectively proven the safety and efficacy of APBI for a closely selected group of patients with favorable early breast cancer.

### *Advantages of Accelerated Partial Breast Irradiation*
1. Reduced volume of radiation, thus reducing normal tissue toxicity
2. Reduced duration of treatment, which is more acceptable to patients
3. Economic benefits, such as a reduced cost of care and insurance claims, a reduced load on treatment machines, etc

### *Techniques*
1. Multicatheter IBT
2. Balloon-based brachytherapy
   a. Single lumen: MammoSite
   b. Multilumen: Contura, SAVI
3. Intraoperative radiotherapy
   a. Intraoperative electron (ELIOT)
   b. Intraoperative kV x-ray (TARGIT)
   c. CT-HDR-IORT (54)
4. EBRT with three-dimensional CRT or IMRT
5. Noninvasive brachytherapy techniques
   a. Gammapod
   b. XOFT electronic breast brachytherapy

### *Dose of Accelerated Partial Breast Irradiation*
1. Brachytherapy: 34 Gy in 10 fractions, delivered in 2 fractions per day of 3.4 Gy each at 6-hour intervals. The treatment is effectively complete in 1 week.
2. Alternative schedule: 40 Gy in 8 fractions, delivered in 2 fractions per day at 6-hour intervals.

***Patient Selection for Accelerated Partial Breast Irradiation.*** The most crucial factor to successful APBI is appropriate patient selection. In general, a favorable early-stage breast cancer patient who has undergone BCS and has a detailed histopathology report available should be evaluated for APBI. At least four different collaborative groups have formulated patient selection criteria for successful APBI programs (46,55–57). Table 6.7 summarizes these criteria.

A few randomized trials with APBI have already been completed, and some are currently ongoing. Tables 6.8 and 6.9 summarize the results of these studies. All these studies have conclusively established excellent outcomes with APBI in select groups of patients.

**TABLE 6.7**  Consensus statement for APBI patient-selection criteria

| Factor | ASTRO consensus statement categories (48) | | | GEC-ESTRO consensus statement categories (62) | | | ASBS (63) | | ABS 2013 (64) |
| --- | --- | --- | --- | --- | --- | --- | --- | --- | --- |
| | Suitable | Cautionary | Unsuitable | Low-risk: good candidate | Intermediate-risk: possible candidate | High-risk: contraindicated | Suitable | Unsuitable | Acceptable |
| Age (yrs) | ≥60 | 50–59 | <50 | >50 | >40–50 | ≤40 | ≥45 if invasive carcinoma, ≥50 if DCIS | <45 if invasive carcinoma or LCIS, <50 if DCIS | ≥50 |
| *BRCA1/2* mutation | Not present | n/a | Present | | | | | | |
| Size | ≤2 cm | 2.1–3.0 cm | >3.0 cm | ≤3 cm | ≤3 cm | >3 cm | ≤3 cm | | ≤3 cm |
| T stage | T1 | T0 (DCIS) and T2 | T3/T4 | T1/T2 | T1/T2 | T2 (>3 cm), T3, T4 | Tis (≤3 cm), T1, T2 (≤3 cm) | Tis (>3 cm), T2 (>3 cm), T3–T4 | T1, T2 (≤3 cm) |
| Multicentric | Unicentric | | Present | Unicentric | | Multicentric | | | |
| Multifocal | Clinically unifocal | Clinically unifocal | >3 cm | Unifocal | Multifocal (limited to within 2 cm of the index lesion) | Multifocal (>2 cm from the index lesion) | | | |
| Grade | Any | n/a | n/a | Any | n/a | | | | |
| LVSI | No | Limited | Extensive | No | No | Present | | | |
| ER | Positive | Negative | n/a | Any | n/a | n/a | | | |
| N stage | Negative | n/a | Positive | Negative | pN1mic–N1a | pNx; ≥pN2a (≥4LN+) | N0 | ≥N1 | N0 |

**TABLE 6.7** (*Continued*)

| Factor | ASTRO consensus statement categories (48) | | | GEC-ESTRO consensus statement categories (62) | | | ASBS (63) | | ABS 2013 (64) |
| | Suitable | Cautionary | Unsuitable | Low-risk: good candidate | Intermediate-risk: possible candidate | High-risk: contraindicated | Suitable | Unsuitable | Acceptable |
| --- | --- | --- | --- | --- | --- | --- | --- | --- | --- |
| Nodal surgery | SLNB or ALND | n/a | None performed | SLNB or ALND | ALND (at least 6 LN examined) | | | | |
| Margins | Negative (≥2 mm) | Close (<2 mm) | Positive | Negative (≥2 mm) | Close (<2 mm) | Positive | Negative | Positive | |
| Histology | IDC and other favorable | DCIS ≤3 cm or ILC | DCIS >3 cm | IDC and other favorable histologies | IDC and other favorable histologies or ILC | | Invasive carcinoma or DCIS | | Invasive carcinoma |
| EIC | None | Present and tumor size ≤3 cm | Present and tumor size >3 cm | None | None | Present | | | |
| Associated LCIS | Allowed | n/a | n/a | Allowed | n/a | | | | |
| Neoadjuvant therapy | Not allowed | n/a | Used | No | No | Used | | | |
| Clinical M stage | | | | | | | | | M0 |
| General contraindications to RT | | | | | | | | | None |

*Note*: ALND, axillary lymph node dissection; DCIS, ductal carcinoma in situ; EIC, extensive intraductal carcinoma; IDC, invasive ductal carcinoma; ILC, invasive lobular carcinoma; LCIS, lobular carcinoma in situ; LVSI, lymphovascular space invasion; RT, radiation therapy; SNLB, sentinel lymph node biopsy.

*Source:* Adapted from References 46, 55, 56, 57.

**TABLE 6.8** Completed randomized trials comparing brachytherapy APBI vs. whole-breast irradiation

| Trial name | Location | Patient inclusion criteria | Surgery | Control arm: WBI |
|---|---|---|---|---|
| National Institute of Oncology (65) | Hungary | IDC, pT1, cN0, pN0–1mic, grade ≤ 2, unifocal, no EIC; after year 2001 > 40 yrs | Wide excision, negative margins | 42–50 Gy/21–25 fx |
| TARGIT-A (66) | Multicountry | ≥45 yrs, IDC, T1 and small T2, N0/1, unifocal, no EIC, cN0 | Wide local excision | 40–56 Gy ± 10–16-[...] boost |
| ELIOT (69) | Italy | >45 yrs, tumor < 2.5 cm | Quadrantectomy and ALND or SLNB | 50 Gy/25 fx + 10-Gy[...] boost |
| GEC-ESTRO (67) | Europe | ≥40 yrs, stage 0 (DCIS)-II, no LVSI, no hemangiosis, low- to intermediate-grade DCIS, unifocal, unicentric, no EIC, tumors ≤ 3 cm, ≤ pN1mic | BCS with ≥ 2-mm margins (≥5 mm if DCIS or ILC), ALND or SLNB (optional with DCIS) | 50–50.4 Gy/25–28 fx + 10 Gy/5 fx tum[...] bed boost |

*Note:* APBI, accelerated partial breast irradiation; ALND, axillary lymph node dissection; EIC, extensive intraductal carcinoma; DCIS, ductal carcinoma in situ; HDR, high dose rate; IBTR, ipsilateral breast tumor recurrence; IDC, invasive ductal carcinoma; IORT, intraoperative radiotherapy; LVSI, lymphovascular space invasion; MIB, minimally invasive biopsy; WBI, whole-breast irradiation.

*Source:* Adapted from References 87, 88, 89, 90.

***Brachytherapy in Recurrent Disease.*** Although the standard treatment of a localized recurrence after initial BCT is a mastectomy, brachytherapy can also be helpful. In a small series of 36 patients with ipsilateral localized breast recurrence, Guix et al found a 10-year local control rate of 90% after a repeat wide excision and HDR brachytherapy with 30 Gy in 12 fractions (58).

## Brachytherapy for Esophageal Cancers

Esophageal cancer can be difficult to treat, and its incidence is rising due to an increase in lower-esophageal adenocarcinoma. The need for brachytherapy in

| arm: APBI | Median follow-up | Accrual | Local failure | Notable features | Toxicity |
|---|---|---|---|---|---|
| HDR Gy/7 fx or :trons 50 Gy/ 25 fx | 10 yrs | 258 | 10-yr IBTR: APBI 5.9% vs 5.1% WBI ($P=.50$) | | Excellent–good cosmesis: 81% APBI vs. 63% WBI ($P=.009$) |
| V x-rays: Gy at n/1 fx | Not reported | 2,232 | 5-yr IBTR: 3.3% IORT vs 1.3% WBI ($P=.042$) | If final path review: ILC, EIC, or adverse criterion per local center, then WBI added to APBI | Grade 3–4 skin complications 6 mo after randomization: 0.2% vs. 0.8, IORT vs WBI |
| aoperative :trons: 21 Gy 0% IDL/1 fx | 5.8 yrs | 1,305 | 5-yr IBTR 4.4% IORT vs. 0.4% WBI ($P=.0001$) 5-yr IBTR in same quadrant as primary: 2.5% IORT vs. 0.4% WBI ($P=.0003$) | | Erythema, dryness, hyperpigmentation, and pruritis were all more prevalent with WBI compared to IORT. Fat necrosis 14.6% IORT vs. 6.8% WBI. |
| rstitial HDR iy/8 fx or R 30.3 Gy/7 fx DR 50 Gy at 0.8 Gy/hr | 6.6 years | 1184 | 1.44% with APBI vs. 0.92% with WBI | Multicatheter interstitial brachytherapy noninferior to WBI | Grade 2–3 late skin toxicity 3.2% vs. 5.7 %, Grade 2–3 subcutaneous late toxicity 7.6% vs. 6.3% with APBI vs. WBI. No severe fibrosis at 5 yrs with APBI. No grade 4 late effects. |

today's treatment protocols is mostly palliative. Historically, however, esophageal cancers were treated with endoluminal brachytherapy in combination with EBRT and/or chemotherapy.

Esophageal brachytherapy is performed by introducing a nasogastric tube or a special esophageal brachytherapy applicator. The tumor along with a 2-cm to 5-cm proximal and distal margin is treated. The dose is usually prescribed at 1 cm from the center of the source.

**TABLE 6.9** Ongoing randomized trial of brachytherapy APBI vs. whole-breast irradiation

| Trial name | Location | Patient inclusion criteria | Surgery | Control arm: WBI | Test arm: APBI | Date opened/ closed | Target accrual | Primary end point | Secondary end points |
|---|---|---|---|---|---|---|---|---|---|
| NSABP B-39/ RTOG 0413 (68) | United States | ≥18 yrs, stage 0 (DCIS), I or II, tumor ≤ 3 cm, unifocal, unicentric, ≤3 positive LNs (closed to low risk in 2007) | BCS with negative margins (at ink); ALND (≥6 LN sampled if LN+) or SLNB for invasive carcinoma | 50–50.4 Gy/ 25–28 fx ±10–16.2 Gy/ 5–9 fx tumor bed boost | 3D-CRT 38.5 Gy/10 fx *or* multicatheter brachytherapy 34 Gy/10 fx *or* intracavitary brachytherapy 34 Gy/10 fx | 2005/2013 | 4,300 | IBTR | OS, RFS, DMFS, toxicity, cosmesis (MD- and pt-reported), QOL |

*Note:* ALND, axillary lymph node dissection; APBI, accelerated partial breast irradiation; BCS, breast-conserving surgery; CRT, chemoradiotherapy; DFMS, distant metastasis free survival; EIC, extensive intraductal carcinoma; IBTR, ipsilateral breast tumor recurrence; LN, lymph node; NSABP, National Surgical Adjuvant Breast and Bowel Project; OS, overall survival; ROTG, Radiation Therapy Oncology Group; RFS, recurrence-free survival; QOL, quality of life; SNLB, sentinel lymph node biopsy; WBI, whole-breast irradiation.

*Source:* Adapted from Shah NM, Tenenholz T, Arthur D, et al. MammoSite and interstitial brachytherapy for accelerated partial breast irradiation: factors that affect toxicity and cosmesis. *Cancer.* 2004;101(4):727–734.

## Indications of Esophageal Brachytherapy

*As Part of Radical Treatment.* Radical brachytherapy for very superficial mucosal tumors can be treated with radical brachytherapy alone. Maingon et al reported on 13 patients who were treated with radical HDR brachytherapy alone for superficial T1 tumors (59). The average brachytherapy dose was 54 ± 10 Gy. After a mean follow-up of 31 months (24–96), the arm receiving HDR alone had an OS of 43%.

The vast majority of radical brachytherapy treatments are usually to escalate the dose of EBRT, with or without chemotherapy. When used before EBRT, brachytherapy can rapidly relieve dysphagia. The ABS recommends a dose of 10 Gy in two fractions after 50 Gy of EBRT (60). Different studies employing a brachytherapy boost with EBRT have used a wide range of dose fractions from 3 Gy to 8 Gy, with the total dose varying from 12 Gy to 18 Gy. The outcomes of treatment vary widely (61–65). One concern with HDR brachytherapy is the development of a fistula or a stricture due to an inhomogeneous dose distribution to the mucosal surface (66). However, this risk can be significantly mitigated by using applicators that are at least 6 mm, as well as centered applicators.

*Palliative Brachytherapy.* The vast majority of esophageal brachytherapy treatments are used for symptom palliation. Endoluminal brachytherapy is very effective at rapidly controlling and relieving symptoms of dysphagia. In a large prospective International Atomic Energy Agency (IAEA) multicenter randomized trial involving 219 patients, a combination of EBRT and brachytherapy showed much greater symptom relief. Dysphagia, odynophagia, chest pain, and regurgitation were significantly improved (67). Other studies have documented similar benefits with brachytherapy when used for palliative purposes (68–71).

### Brachytherapy for Sarcomas

Soft tissue sarcomas are another important area employing widespread brachytherapy use, usually in the extremities, where an implant is technically feasible. A temporary interstitial implant with a flexible catheter is the standard of care. This treatment is delivered using the LDR or HDR technique, although recently a permanent mesh implant for sarcomas of the retroperitoneum, pelvis, and chest has been reported (72).

### Indications for Brachytherapy

1. As monotherapy: Brachytherapy can be used for patients with a high-grade extremity or trunk sarcoma with clear postoperative margins (73).
2. As a combination with EBRT: The ABS recommends brachytherapy for recurrent sarcomas without a history of prior radiation (73). Overall, the

indications can be summarized as: a high-grade tumor, close margins, a deep-seated tumor greater than 5 cm in size, and a recurrent sarcoma.

3. In a select group of pediatric patients to avoid radiation to critical structures (74).

## Techniques

The available techniques for sarcoma brachytherapy are:

1. LDR interstitial implant
2. HDR interstitial implant
3. Permanent seed/mesh implant
4. Surface mold
5. Intraoperative brachytherapy boost

Catheters may be implanted in parallel or perpendicular to the surgical incision depending on the location of the tumor and the neurovascular and lymphatic relationship. The target for brachytherapy is usually the surgical bed plus a 2-cm margin in craniocaudal directions and a 1-cm to 2-cm margin in radial directions (73,75). The scar and drain sites are not included in the brachytherapy target volume. CT-based volumetric planning is recommended.

Doses from the recent ABS guidelines are summarized in Table 6.10. With LDR or PDR, a dose rate of 0.45 Gy to 0.50 Gy per hour is used. The HDR technique typically delivers two fractions daily at 6-hour intervals, with 2 Gy to 4 Gy per fraction.

The results of brachytherapy for primary soft tissue sarcomas are variable, and local control rates were reported to be 50% to 100% according to different studies (76–78). However, these studies were nonrandomized. In another nonrandomized comparison between IMRT and brachytherapy, Alektiar et al have documented inferior local control with LDR brachytherapy (92% vs. 81%). However, the median dose with postoperative IMRT was 63 Gy, which was more than the median brachytherapy dose of 45 Gy.

Pediatric patients need special mention. EBRT often leads to long-term morbidity and limb deformity, including fibrosis. Careful brachytherapy can provide excellent cosmetic and functional outcomes (74).

### Endobronchial Brachytherapy

The concept of endobronchial brachytherapy (EBBT) is similar to esophageal brachytherapy, since the bronchus is essentially a luminal structure like the esophagus. However, endobronchial brachytherapy is technically much more challenging.

**TABLE 6.10**  Brachytherapy dose for sarcomas

| Brachytherapy alone | | Brachytherapy and EBRT combination | |
| --- | --- | --- | --- |
| Brachytherapy technique | Dose (Gy) | EBRT dose (Gy) | Brachytherapy dose (Gy) |
| LDR | 45–50 | 45–50 | 15–25 |
| HDR | 30–54 | 45–50 | 12–20 |
| PDR | 45–50 | 45–50 | 15–25 |

*Note:* EBRT, external beam radiation therapy.

## Indications

1. EBBT can be used both in radical treatment and for the palliation of symptoms from endobronchial growth. When used for radical treatment, EBBT can be used as the sole modality or in combination with EBRT to boost the residual endobronchial or mucosal lesion.
2. More commonly, the palliation of cough, obstruction, dyspnea, hemoptysis, and pain are achieved with EBBT.
3. Patients with significant endobronchial growth who are not candidates for surgery or EBRT may benefit from EBBT.

## Technique and Dose Solution

Commonly, HDR brachytherapy is the technique conducted. The endobronchial tumor along with a 1-cm to 2-cm longitudinal margin is treated to a depth of 1 cm. The dose can be delivered once a week or in a single fraction for palliation. The ABS recommends the following dose fractionation scheme for EBBT after radical EBRT: 10 Gy to 15 Gy in two to three fractions of HDR treatment. For palliation, a dose rate of 5 Gy per fraction to 15 Gy per fraction can be used:

- 30 Gy in six fractions
- 24 Gy in four fractions
- 22.5 Gy in three fractions
- 14.2 to 20 Gy in two fractions
- 15 Gy in one fraction
- 10 Gy in one fraction

Skowronek et al, in a large retrospective series of 648 patients treated with either 22.5 Gy in three weekly fractions of 7.5 Gy each or a single fraction of 10 Gy, have demonstrated similar symptom palliation with either schedule (79).

## CONCLUSIONS

Brachytherapy has its own role in the management of many malignancies at some part of the disease. The role of brachytherapy in other malignancies, such as head and neck cancers, anorectal malignancies, biliary malignancies, ocular malignancies, brain tumors, and metastatic disease, are also established. Technical expertise is central to the success of any brachytherapy program. The highly conformal dose distribution with its high dose gradient is definitely not achievable with other treatment modalities, but it does require attention to detail in terms of quality and safety. The appropriate selection of patients and techniques is also very important for achieving success.

## References


1. Belot, J. Resolvent action on epithelial neoplasm. In:. *Radiotherapy in Skin Disease,* trans. WD Butcher. London: Rebman; 1905:380.

2. Delregato JA, Cox JD. Transvaginal roentgen therapy in the conservative management of carcinoma in situ of the uterine cervix. *Radiology.* 1965;84:1090–1095.

3. Viswanathan AN. Uterine cervix. In: Halperin EC, Wazer DE, Perez CA, Brady LW et al, eds. *Principles and Practice of Radiation Oncology.* Philadelphia: Lippincott Williams and Wilkins; 2013:1355–1425.

4. Grigsby PW, Perez CA. Radiotherapy alone for medically inoperable carcinoma of the cervix: stage IA and carcinoma in situ. *Int J Radiat Oncol Biol Phys.* 1991;21(2):375–378.

5. Ogino I, Kitamura T, Okajima H, et al. High-dose-rate intracavitary brachytherapy in the management of cervical and vaginal intraepithelial neoplasia. *Int J Radiat Oncol Biol Phys.* 1998;40(4):881–887.

6. Kim YB, Kim YT, Cho NH, et al. High-dose-rate intracavitary radiotherapy in the management of cervical intraepithelial neoplasia 3 and carcinoma in situ presenting with poor histologic factors after undergoing excisional procedures. *Int J Radiat Oncol Biol Phys.* 2012;84(1):e19-e22. doi:10.1016/j.ijrobp.2012.02.045

7. Sharma DN, Rath GK, Kumar S, et al. Postoperative radiotherapy following inadvertent simple hysterectomy versus radical hysterectomy for cervical carcinoma. *Asian Pac J Cancer Prev.* 2011;12(6):1537–1541.

8. Andras EJ, Fletcher GH, Rutledge F. Radiotherapy of carcinoma of the cervix following simple hysterectomy. *Am J Obstet Gynecol.* 1973;115(5):647–655.

9. Kolstad P. Follow-up study of 232 patients with stage Ia1 and 411 patients with stage Ia2 squamous cell carcinoma of the cervix (microinvasive carcinoma). *Gynecol Oncol.* 1989;33(3):265–272.

10. Hamberger AD, Fletcher GH, Wharton JT. Results of treatment of early stage I carcinoma of the uterine cervix with intracavitary radium alone. *Cancer.* 1978;41(3):980–985.

11. Nag S, Chao C, Erickson B, et al. The American Brachytherapy Society recommendations for low-dose-rate brachytherapy for carcinoma of the cervix. *Int J Radiat Oncol Biol Phys.* 2002;52(1):33–48.

12. Small W Jr, Beriwal S, Demanes DJ, et al. American Brachytherapy Society consensus guidelines for adjuvant vaginal cuff brachytherapy after hysterectomy. *Brachytherapy.* 2012;11(1):58–67. doi:10.1016/j.brachy.2011.08.005

13. Gerbaulet A, Maher M, Haie-Meder C, et al. Cancer of the cervix (K. Morita): the Paris method. In: Vahrson HV, ed. *Radiation Oncology of Gynecological Cancers*. New York: Springer; 1997:198–205.

14. Gerbaulet AL, Kunkler IH, Kerr GR, et al. Combined radiotherapy and surgery: local control and complications in early carcinoma of the uterine cervix: the Villejuif experience, 1975–84. *Radioth Oncol*. 1992;23(2):66–73.

15. Landoni F, Maneo A, Colombo A, et al. Randomised study of radical surgery versus radiotherapy for stage Ib-IIa cervical cancer. *Lancet*. 1997;350(9077):535–540.

16. Keys HM, Bundy BN, Stehman FB, et al. Cisplatin, radiation, and adjuvant hysterectomy compared with radiation and adjuvant hysterectomy for bulky stage IB cervical carcinoma. *N Engl J Med*. 1999;340:1154–1161.

17. Rose PG, Ali S, Watkins E, et al. Long-term follow-up of a randomized trial comparing concurrent single agent cisplatin, cisplatin-based combination chemotherapy, or hydroxyurea during pelvic irradiation for locally advanced cervical cancer: a Gynecologic Oncology Group Study. *J Clin Oncol*. 2007;25(19):2804–2810.

18. Eifel PJ, Winter K, Morris M, et al. Pelvic irradiation with concurrent chemotherapy versus pelvic and para-aortic irradiation for high-risk cervical cancer: an update of radiation therapy oncology group trial (RTOG) 90–01. *J Clin Oncol*. 2004;22(5):872–880.

19. Rose PG, Bundy BN, Watkins EB, et al. Concurrent cisplatin-based radiotherapy and chemotherapy for locally advanced cervical cancer. *N Engl J Med*. 1999;340(15): 1144–1153.

20. Sedlis A, Bundy BN, Rotman MZ, et al. A randomized trial of pelvic radiation therapy versus no further therapy in selected patients with stage IB carcinoma of the cervix after radical hysterectomy and pelvic lymphadenectomy: a Gynecologic Group Study. *Gynecol Oncol*. 1999;73(2):177–183.

21. Pötter R, Haie-Meder C, Van Limbergen E, et al. Recommendations from gynaecological (GYN) GEC ESTRO working group (II): concepts and terms in 3D image-based treatment planning in cervix cancer brachytherapy-3D dose volume parameters and aspects of 3D image-based anatomy, radiation physics, radiobiology. *Radiother Oncol*. 2006;78(1):67–77.

22. Sharma DN, Rath GK, Thulkar S, et al. High-dose rate interstitial brachytherapy using two weekly sessions of 10 Gy each for patients with locally advanced cervical carcinoma. *Brachytherapy*. 2011;10(3):242–248. doi:10.1016/j.brachy.2010.09.001

23. Murakami N, Kato T, Miyamoto Y, et al. Salvage high-dose-rate interstitial brachytherapy for pelvic recurrent cervical carcinoma after hysterectomy. *Anticancer Res*. 2016; 36(5):2413–2421.

24. Grigsby PW, Portelance L, Williamson JF. High dose ratio (HDR) cervical ring applicator to control bleeding from cervical carcinoma. *Int J Gynecol Cancer*. 2002;12(1):18–21.

25. Creutzberg CL, van Putten WL, Koper PC, et al. Surgery and postoperative radiotherapy versus surgery alone for patients with stage-1 endometrial carcinoma: multicentre randomised trial. PORTEC Study Group. Postoperative Radiation Therapy in Endometrial Carcinoma. *Lancet*. 2000;355(9213):1404–1411.

26. Keys HM, Roberts JA, Brunetto VL, et al. A phase III trial of surgery with or without adjunctive external pelvic radiation therapy in intermediate risk endometrial adenocarcinoma: a Gynecologic Oncology Group study. *Gynecol Oncol*. 2004;92(3):744–751.

27. Blake P, Swart AM, Otron J, et al. Adjuvant external beam radiotherapy in the treatment of endometrial cancer (MRC ASTEC and NCIC CTG EN.5 randomised trials): pooled trial results, systematic review, and meta-analysis. *Lancet*. 2009;373(9658): 137–146.

28. Sorbe B, Nordström B, Mäenpää J, et al. Intravaginal brachytherapy in FIGO stage I low-risk endometrial cancer: a controlled randomized study. *Int J Gynecol Cancer.* 2009;19(5):873–878.

29. Nout RA, Smit VT, Putter H, et al. PORTEC Study Group. Vaginal brachytherapy versus pelvic external beam radiotherapy for patients with endometrial cancer of high-intermediate risk (PORTEC–2): an open-label, non-inferiority, randomised trial. *Lancet.* 2010;375(9717):816–823.

30. Landrum LM, Nugent EK, Zuna RE, et al. Phase II trial of vaginal cuff brachytherapy followed by chemotherapy in early stage endometrial cancer patients with high-intermediate risk factors. *Gynecol Oncol.* 2014;132(1):50–54. doi:10.1016/j.ygyno.2013.11.005

31. McMeekin DS, Filiaci VL, Aghajanian C, et al. A randomized phase III trial of pelvic radiation therapy (PXRT) versus vaginal cuff brachytherapy followed by paclitaxel/carboplatin chemotherapy (VCB/C) in patients with high risk (HR), early stage endometrial cancer (EC): a Gynecologic Oncology Group trial. *Gynecol Oncol.* 2014;134(2):438.

32. Beriwal S, Demanes DJ, Erickson B, et al. American Brachytherapy Society consensus guidelines for interstitial brachytherapy for vaginal cancer. *Brachytherapy.* 2012;11(1):68–75. doi:10.1016/j.brachy.2011.06.008

33. Zamboglou N, Tselis N, Baltas D, et al. High–dose-rate interstitial brachytherapy as monotherapy for clinically localized prostate cancer: treatment evolution and mature results. *Int J Radiat Oncol Biol Phys.* 2013;85(3):672–678. doi:10.1016/j.ijrobp.2012.07.004

34. Sánchez-Gómez LM, Polo-deSantos M, Rodríguez-Melcón JI, et al. High-dose rate brachytherapy as monotherapy in prostate cancer: a systematic review of its safety and efficacy. *Actas Urol Esp.* 2016;pii:S0210-S4806(16)30101-30102. doi:10.1016/j.acuro.2016.06.001

35. Davis BJ, Horwitz EM, Lee WR, et al. American Brachytherapy Society consensus guidelines for transrectal ultrasound-guided permanent prostate brachytherapy. *Brachytherapy.* 2012;11(1):6–19. doi:10.1016/j.brachy.2011.07.005

36. Ash D, Flynn A, Battermann J, et al. ESTRO/EAU/EORTC recommendations on permanent seed implantation for localized prostate cancer. *Radiother Oncol.* 2000;57(3):315–321.

37. Potters L, Morgenstern C, Calugaru E, et al. 12-year outcomes following permanent prostate brachytherapy in patients with clinically localized prostate cancer. *J Urol.* 2008;179(suppl 5):S20-S24. doi:10.1016/j.juro.2008.03.133

38. Sylvester JE, Grimm PD, Wong J, et al. Fifteen-year biochemical relapse-free survival, cause-specific survival, and overall survival following I(125) prostate brachytherapy in clinically localized prostate cancer: Seattle experience. *Int J Radiat Oncol Biol Phys.* 2011;81(2):376–381. doi:10.1016/j.ijrobp.2010.05.042

39. Zelefsky MJ, Chou JF, Pei X, et al. Predicting biochemical tumor control after brachytherapy for clinically localized prostate cancer: the Memorial Sloan-Kettering Cancer Center experience. *Brachytherapy.* 2012;11(4):245–249. doi:10.1016/j.brachy.2011.08.003

40. Vargas C, Swartz D, Vashi A, et al. Long-term outcomes and prognostic factors in patients treated with intraoperatively planned prostate brachytherapy. *Brachytherapy.* 2013;12(2):120–125. doi:10.1016/j.brachy.2012.08.002

41. Buckstein M, Carpenter TJ, Stone NN, et al. Long-term outcomes and toxicity in patients treated with brachytherapy for prostate adenocarcinoma younger than 60 years of age at treatment with minimum 10 years of follow-up. *Urology.* 2013;81(2):364–368. doi:10.1016/j.urology.2012.08.112

42. Morris WJ, Keyes M, Spadinger I, et al. Population-based 10-year oncologic outcomes after low-dose-rate brachytherapy for low-risk and intermediate-risk prostate cancer. *Cancer.* 2013;119(8):1537–1546. doi:10.1002/cncr.27911

43. Morris WJ, Tyldesley S, Pai HH, et al. ASCENDE-RT: A multicenter, randomized trial of dose-escalated external beam radiation therapy (EBRT-B) versus low-dose-rate brachytherapy (LDR-B) for men with unfavorable-risk localized prostate cancer. *J Clin Oncol.* 2015;33(suppl 7):abstract 3.

44. Orio PF III, Nguyen PL, Buzurovic I, et al. The decreased use of brachytherapy boost for intermediate and high-risk prostate cancer despite evidence supporting its effectiveness. *Brachytherapy.* 2016;pii:S1538-S4721(16)30457-30453. doi: 0.1016/j.brachy.2016.05.001

45. Sharma DN, Deo SV, Rath GK, et al. Perioperative high-dose-rate interstitial brachytherapy boost for patients with early breast cancer. *Tumori.* 2013;99(5):604–610. doi:10.1700/1377.15310

46. Smith BD, Arthur DW, Buchholz TA, et al. Accelerated partial breast irradiation consensus statement from the American Society for Radiation Oncology (ASTRO). *Int J Radiat Oncol Biol Phys.* 2009;74(4):987–1001. doi:10.1016/j.ijrobp.2009.02.031

47. Nag S, Kuske RR, Vicini FA, et al. Brachytherapy in the treatment of breast cancer. *Oncology (Williston Park).* 2001;15(2):195–202, 205–207.

48. Strnad V, Hannoun-Levi JM, Guinot JL, et al. Recommendations from GEC ESTRO Breast Cancer Working Group (I): target definition and target delineation for accelerated or boost partial breast irradiation using multicatheter interstitial brachytherapy after breast conserving closed cavity surgery. *Radiother Oncol.* 2015;115(3):342–348. doi:10.1016/j.radonc.2015.06.010

49. Major T, Gutiérrez C, Guix B, et al. Recommendations from GEC ESTRO Breast Cancer Working Group (II): target definition and target delineation for accelerated or boost partial breast irradiation using multicatheter interstitial brachytherapy after breast conserving open cavity surgery. *Radiother Oncol.* 2016;118(1):199–204. doi:10.1016/j.radonc.2015.12.006

50. Fritz P, Berns C, Anton HW, et al. PDR brachytherapy with flexible implants for interstitial boost after breast-conserving surgery and external beam radiation therapy. *Radiother Oncol.* 1997;45(1):23–32.

51. Beato Tortajada I, Guinot Rodríguez JL, Arribas Alpuente L, et al. Single fraction boost with high dose rate interstitial brachytherapy in conservative treatment of breast carcinoma. *Clin Transl Oncol.* 2005;7(9):404–408.

52. Fisher B, Anderson S, Bryant J, et al. Twenty-year follow-up of a randomized trial comparing total mastectomy, lumpectomy, and lumpectomy plus irradiation for the treatment of invasive breast cancer. *N Engl J Med.* 2002;347(16):1233–1241.

53. Veronesi U, Marubini E, Mariani L, et al. Radiotherapy after breast-conserving surgery in small breast carcinoma: long-term results of a randomized trial. *Ann Oncol.* 2001;12(7):997–1003.

54. Showalter SL, Petroni G, Trifiletti DM, et al. A novel form of breast intraoperative radiation therapy with CT-guided high-dose-rate brachytherapy: results of a prospective phase 1 clinical trial. *Int J Radiat Oncol Biol Phys.* 2016;96(1):46–54. doi:10.1016/j.ijrobp.2016.04.035

55. Polgár C, Van Limbergen E, Pötter R, et al. Patient selection for accelerated partial-breast irradiation (APBI) after breast-conserving surgery: recommendations of the Groupe Europeen de Curietherapie-European Society for Therapeutic Radiology and Oncology (GEC-ESTRO) breast cancer working group based on clinical evidence (2009). *Radiother Oncol.* 2010;94(3):264–273.

56. Consensus statement for accelerated partial breast irradiation. American Society of Breast Surgeons. 2011. Accessed October 23, 2016. https://www.breastsurgeons.org/new_layout/about/statements/PDF_Statements/APBI.pdf

57. Shah C, Vicini F, Wazer DE, et al. American Brachytherapy Society guidelines for accelerated partial breast irradiation. 2012. *Brachytherapy.* 2013;12(4):267–277. doi:10.1016/j.brachy.2013.02.001

58. Guix B, Lejárcegui JA, Tello JI, et al. Exeresis and brachytherapy as salvage treatment for local recurrence after conservative treatment for breast cancer: results of a ten-year pilot study. *Int J Radiat Oncol Biol Phys.* 2010;78(3):804–810. doi:10.1016/j.ijrobp.2009.08.009

59. Maingon P, d'Hombres A, Truc G, et al. High dose rate brachytherapy for superficial cancer of the esophagus. *Int J Radiat Oncol Biol Phys.* 2000;46(1):71–76.

60. Gaspar LE, Nag S, Herskovic A, et al. American Brachytherapy Society (ABS) consensus guidelines for brachytherapy of esophageal cancer. Clinical Research Committee, American Brachytherapy Society, Philadelphia, PA. *Int J Radiat Oncol Biol Phys.* 1997;38(1):127–132.

61. Sur RK, Singh DP, Sharma SC, et al. Radiation therapy of esophageal cancer: role of high dose rate brachytherapy. *Int J Radiat Oncol Biol Phys.* 1992;22(5):1043–1046.

62. Gaspar LE, Winter K, Kocha WI, et al. A phase I/II study of external beam radiation, brachytherapy, and concurrent chemotherapy for patients with localized carcinoma of the esophagus (Radiation Therapy Oncology Group Study 9207): final report. *Cancer.* 2000;88(5):988–995.

63. Yin W. Radiotherapy of carcinoma of oesophagus in China. *Chin Med J.* 1997;110(4):289–293.

64. Ishikawa H, Sakurai H, Yamakawa M, et al. Clinical outcomes and prognostic factors for patients with early esophageal squamous cell carcinoma treated with definitive radiation therapy alone. *J Clin Gastroenterol.* 2005;39(6):495–500.

65. Yamada K, Murakami M, Okamoto Y, et al. Treatment results of chemoradiotherapy for clinical stage I (T1N0M0) esophageal carcinoma. *Int J Radiat Oncol Biol Phys.* 2006;64(4):1106–1111.

66. Kumar S, Dimri K, Khurana R, et al. A randomised trial of radiotherapy compared with cisplatin chemo-radiotherapy in patients with unresectable squamous cell cancer of the esophagus. *Radiother Oncol.* 2007;83(2):139–147.

67. Rosenblatt E, Jones G, Sur RK, et al. Adding external beam to intra-luminal brachytherapy improves palliation in obstructive squamous cell oesophageal cancer: a prospective multi-centre randomized trial of the International Atomic Energy Agency. *Radiother Oncol.* 2010;97(3):488–494.

68. Sur R, Donde B, Falkson C, et al. Randomized prospective study comparing high-dose-rate intraluminal brachytherapy (HDRILBT) alone with HDRILBT and external beam radiotherapy in the palliation of advanced esophageal cancer. *Brachytherapy.* 2004;3(4):191–195.

69. Sur R, Kochar R, Negi P, et al. High dose rate intraluminal brachytherapy in palliation of esophageal carcinoma. *Endocuriether Hypertherm Oncol.* 1994;10:25–29.

70. Sur RK, Levin CV, Donde B, et al. Prospective randomized trial of HDR brachytherapy as a sole modality in palliation of advanced esophageal carcinoma: an International Atomic Energy Agency study. *Int J Radiat Oncol Biol Phys.* 2002;53(1):127–133.

71. Sur RK, Donde B, Levin VC, et al. Fractionated high dose rate intraluminal brachytherapy in palliation of advanced esophageal cancer. *Int J Radiat Oncol Biol Phys.* 1998;40(2):447–453.

72. Fairweather M, Wang J, Devlin PM, et al. Safety and efficacy of radiation dose delivered via iodine-125 brachytherapy mesh implantation for deep cavity sarcomas. *Ann Surg Oncol.* 2015;22(5):1455–1463. doi:10.1245/s10434-014-4171-y

73. Holloway CL, Delaney TF, Alektiar KM, et al. American Brachytherapy Society (ABS) consensus statement for sarcoma brachytherapy. *Brachytherapy.* 2013;12(3):179–190. doi:10.1016/j.brachy.2012.12.002

74. Laskar S, Bahl G, Muckaden MA, et al. Interstitial brachytherapy for childhood soft tissue sarcoma. *Pediatr Blood Cancer.* 2007;49(5):649–655.

75. Nag S, Shasha D, Janjan N, et al. The American Brachytherapy Society recommendations for brachytherapy of soft tissue sarcomas. *Int J Radiat Oncol Biol Phys.* 2001;49(4): 1033–1043.

76. Koizumi M, Inoue T, Yamazaki H, et al. Perioperative fractionated high-dose rate brachytherapy for malignant bone and soft tissue tumors. *Int J Radiat Oncol Biol Phys.* 1999;43(5):989–993.

77. Chun M, Kang S, Kim BS, et al. High dose rate interstitial brachytherapy in soft tissue sarcoma: technical aspects and results. *Jpn J Clin Oncol.* 2001;31(6):279–283.

78. Rachbauer F, Sztankay A, Kreczy A, et al. High-dose-rate intraoperative brachytherapy (IOHDR) using flab technique in the treatment of soft tissue sarcomas. *Strahlenther Onkol.* 2003;179(7):480–485.

79. Skowronek J, Kubaszewska M, Kanikowski M, et al. HDR endobronchial brachytherapy (HDRBT) in the management of advanced lung cancer—comparison of two different dose schedules. *Radiother Oncol.* 2009;93(3):436–440.

80. Perez CA, Taylor ME, Halverson K, et al. Brachytherapy or electron beam boost in conservation therapy of carcinoma of the breast: a nonrandomized comparison. *Int J Radiat Oncol Biol Phys.* 1996;34(5):995–1007.

81. Resch A, Pötter R, Van Limbergen E, et al. Long-term results (10 years) of intensive breast conserving therapy including a high-dose and large-volume interstitial brachytherapy boost (LDR/HDR) for T1/T2 breast cancer. *Radiother Oncol.* 2002;63(1): 47–58.

82. Polgár C, Fodor J, Orosz Z, et al. Electron and high-dose-rate brachytherapy boost in the conservative treatment of stage I-II breast cancer first results of the randomized Budapest boost trial. *Strahlenther Onkol.* 2002;178(11):615–623.

83. Budrukkar AN, Sarin R, Shrivastava SK, et al. Cosmesis, late sequelae and local control after breast-conserving therapy: influence of type of tumour bed boost and adjuvant chemotherapy. *Clin Oncol (R Coll Radiol).* 2007;19(8):596–603.

84. Gitt A, Böse-Ribeiro H, Nieder C, et al. Treatment Results of MammoSite catheter in combination with whole-breast irradiation. *Anticancer Res.* 2016;36(1):355–360.

85. Hennequin C, Durdux C, Espie M, et al. High-dose-rate brachytherapy for early breast cancer: an ambulatory technique. *Int J Radiat Oncol Biol Phys.* 1999;45(1):85–90.

86. Neumanova R, Petera J, Frgala T, et al. Long-term outcome with interstitial brachytherapy boost in the treatment of women with early-stage breast cancer. *Neoplasma.* 2007;54(5):413–423.

87. Polgar C, Fodor J, Major T, et al. Breast-conserving therapy with partial or whole breast irradiation: ten-year results of the Budapest randomized trial. *Radiother Oncol.* 2013;108(2):197–202.

88. Vaidya JS, Wenz F, Bulsara M, et al. Risk-adapted targeted intraoperative radiotherapy versus whole-breast radiotherapy for breast cancer: 5-year results for local control and overall survival from the TARGIT—a randomised trial. *Lancet.* 2014;383(9917):603–613. doi:10.1016/S0140-6736(13)61950-9

89. Strnad V, Ott OJ, Hildebrandt G, et al. 5-year results of accelerated partial breast irradiation using sole interstitial multicatheter brachytherapy versus whole-breast irradiation

with boost after breast-conserving surgery for low-risk invasive and in-situ carcinoma of the female breast: a randomised, phase 3, non-inferiority trial. *Lancet.* 2016;387(10015): 229–238. doi:10.1016/S0140-6736(15)00471-7

90. Shah NM, Tenenholz T, Arthur D, et al. MammoSite and interstitial brachytherapy for accelerated partial breast irradiation: factors that affect toxicity and cosmesis. *Cancer.* 2004;101(4):727–734.

# Proton Beam Therapy 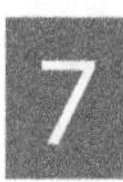

*Ryan Rhome and Rahul R. Parikh*

## INTRODUCTION TO PROTON THERAPY

As with all treatments in clinical oncology, the ultimate goal of radiation therapy is to maximize effective tumor dose while minimizing toxicity to surrounding normal structures. Using photon-based therapy, this has been achieved incrementally by improvements in patient simulation, immobilization, image guidance, tumor sensitization, and conformal planning techniques. The use of charged particles, such as in *proton therapy* (PT), is another advance toward this common goal. In this chapter we will discuss the characteristics of PT that make it both desirable and technically challenging as well as review the available evidence for its efficacy, toxicity, and cost-effectiveness.

## PHYSICAL AND BIOLOGICAL CHARACTERISTICS

Traditional photon-based radiation with x-rays delivers energy as an absorbed dose as the rays pass through the patient, interacting with the atoms comprising various tissues. The beam is attenuated in variable ways based on the type and the amount of tissue it interacts with, ultimately depositing a predetermined dose to the target prior to continuing along the path. This results in a significant amount of energy being delivered to normal tissues proximal and distal to the tumor, which can affect the dose-limiting toxicities that ultimately alter the therapeutic ratio. Unlike the x-ray therapy commonly employed in radiation therapy centers, PT offers an opportunity to exploit the behavior of accelerated particles to deliver the desirable dose with a theoretical sparing of adjacent tissues.

Protons as discussed here consist of a hydrogen atom that is charged due to the loss of an electron. The kinetic energy deposited by a particle entering a medium is inversely proportional to the square of the velocity (1). The mass of a proton is $1.67 \times 10^{-27}$ kg, or about 1,800 times more than an electron. As charged particles with mass, such as protons, slow down while passing through tissue, the probability of ionization events increases. This transfer is known as *linear energy transfer* (LET). The deposition of this energy rapidly reaches a narrow maximum before abruptly falling off, resulting in the characteristic Bragg peak described over 100 years ago (2). This steep dose gradient at the end of a beam is the basis of the proposed therapeutic gain of PT.

Radiobiologically, therapeutic protons show some key similarities and differences compared to photons. *Relative biological effectiveness* (RBE) refers to a ratio of the dose of x-rays required for a specific effect to the dose of a test particle required for that same effect, which for our purposes refers to protons. Although the RBE will vary with tissue type, beam energy, and fraction size, the average generic accepted RBE for protons is about 1.1 based on in vivo data (3). They conclude that RBE likely increases near the distal edge of the Bragg peak (up to 1.35) and then rises to 1.7 in the falloff, though these numbers have been debated and are possibly underestimated based on some in vitro data (4,5). Doses in treatment planning typically will take this average RBE of 1.1 into account.

Another parameter often described for different treatment modalities is the oxygen enhancement ratio (OER). This quantity is necessary due to the differential tumor effects, with some treatments given in hypoxic compared to aerated environments. The OER is a ratio of the dose required for a given effect in the presence of oxygen compared to the dose for that effect in hypoxia and reflects the dependence of cell killing and repair on oxygenation. The OER is energy, cell-cycle, and dose-rate dependent but is generally accepted to be 2.5 to 3.5 for photons. Similar if not slightly lower OERs of 2 to 3 have been suggested for protons, though the ranges often overlap (6–8). This slight OER reduction likely reflects more direct DNA damage from protons compared to photons.

## TECHNICAL CONSIDERATIONS

The protons are usually generated by applying a high-voltage current to hydrogen gas, which removes the electrons. To generate the energies required for therapy (up to 250 MeV), either a cyclotron or a synchrotron accelerates the protons. With cyclotrons, the beam is monoenergetic and therefore must be subjected to energy degradation if a lower energy beam is required. Magnets divert the beam from its

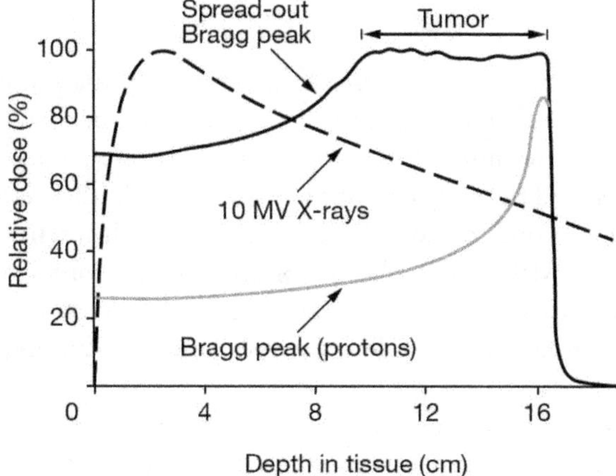


**FIGURE 7.1** Depiction of the dose-depth relationship between 100-MV x-rays, a single-proton Bragg peak, and the SOBP used to treat the full target thickness

*Note:* SOPB, spread-out Bragg peak.

*Source:* Originally published by Yock TI, Tarbell NJ. Technology insight: proton beam radiotherapy for treatment in pediatric brain tumors. *Nat Clin Pract Oncol.* 2004;1(2):97–103, quiz 101.

continuous acceleration and direct it into the rooms where patients are receiving treatment. In contrast, synchrotrons allow selectable energies.

The Bragg peak results in a deposition of the maximum dose that is approximately 1 cm wide if not otherwise modified, which is smaller than many tissue targets for PT. To allow for the treatment of larger structures, a spread-out Bragg peak (SOBP) must be generated by staggering the thicknesses of range modulation devices to result in a uniform dose deposition of adequate size and distal falloff. A typical dose buildup and falloff of a single Bragg peak and an SOBP are shown in Figure 7.1 and compared to photons (originally published by Yock et al) (9).

The dose profile is modified with either the scattering technique or the scanning technique. With scattering, the beam is spread by a single filter or a double filter, with the latter producing a flatter profile laterally. One should note that neutron production increases using this process, but several retrospective studies and modeling data have failed to show any increase in secondary malignancies. Some have suggested this rate is improved with PT (10–13).

The scanning technique modifies the initial pencil beam by magnetically guiding it across the field to ultimately create a larger uniform SOBP at treatment depth. When the proton beam is modulated while being moved, this technique is called *intensity-modulated proton therapy* (IMPT).

## PITFALLS AND POTENTIAL UNCERTAINTIES

Proton therapy in general is sensitive to patient setup inaccuracies given the abrupt falloff of dose distal to the SOBP. Furthermore, normal organ motion, such as breathing, can cause a decrease in dose uniformity, especially for gaussian beam shapes, and options for tumor tracking would theoretically improve targeting in areas prone to movement (14–17). As with intensity- modulated radiation therapy (IMRT) with photons or other highly conformal techniques, IMPT is sensitive to variations in patient setup, organ motion, and interfraction tumor differences, which can lead to target misses and possibly normal tissue toxicities.

Another potential pitfall to consider with PT is the RBE uncertainty, particularly at the end of the range, which may lead to an under- or overestimation of the dose (18). Several approaches have been suggested to improve this uncertainty, including tapering the distal Bragg peak edge, improving modeling, implementing robustness measures, and using imaging to substantiate the anticipated range (19–22).

## CLINICAL DATA: TOXICITY

The basis of improved toxicity in the use of proton therapy is the steep dose falloff after the Bragg peak and the lower integral dose compared to photon therapy. This improvement in dosimetry has been corroborated by varying degrees in multiple disease sites and populations, including head and neck (23–25), orbit (26), breast (27), lung (28–30), thymoma (31), lymphoma (32,33), pancreas (34), esophagus (35–37), central nervous system (38), prostate (39,40), and various pediatric malignancies (41,42). Many of these studies were aimed at evaluating dose plans on the basis of target conformality and dose to adjacent organs at risk (OAR). Figure 7.2 shows a representative prostate treatment plan for IMRT compared with PT, and Figure 7.3 shows the comparative dosimetry of radiation therapy for anterior mediastinal Hodgkin lymphoma, both originally presented in the sixth edition of *Principles of Radiation Therapy* by Perez and Brady.

Although dosimetric evaluation is important, it is primarily hypothesis-generating in the absence of clinical correlation. The gold standard to demonstrate improved toxicities with proton therapy compared to photon therapy would be a comparative randomized clinical trial, but these are rare (43). Many single-institution reports on toxicity exist, usually without comparison arms or compared to historical controls. Regarding the clinical experience of protons, we look at toxicity profiles from trials ideally designed to assess the comparative

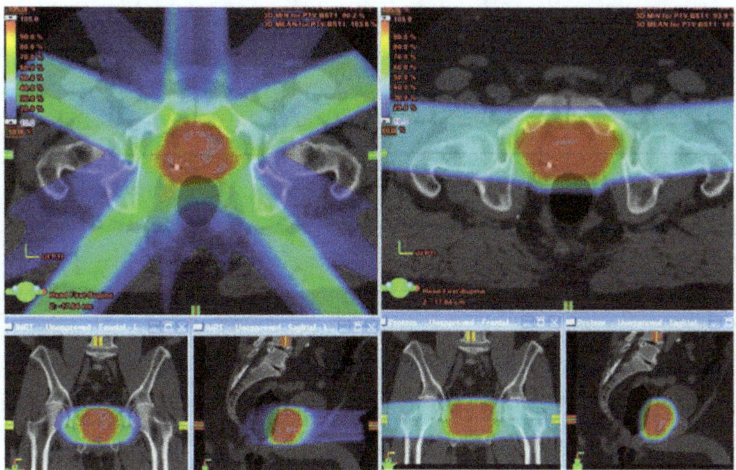

**FIGURE 7.2** Representative dosimetric plans for IMRT and proton therapy for the treatment of prostate cancer

*Note:* IMRT, intensity-modulated radiation therapy.

*Source:* Reprinted with permission of Halperin EC, Brady LW, Perez CA, et al. *Principles and Practices of Radiation Oncology.* 6th edition. Wolters Kluwer Health and Lippincott Williams and Wilkins; 2013.

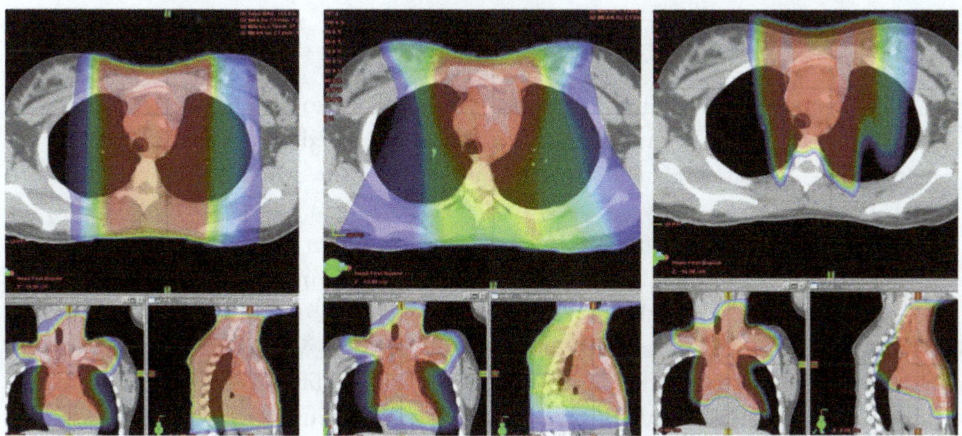

**FIGURE 7.3** Representative dosimetric plans for radiation therapy for an anterior mediastinal Hodgkin lymphoma with three-dimensional CRT, IMRT, and proton therapy

*Note:* IMRT, intensity-modulated radiation therapy.

*Source:* Reprinted with permission of Halperin EC, Brady LW, Perez CA, et al. *Principles and Practices of Radiation Oncology.* 6th edition. Wolters Kluwer Health and Lippincott Williams and Wilkins; 2013.

toxicity of standard techniques. Shipley et al (44) found a significant increase in grade 1 and 2 rectal bleeding (32% vs. 12%) in localized prostate patients treated with a conformal proton boost compared to conventional photons, though this group also received a higher target dose and was not truly designed to compare the two modalities. Pooled single-arm prospective trials have shown a low incidence of grade 3 genitourinary (1.9%) and gastrointestinal (<0.5%) toxicities in patients treated for localized prostate cancer, but this was not compared to photon-based treatments (45). On the other hand, a large population-based analysis of toxicity coding in the Surveillance, Epidemiology, and End Results (SEER)-Medicare database suggested that localized prostate patients were coded as having a higher incidence of gastrointestinal morbidity (or gastrointestinal evaluation; ie, colonoscopy) if they received PT compared to IMRT (46). One should interpret all current outcomes data with caution because nonrandomized, single-institution (or observational) data sets may be subject to selection bias, reporting bias, and/or incomplete data.

Given the rarity of conditions such as pediatric malignancies, ocular tumors, and skull base tumors, it would be difficult to show true comparative level I evidence for improved toxicities, so a lower level of evidence may justify the use of PT in these cases. For example, a study of sinonasal tumors treated with the equivalent of nearly 70 Gy with PT reported an acceptable level of visual complications (15.8% grade 2+) given the dose and tumor location (47).

## CLINICAL DATA: EFFICACY

The notion that PT will improve toxicity profiles due to the physical dose characteristics of proton beams has been previously discussed. A correlative hypothesis, then, is that improved toxicity could allow for dose escalation, which has been shown in many disease sites to confer at least a local control benefit. Alternatively, demonstrating equivalent efficacy but an improved toxicity rate may still yield a clinically meaningful improvement in the therapeutic ratio. These are similar hypotheses to those advocating for the implementation of IMRT, and some have argued that this modality was widely adopted without the need for randomized trials showing clinical benefit. Randomized clinical trials evaluating the true comparative efficacy of PT are uncommon (43,48). Two well-known trials have examined the addition of a PT boost to photon therapy as a means of dose escalation in prostate cancer, but the benefit is likely more a function of dose escalation, rather than radiation modality (44,49). The mixed modalities make it difficult to cite this as evidence of the improved efficacy of protons compared to photons.

Lower level evidence studies in certain disease sites have shown enough promise in improved therapeutic ratio due to the proximity to critical OARs that the adoption of PT has been met with less skepticism. This includes a partially prospective series of treatment for uveal melanomas compared to iodine brachytherapy (50). Others argue that in the setting of pediatric malignancies, where the induction of a secondary malignancy and late effects such as cardiac toxicity may occur, improvements in dosimetry evaluation could make it difficult to ethically randomize children to treatment with photon-based therapies. A recent systematic review was able to identify two comparative case series on pediatric tumors (51). The first retrospectively compared retinoblastoma patients treated with PT to those treated with photon therapy. It showed a significantly lower rate of in-field second malignancy in the PT group (0% vs. 14%) (52). Another examined the outcomes and toxicity of childhood craniopharyngiomas treated with PT compared to a cohort treated with photon therapy and demonstrated no significant differences between overall survival or local failure (53). The remaining studies featured in the systematic review examined noncomparative outcomes in 15 different pediatric malignancies, with the ultimate conclusion that prospective clinical trials are needed (52). With skull base tumors, actuarial local control of skull base chondrosarcomas treated with PT ranges from 57% to 98% and has allowed for significant dose escalation, but clinical studies have not directly compared PT's effectiveness with photon therapy (54–57).

A phase III study (RTOG 1308, NCT01993810) is currently accruing stage II through IIIB non–small cell lung cancer patients and randomizing their treatment to either photon- or PT-based radiation with concurrent chemotherapy. This trial will be important for many reasons and will be able to assess comparative efficacy and toxicity in the setting of multimodality therapy, at least for this particular disease site. A randomized clinical trial has opened accruing nonmetastatic breast cancer patients to treatment with either PT or photon radiation therapy with the goal of assessing survival, quality of life, cardiac mortality, and other disease-specific outcomes. Of course, the results of this trial will take many years to mature, but this experimental design is vital to truly address these unanswered questions. For reference, all current, ongoing randomized phase III clinical trials employing PT are summarized in Table 7.1, though many more phase I or II trials are open. Physicians are highly encouraged to enroll all patients treated with PT in these clinical trials to ascertain the therapy's effectiveness.

## COST-EFFECTIVENESS

In addition to the need to show at least equivalent efficacy with improved toxicity with PT, determining if these gains are worth the cost of delivering the treatment from a public health and resource utilization standpoint is an

**TABLE 7.1** Summary of all current, ongoing phase II/III randomized clinical trials employing PT

| Disease site | Patient population | Design | Primary end point | Expected enrollment | Trial name | Trial identifier |
|---|---|---|---|---|---|---|
| Prostate | Low- or intermediate-risk prostate cancer | PT vs. IMRT | Patient reported GI toxicity at 6 months | 350 | PartiQOL | NCT01617161 |
| | Intermediate-risk prostate cancer | Mildly hypofractionated PT (70 Gy/28 fx) +/−androgen deprivation | Freedom from failure | 192 | | NCT01492972 |
| | Low-risk prostate cancer | Hypofractionated PT (38 Gy/5 fx) vs. 79.2 Gy/44 fx) | Freedom from failure | 192 | | NCT01230866 |
| Breast | Nonmetastatic invasive breast cancer | PT vs. photon therapy | Reduction of cardiovascular events at 10 years | 1720 | RADCOMP | NCT02603341 |
| Liver | Medium-to-large hepatocellular carcinoma | PT vs. RFA | Local control at 3 years | 166 | | NCT02640924 |
| | Recurrent or residual small hepatocellular carcinoma | PT (66 Gy/10 fx) vs. RFA | Local progression-free survival | 144 | APROH | NCT01963429 |
| Lung | Inoperable stage IIA–IIIB NSCLC | PT vs. photon therapy, with image guidance and concurrent chemotherapy | Overall survival | 560 | RTOG 1308 | NCT01993810 |

**TABLE 7.1** (*Continued*)

| Disease site | Patient population | Design | Primary end point | Expected enrollment | Trial name | Trial identifier |
|---|---|---|---|---|---|---|
| Brain | Glioblastoma, newly diagnosed | Randomized phase II, dose-escalated (75 Gy/ 30 fx) photon IMRT vs. PT, with temozolomide | Overall survival | 576 | NRG-BN001 | NCT02179086 |
| Head and neck | Stage III–IV oropharyngeal SCC | IMPT vs. IMRT, 70 Gy+chemo at discretion | Rate of grade 3–5 late toxicities | 360 | | NCT01893307 |
| Skull base | Skull base chordoma | PT vs. carbon ion therapy | Localprogression-free survival | 319 | Heidelberg University | NCT01182753 |
| Esophagus | Esophageal SCC or adenocarcinoma | PT vs. IMRT | Progression- free survival and total toxicity burden | 180 | | NCT01512589 |
| Various | Radioresistant tumors (chordoma, ACC, sarcoma) | PT or IMRT vs. carbon ion therapy | Progression- free survival | 250 | ETOILE | NCT02838602 |

*Note:* ACC, adenoid cystic carcinoma; fx=fractions; GI, gastrointestinal; IMPT, intensity-modulated proton therapy; IMRT, intensity-modulated radiation therapy; NSCLC, non–small cell lung cancer; PT, proton therapy; RFA, radiofrequency ablation; SCC, squamous cell carcinoma.

important aspect of any treatment intervention. In the attempt to quantify cost-effectiveness, the focus has been on long-term outcomes in either pediatric populations (58) or common conditions with a long expected overall survival, such as early-stage breast cancer (59). One such recent study employed a cost-effectiveness model to assess whether the improved cardiac toxicities in early-stage breast cancer warranted the use of PT. In certain scenarios, as the model identified, the savings in avoiding the long-term cardiac comorbidities associated with a significant healthcare resource drain outweighed the cost of PT. In contrast, other common conditions, such as prostate cancer, have been examined, and these models have not found an obvious overall cost benefit to PT (60).

These attempts aim to justify the cost of PT from a public health point of view. However, there may be difficulty covering the large up-front cost and potential debt to any one institution or cooperative group funding the construction and operation of a modern PT facility (61). To justify the facility cost of treating relatively rare malignancies, such as skull base or pediatric tumors, treating a certain percentage of patients with more common diseases, such as prostate cancer or breast cancer, may be necessary (62). Nevertheless, with limited data on its cost-effectiveness on the population level already detailed, reimbursement for PT delivery may not be able to keep pace with the worldwide need (63,64).

Ultimately, PT has certainly revolutionized the radiation oncologist's toolbox and now offers patients a level of hope that has never existed in such a widespread nature. With approximately 20 operational PT facilities in the United States, more than 26 additional centers in 13 other countries, and 40 more in planning or under construction worldwide, this treatment modality is sure to be included in the multidisciplinary discussion of our cancer patients.

## References


1. Lomax AJ. Charged particle therapy: the physics of interaction. *Cancer J.* 2009;15(4): 285–291.
2. Brown A, Suit H. The centenary of the discovery of the Bragg peak. *Radiother Oncol.* 2004;73(3):265–268.
3. Paganetti H, Niemierko A, Ancukiewicz M, et al. Relative biological effectiveness (RBE) values for proton beam therapy. *Int J Radiat Oncol Biol Phys.* 2002;53(2):407–421.
4. Cuaron JJ, Chang C, Lovelock M, et al. Exponential increase in relative biological effectiveness along distal edge of a proton Bragg peak as measured by deoxyribonucleic acid double-strand breaks. *Int J Radiat Oncol Biol Phys.* 2016;95(1):62–69.
5. Marshall TI, Chaudhary P, Michaelidesova A, et al. Investigating the implications of a variable RBE on proton dose fractionation across a clinical pencil beam scanned spread-out Bragg peak. *Int J Radiat Oncol Biol Phys.* 2016;95(1):70–77.

6. Williams JR, Gould RG, Flynn D, et al. Relative survival of hybrid X-ray-resistant, and normally sensitive mammalian cells exposed to X rays and protons under aerobic and hypoxic conditions. *Radiat Res.* 1978;73(3):585–590.

7. Raju MR, Amols HI, Bain E, et al. A heavy particle comparative study. Part III: OER and RBE. *Br J Radiol.* 1978;51(609):712–719.

8. Iwata H, Ogino H, Hashimoto S, et al. Spot scanning and passive scattering proton therapy: relative biological effectiveness and oxygen enhancement ratio in cultured cells. *Int J Radiat Oncol Biol Phys.* 2016;95(1):95–102.

9. Yock TI, Tarbell NJ. Technology insight: proton beam radiotherapy for treatment in pediatric brain tumors. *Nat Clin Pract Oncol.* 2004;1(2):97–103, quiz 101.

10. Miralbell R, Lomax A, Cella L, et al. Potential reduction of the incidence of radiation-induced second cancers by using proton beams in the treatment of pediatric tumors. *Int J Radiat Oncol Biol Phys.* 2002;54(3):824–829.

11. Newhauser WD, Fontenot JD, Mahajan A, et al. The risk of developing a second cancer after receiving craniospinal proton irradiation. *Phys Med Biol.* 2009;54(8):2277–2291.

12. Fontenot JD, Lee AK, Newhauser WD. Risk of secondary malignant neoplasms from proton therapy and intensity-modulated x-ray therapy for early-stage prostate cancer. *Int J Radiat Oncol Biol Phys.* 2009;74(2):616–622.

13. Taddei PJ, Howell RM, Krishnan S, et al. Risk of second malignant neoplasm following proton versus intensity-modulated photon radiotherapies for hepatocellular carcinoma. *Phys Med Biol.* 2010;55(23):7055–7065.

14. Phillips MH, Pedroni E, Blattmann H, et al. Effects of respiratory motion on dose uniformity with a charged particle scanning method. *Phys Med Biol.* 1992;37(1):223–234.

15. van de Water S, Kreuger R, Zenklusen S, et al. Tumour tracking with scanned proton beams: assessing the accuracy and practicalities. *Phys Med Biol.* 2009;54(21):6549–6563.

16. Seiler PG, Blattmann H, Kirsch S, et al. A novel tracking technique for the continuous precise measurement of tumour positions in conformal radiotherapy. *Phys Med Biol.* 2000;45(9):N103-N110.

17. Bert C, Grozinger SO, Rietzel E. Quantification of interplay effects of scanned particle beams and moving targets. *Phys Med Biol.* 2008;53(9):2253–2265.

18. Woodward WA, Amos RA. Proton radiation biology considerations for radiation oncologists. *Int J Radiat Oncol Biol Phys.* 2016;95(1):59–61.

19. Underwood T, Paganetti H. Variable proton relative biological effectiveness: how do we move forward? *Int J Radiat Oncol Biol Phys.* 2016;95(1):56–58.

20. Parodi K, Paganetti H, Shih HA, et al. Patient study of in vivo verification of beam delivery and range, using positron emission tomography and computed tomography imaging after proton therapy. *Int J Radiat Oncol Biol Phys.* 2007;68(3):920–934.

21. Knopf A, Parodi K, Paganetti H, et al. Quantitative assessment of the physical potential of proton beam range verification with PET/CT. *Phys Med Biol.* 2008;53(15):4137–4151.

22. Malyapa R, Lowe M, Bolsi A, et al. Evaluation of robustness to setup and range uncertainties for head and neck patients treated with pencil beam scanning proton therapy. *Int J Radiat Oncol Biol Phys.* 2016;95(1):154–162.

23. Cozzi L, Fogliata A, Lomax A, et al. A treatment planning comparison of 3D conformal therapy, intensity modulated photon therapy and proton therapy for treatment of advanced head and neck tumours. *Radiother Oncol.* 2001;61(3):287–297.

24. Lomax AJ, Goitein M, Adams J. Intensity modulation in radiotherapy: photons versus protons in the paranasal sinus. *Radiother Oncol.* 2003;66(1):11–18.

25. Chera BS, Malyapa R, Louis D, et al. Proton therapy for maxillary sinus carcinoma. *Am J Clin Oncol.* 2009;32(3):296–303.

26. Weber DC, Bogner J, Verwey J, et al. Proton beam radiotherapy versus fractionated stereotactic radiotherapy for uveal melanomas: a comparative study. *Int J Radiat Oncol Biol Phys.* 2005;63(2):373–384.

27. Lomax AJ, Cella L, Weber D, et al. Potential role of intensity-modulated photons and protons in the treatment of the breast and regional nodes. *Int J Radiat Oncol Biol Phys.* 2003;55(3):785–792.

28. Chang JY, Liu HH, Komaki R. Intensity modulated radiation therapy and proton radiotherapy for non-small cell lung cancer. *Curr Oncol Rep.* 2005;7(4):255–259.

29. Zhang X, Li Y, Pan X, et al. Intensity-modulated proton therapy reduces the dose to normal tissue compared with intensity-modulated radiation therapy or passive scattering proton therapy and enables individualized radical radiotherapy for extensive stage IIIB non-small-cell lung cancer: a virtual clinical study. *Int J Radiat Oncol Biol Phys.* 2010;77(2):357–366.

30. Hoppe BS, Flampouri S, Henderson RH, et al. Proton therapy with concurrent chemotherapy for non-small-cell lung cancer: technique and early results. *Clin Lung Cancer.* 2012;13(5):352–358.

31. Parikh RR, Rhome R, Hug E, et al. Adjuvant proton beam therapy in the management of thymoma: a dosimetric comparison and acute toxicities. *Clin Lung Cancer.* 2016; 17(5):362–366.

32. Chera BS, Rodriguez C, Morris CG, et al. Dosimetric comparison of three different involved nodal irradiation techniques for stage II Hodgkin's lymphoma patients: conventional radiotherapy, intensity-modulated radiotherapy, and three-dimensional proton radiotherapy. *Int J Radiat Oncol Biol Phys.* 2009;75(4):1173–1180.

33. Hoppe BS, Flampouri S, Su Z, et al. Consolidative involved-node proton therapy for stage IA-IIIB mediastinal Hodgkin lymphoma: preliminary dosimetric outcomes from a phase II study. *Int J Radiat Oncol Biol Phys.* 2012;83(1):260–267.

34. Bouchard M, Amos RA, Briere TM, et al. Dose escalation with proton or photon radiation treatment for pancreatic cancer. *Radiother Oncol.* 2009;92(2):238–243.

35. Welsh J, Gomez D, Palmer MB, et al. Intensity-modulated proton therapy further reduces normal tissue exposure during definitive therapy for locally advanced distal esophageal tumors: a dosimetric study. *Int J Radiat Oncol Biol Phys.* 2011;81(5):1336–1342.

36. Makishima H, Ishikawa H, Terunuma T, et al. Comparison of adverse effects of proton and X-ray chemoradiotherapy for esophageal cancer using an adaptive dose-volume histogram analysis. *J Radiat Res.* 2015;56(3):568–576.

37. Chuong MD, Hallemeier CL, Jabbour SK, et al. Improving outcomes for esophageal cancer using proton beam therapy. *Int J Radiat Oncol Biol Phys.* 2016;95(1):488–497.

38. Baumert BG, Norton IA, Lomax AJ, et al. Dose conformation of intensity-modulated stereotactic photon beams, proton beams, and intensity-modulated proton beams for intracranial lesions. *Int J Radiat Oncol Biol Phys.* 2004;60(4):1314–1324.

39. Chera BS, Vargas C, Morris CG, et al. Dosimetric study of pelvic proton radiotherapy for high-risk prostate cancer. *Int J Radiat Oncol Biol Phys.* 2009;75(4):994–1002.

40. Trofimov A, Nguyen PL, Coen JJ, et al. Radiotherapy treatment of early-stage prostate cancer with IMRT and protons: a treatment planning comparison. *Int J Radiat Oncol Biol Phys.* 2007;69(2):444–453.

41. Boehling NS, Grosshans DR, Bluett JB, et al. Dosimetric comparison of three-dimensional conformal proton radiotherapy, intensity-modulated proton therapy, and intensity-modulated radiotherapy for treatment of pediatric craniopharyngiomas. *Int J Radiat Oncol Biol Phys.* 2012;82(2):643–652.

42. Beltran C, Roca M, Merchant TE. On the benefits and risks of proton therapy in pediatric craniopharyngioma. *Int J Radiat Oncol Biol Phys.* 2012;82(2):e281-e287.

43. Glatstein E, Glick J, Kaiser L, et al. Should randomized clinical trials be required for proton radiotherapy? an alternative view. *J Clin Oncol.* 2008;26(15):2438–2439.

44. Shipley WU, Verhey LJ, Munzenrider JE, et al. Advanced prostate cancer: the results of a randomized comparative trial of high dose irradiation boosting with conformal protons compared with conventional dose irradiation using photons alone. *Int J Radiat Oncol Biol Phys.* 1995;32(1):3–12.

45. Mendenhall NP, Li Z, Hoppe BS, et al. Early outcomes from three prospective trials of image-guided proton therapy for prostate cancer. *Int J Radiat Oncol Biol Phys.* 2012; 82(1):213–221.

46. Sheets NC, Goldin GH, Meyer AM, et al. Intensity-modulated radiation therapy, proton therapy, or conformal radiation therapy and morbidity and disease control in localized prostate cancer. *JAMA.* 2012;307(15):1611–1620.

47. Weber DC, Chan AW, Lessell S, et al. Visual outcome of accelerated fractionated radiation for advanced sinonasal malignancies employing photons/protons. *Radiother Oncol.* 2006;81(3):243–249.

48. Goitein M, Cox JD. Should randomized clinical trials be required for proton radiotherapy? *J Clin Oncol.* 2008;26(2):175–176.

49. Zietman AL, DeSilvio ML, Slater JD, et al. Comparison of conventional-dose vs high-dose conformal radiation therapy in clinically localized adenocarcinoma of the prostate: a randomized controlled trial. *JAMA.* 2005;294(10):1233–1239.

50. Char DH, Kroll S, Phillips TL, et al. Late radiation failures after iodine 125 brachytherapy for uveal melanoma compared with charged-particle (proton or helium ion) therapy. *Ophthalmology.* 2002;109(10):1850–1854.

51. Leroy R, Benahmed N, Hulstaert F, et al. Proton therapy in children: a systematic review of clinical effectiveness in 15 pediatric cancers. *Int J Radiat Oncol Biol Phys.* 2016;95(1): 267–278.

52. Sethi RV, Shih HA, Yeap BY, et al. Second nonocular tumors among survivors of retinoblastoma treated with contemporary photon and proton radiotherapy. *Cancer.* 2014; 120(1):126–133.

53. Bishop AJ, Greenfield B, Mahajan A, et al. Proton beam therapy versus conformal photon radiation therapy for childhood craniopharyngioma: multi-institutional analysis of outcomes, cyst dynamics, and toxicity. *Int J Radiat Oncol Biol Phys.* 2014;90(2):354–361.

54. Indelicato DJ, Rotondo RL, Begosh-Mayne D, et al. A prospective outcomes study of proton therapy for chordomas and chondrosarcomas of the spine. *Int J Radiat Oncol Biol Phys.* 2016;95(1):297–303.

55. Munzenrider JE, Liebsch NJ. Proton therapy for tumors of the skull base. Strahlentherapie und Onkologie: Organ der Deutschen Rontgengesellschaft. 1999;175(suppl 2):57–63.

56. Hug EB, Loredo LN, Slater JD, et al. Proton radiation therapy for chordomas and chondrosarcomas of the skull base. *J Neurosurg.* 1999;91(3):432–439.

57. Brada M, Pijls-Johannesma M, De Ruysscher D. Proton therapy in clinical practice: current clinical evidence. *J Clin Oncol.* 2007;25(8):965–970.

58. Mailhot Vega RB, Kim J, Bussiere M, et al. Cost effectiveness of proton therapy compared with photon therapy in the management of pediatric medulloblastoma. *Cancer.* 2013; 119(24):4299–4307.

59. Mailhot Vega RB, Ishaq O, Raldow A, et al. Establishing cost-effective allocation of proton therapy for breast irradiation. *Int J Radiat Oncol Biol Phys.* 2016;95(1):11–18.

60. Konski A, Speier W, Hanlon A, et al. Is proton beam therapy cost effective in the treatment of adenocarcinoma of the prostate? *J Clin Oncol.* 2007;25(24):3603–3608.

61. Johnstone PA, Kerstiens J, Richard H. Proton facility economics: the importance of "simple" treatments. *J Am Coll Radiol.* 2012;9(8):560–563.

62. Johnstone PA, Kerstiens J. Doing poorly by doing good: the bottom line of proton therapy for children. *J Am Coll Radiol.* 2014;11(10):995–997.

63. Kerstiens J, Johnstone PA. Proton therapy expansion under current United States reimbursement models. *Int J Radiat Oncol Biol Phys.* 2014;89(2):235–240.

64. Johnstone PA, Kerstiens J. Reconciling reimbursement for proton therapy. *Int J Radiat Oncol Biol Phys.* 2016;95(1):9–10.

# Intraoperative Radiation Therapy    8

*Daniel J. Tandberg, Christopher G. Willett,*
*Manisha Palta, and Brian G. Czito*

## INTRODUCTION

Intraoperative radiation therapy (IORT) is the delivery of high-dose radiation in a single fraction at the time of surgery. By shielding dose-limiting sensitive structures and directly targeting the radiation to the tumor bed, IORT allows dose escalation without significantly increasing normal tissue toxicity. As the radiation dose is increased, the likelihood of local tumor control increases. Various techniques and technologies have been employed to deliver IORT, including intraoperative electron irradiation (IOERT) and intraoperative high–dose rate brachytherapy (HDR-IORT) as well as orthovoltage techniques (kV-IORT). IORT is often used in combination with external beam radiation therapy (EBRT), with or without chemotherapy, and surgical resection.

IORT is commonly integrated into the multimodality treatment of locally advanced or recurrent abdominal and pelvis malignancies. Often in these situations, anatomic or normal tissue constraints limit the use of resection and EBRT. The addition of IORT to conventional treatment has been shown to improve local control, as well as potentially survival, in many disease sites. IORT is also being explored as an alternative to standard whole-breast EBRT in breast conservation therapy for women with early-stage breast cancer.

This chapter reviews the rationale and radiobiology of IORT, the technical applications and logistics of IORT, and the clinical results of IORT (with or without EBRT) in different disease sites.

## RATIONALE

A major goal of radiation therapy is to maximize the dose to the tumor volume while minimizing the dose to the adjacent normal tissues. By maximizing the therapeutic ratio, the probability of local disease control is increased without significantly increasing the incidence of normal tissue complications. IORT is an effective method to maximize this therapeutic ratio. This can be achieved by two means. First, by delivering radiation during surgery, dose-limiting normal structures can be excluded from the treatment field by operative mobilization or direct shielding. Second, the volume of the irradiation "boost" field can be decreased by direct tumor/tumor bed visualization and conformal treatment. This allows for a very focal delivery of high-dose irradiation.

IORT is often utilized in combination with fractionated EBRT (with or without concomitant chemotherapy) and resection. The rationale is that EBRT fields encompass the primary tumor and surrounding tissues harboring potential microscopic disease. In contrast to a large single fraction of irradiation, fractionated radiation (EBRT) is radiobiologically advantageous in promoting tumor control while minimizing late normal tissue injury. However, in many disease sites, the proximity of the tumor to sensitive normal structures limits the EBRT radiation dose that can be delivered safely.

Shrinking field irradiation, otherwise known as *boost* treatments, has been used for dose escalation in many disease sites, including head and neck, breast, gastrointestinal, and cervical cancers, with excellent local control and acceptable morbidity to dose-limiting normal tissues. EBRT, interstitial, and intracavitary brachytherapy, as well as superficial electrons, have all been used to deliver boost radiation treatments. For selected intra-abdominal, pelvic, thoracic, breast, and other malignancies, IORT is used for localized dose escalation while optimizing normal tissue protection. As would be expected, IORT seems most beneficial in cancers in which local disease control is crucial for long-term survival.

## THE BIOLOGY OF INTRAOPERATIVE RADIATION THERAPY

In classical radiobiology the "4 R's" (normal tissue repair, tumor reoxygenation, tumor cell cycle redistribution, and normal tissue repopulation) can be used to explain the preferential therapeutic advantage for normal tissues relative to tumor tissue with conventionally fractionated EBRT. With the single, large fraction of radiation delivered with IORT, these advantages are lost. Thus, if normal structures were to remain within the IORT treatment field, the risk of late effects may increase. With both fractionated EBRT and IORT, tumor

**TABLE 8.1**  Estimated biologically equivalent EBRT doses (2 Gy per day) of varying IORT doses

| IORT dose | 10 Gy | 15 Gy | 20 Gy |
|---|---|---|---|
| Normal tissue (acute) ($\alpha/\beta=7$) | 20 Gy | 37 Gy | 60 Gy |
| Tumor ($\alpha/\beta=10$) | 17 Gy | 31 Gy | 50 Gy |
| Normal tissue (late) ($\alpha/\beta=2$) | 30 Gy | 65 Gy | 120 Gy |

*Note:* EBRT, external beam radiation therapy; IORT, intraoperative radiation therapy.

response has been shown to correlate with the hypoxic fraction of cells. With fractionated radiation the impact of hypoxia is diminished due to reoxygenation between treatments. This is not the case with IORT. The differential sensitivity between hypoxic and well-oxygenated cells increases with increasing dose.

Using the linear-quadratic model and alpha/beta calculations ($\alpha/\beta$), biologically equivalent doses to a fractionated EBRT course using 2 Gy per fraction for varying IORT doses can be estimated (Table 8.1). A low alpha/beta ratio is typical of late-responding normal tissues. Thus, IORT has the potential for a higher incidence of late normal tissue effects (1). For example, assuming an alpha/beta of 2 for late-reacting normal tissue, the estimated biologically equivalent EBRT dose for a single 20-Gy dose of IORT would be 120 Gy. Indeed, late normal tissue complications are often the limiting sequelae of IORT administration. However, the exclusion of nontarget tissues from the radiation field by direct inspection, as well as the mobilization and shielding of normal organs, can mitigate many of these disadvantages. Experimental animal data and clinical studies have documented the tolerance of normal tissues to IORT, EBRT, or both modalities combined (2). When combined with EBRT and resection, IORT doses of 10 Gy to 20 Gy provide control for most solid tumors, especially in the setting of microscopic-only residual disease. Further, these dose levels are generally within the maximal tolerable dose range for dose-limiting normal structures.

## INTRAOPERATIVE RADIATION THERAPY TECHNIQUES AND DOSE CONSIDERATIONS

### Physics and Techniques

Technologies to deliver IORT include IOERT, HDR-IORT, and kV-IORT. These methods, including a detailed description of their physics and techniques, have been reviewed in detail in a recently published IORT textbook (3).

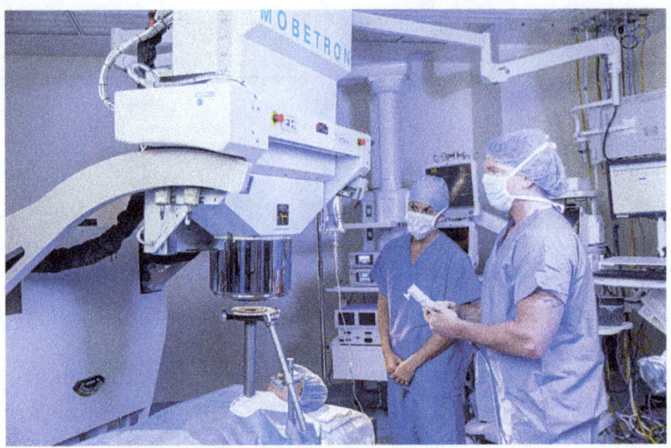

**FIGURE 8.1** Simulated soft-docking procedure for Mobetron unit

*Source:* Courtesy of IntraOp Medical Corporation, Sunnyvale, CA.

IOERT is delivered by a linear accelerator, which generates an electron beam in the dose range of 6 MeV to 15 MeV. In the past patients were often transported from the operating room (OR) to the radiation oncology department, where they were treated with conventional, nonmobile linear accelerators. However, mobile, compact linear accelerators have been developed that can be transported in and out of the operating theater. A shielded OR is not necessary for the operation of these mobile linear accelerators because their maximum energy is 12 MeV, and they do not use bending magnets. Commercially available mobile linear accelerators include the Mobetron (IntraOp Medical Corp., Sunnyvale, CA, 4–12 MeV) (Figure 8.1), the NOVAC 11 (Sordina IORT Technologies S.p.A, Aprilia, Italy, 4–10 MeV) (Figure 8.2A), and the LIAC (Sordina IORT Technologies S.p.A, Aprilia, Italy, 4–10 or 6–12 MeV) (see Figure 8.2B). At the time of surgery, an appropriate IOERT applicator is placed to cover the tumor bed and margins. If necessary, packing or lead shielding is used to limit the dose to critical normal tissues. The linear accelerator is then "docked" to the applicator and the treatment delivered. The NOVAC 11 and the LIAC units are robotic devices that use a hard-docking technique, while the Mobetron uses a soft-docking process that decouples the machine from the applicator. Similar to nonintraoperative electron treatments, the depth of coverage can be controlled through the selection of electron-beam energy and the use of a bolus. For example, the 90% depth dose in water for 4-, 6-, 9-, and 12-MeV electron beams with the Mobetron unit has been shown to be 1.1, 1.9, 2.9, and 3.5 cm, respectively (4).

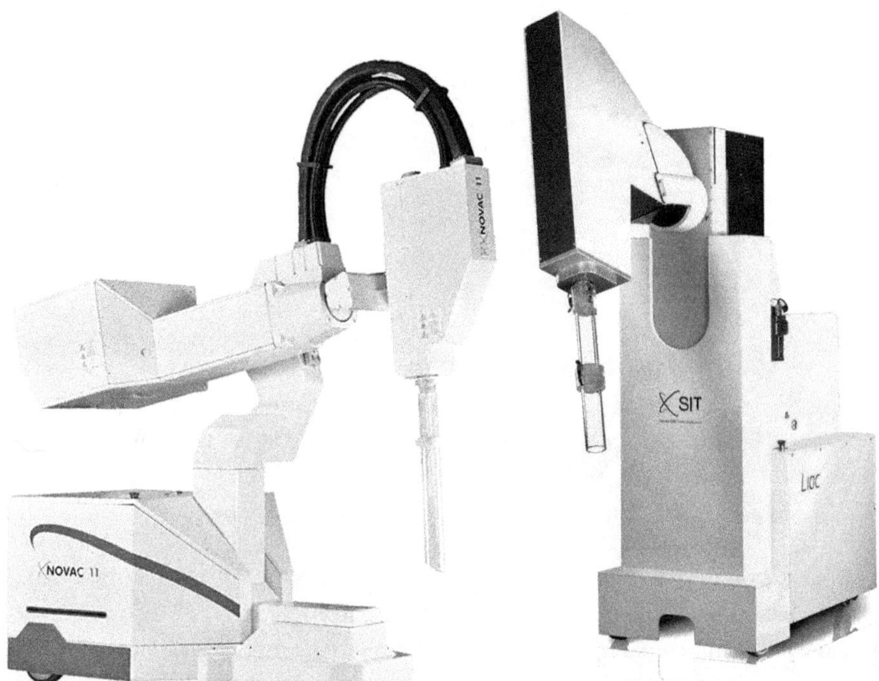

**FIGURE 8.2**  (Left) NOVAC 11 and (Right) LIAC mobile IOERT units

*Note:* IOERT, intraoperative electron irradiation.

*Source:* Courtesy of Sordina IORT Technologies S.p.A, Aprilia, Italy.

HDR–IORT units are remote afterloading devices that utilize a high-energy source (typically iridium-192) to deliver photon radiation. As the maximum depth of effective coverage with HDR–IORT is approximately 0.5 cm deep from the surface of the tumor, this technique is best suited for treatment after a near or total gross resection. Commercially available HDR remote afterloaders are produced by Elekta (Stockholm, Sweden) (Figure 8.3) and Varian Medical Systems (Palo Alto, CA) (Figure 8.4). In contrast to the self-shielded IOERT linear accelerators, HDR–IORT requires room shielding, which may be achieved by retrofitting an existing room or constructing a smaller shielded room adjacent to the operating suite. For HDR–IORT a flexible applicator, such as a Harrison–Anderson–Mick (HAM) applicator (Mick Radio-Nuclear Instruments, Bronx, NY), is secured over the region of interest and connected to the remote afterloader for treatment delivery. Care must be taken to ensure that

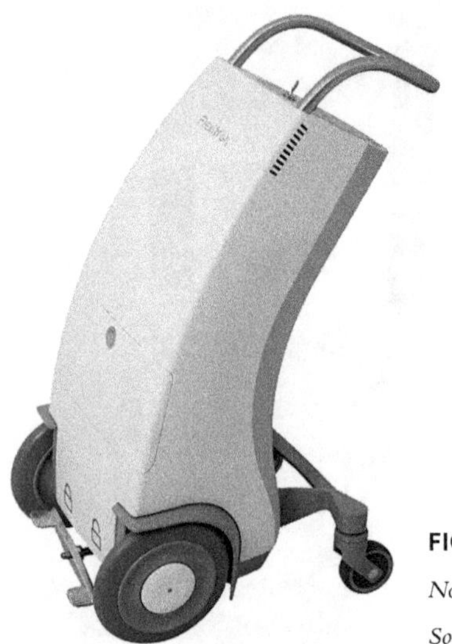

**FIGURE 8.3** Flexitron® HDR brachytherapy afterloader

*Note:* HDR, high dose rate.

*Source:* Courtesy of Elekta, Stockholm, Sweden.

the applicator is in direct contact with the tissue surface in the region of interest, as even a small separation can affect the dose to the target. Similar to IOERT, sensitive tissues are retracted or shielded. For treatment planning, the source position and the dwell times are optimized by computer to deliver a uniform dose to the region of interest. Clinical treatment times vary and depend on the dose prescription, the source strength, and the target size.

Commercially available kV-IORT devices include the INTRABEAM system (Carl Zeiss Meditec, Dublin, CA, 30–50 kV) and the Xoft® Axxent® Electronic Brachytherapy System® (iCAD, Inc., San Jose, CA, 20–50 kV) (Figure 8.5). The INTRABEAM device has a miniature x-ray source at the end of a 10-cm probe. The Axxent system is an electronic brachytherapy device with a microminiature x-ray tube located within a flexible, disposable sheath. The units are mobile and do not require the use of a shielded OR. Based on the spherical dose distribution and the steep dose gradient, ideal targets for kV-IORT include spherical targets with a maximum tissue treatment radius of 1 cm to 2 cm. The INTRABEAM system uses spherical applicators, while the Axxent uses spherical or ellipsoidal balloons for treatment delivery. Applicators have also been developed to treat the vaginal stump as well as superficial skin tumors. KV-IORT has been used most extensively for the IORT treatment of breast cancer, with most studies using the INTRABEAM device.

A detailed description of the relative advantages and disadvantages of IOERT, HDR-IORT, and kV-IORT has been discussed elsewhere and is beyond the

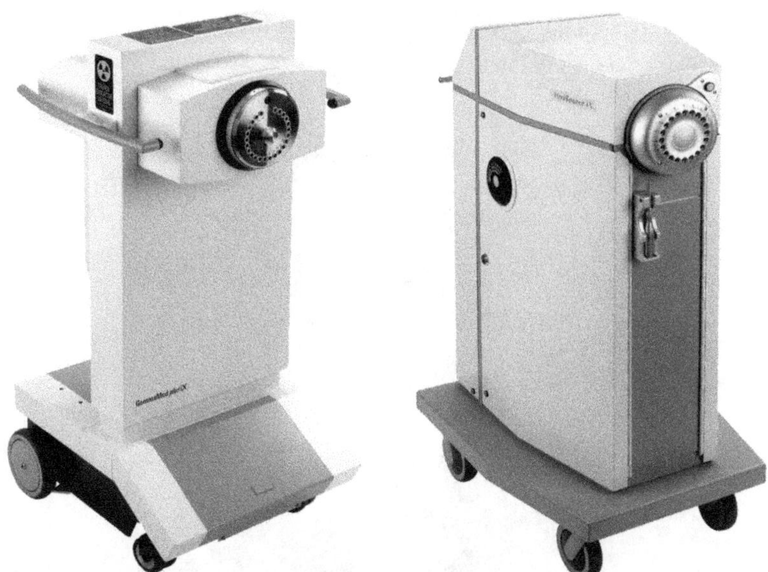

**FIGURE 8.4** GammaMed® HDR/PDR brachytherapy afterloader

*Note:* HDR, high dose rate; PDR, pulsed dose rate.

*Source:* Courtesy of Varian Medical Systems, Palo Alto, CA.

scope of this chapter (Table 8.2) (5). The advantages of IOERT compared to HDR-IORT include better dose homogeneity, faster treatment time, and the ability to select different electron energies for treating both superficial and deeper-seated targets. Less shielding is also required in the OR. The potential disadvantages of IOERT include a decreased surface radiation dose and difficulty treating large or curved body surfaces (eg, large pelvic sidewall fields, the lateral abdominal wall, and the thoracic cage), which may require separate, matching fields with IOERT-based applicators. Although HDR-IORT is generally only appropriate for targets less than or equal to 0.5 cm in thickness, the surface radiation dose is high, and the flexible HAM applicator used in HDR-IORT allows the treatment of large or curved surfaces with a single treatment. kV-IORT does not require a shielded room but needs a small target volume with minimal depth. A comprehensive IORT program would ideally have IOERT and HDR-IORT, as well as perioperative brachytherapy, available to treat all disease sites and situations. These modalities should be viewed as complementary and not competitive.

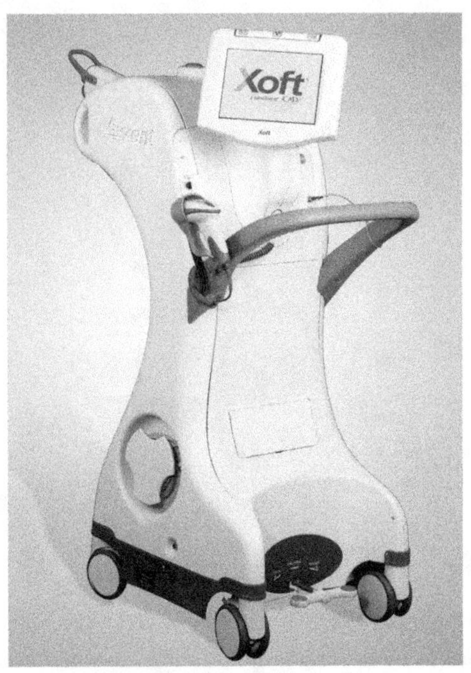
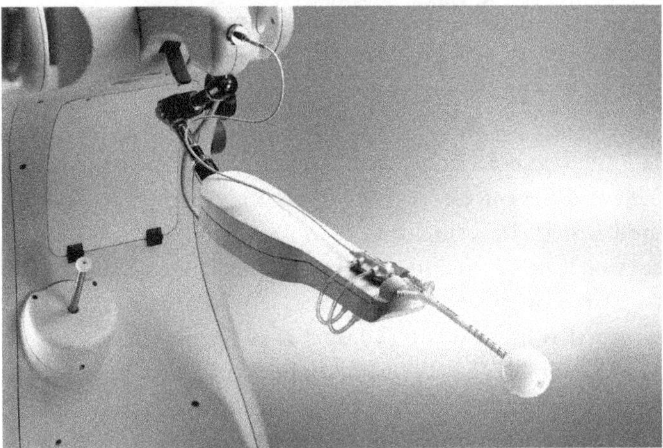

**FIGURE 8.5** (Top) Xoft® Axxent® Electronic Brachytherapy System® controller; (Bottom) Axxent spherical balloon applicator attached to controller

Courtesy of iCAD, Inc., San Jose, CA.

**TABLE 8.2**  Potential differences between IOERT, HDR-IORT, and kV-IORT

|  | IOERT | HDR-IORT | kV-IORT |
|---|---|---|---|
| Actual treatment time | 2–4 min | 5–30 min | 30–45 min |
| Total procedure time | 30–45 min | 45–120 min | 45–120 min |
| Treatment sites | Accessible locations | All areas where depth at risk is ≤0.5–1.0 cm from surface of applicator | Areas where depth at risk is ≤0.5–1.0 cm from surface of applicator; small target volumes only |
| Surface dose | Lower (75–93%) | Higher (200%) | Highest (300%) |
| Dose at depth (2 cm) | Higher (70–100%) | Lower (30%) | Lowest (20%) |
| Dosimetric homogeneity (surface to depth) | ≤10% variation | ≥100% variation | ≥150% variation |

*Note:* HDR-IORT, intraoperative high–dose rate brachytherapy; IOERT, intraoperative electron irradiation; IORT, intraoperative radiation therapy.

*Source:* Adapted from Nag S, Willett C, Gunderson L, et al. IORT with electron-beam, high dose rate brachytherapy or low-kV/Electronic brachytherapy: methodological comparisons. In: Gunderson L, Willett C, Harrison L, Calvo F, eds. *Intraoperative Irradiation—Techniques and Results.* 2nd ed. New York: Humana Press; 2011.

## Dose Considerations

IORT is given as a single fraction during surgery. The prescribed dose should be based on the extent of residual disease at resection, the amount of EBRT delivered previously, and the type and volume of normal tissue irradiated. When given after conventionally fractionated EBRT of 45 Gy to 54 Gy, the IORT dose usually varies from 10 Gy to 20 Gy. For patients with microscopic residual or close margins, the IORT dose is usually 10 Gy to 12.5 Gy. For gross residual disease 15 Gy to 20 Gy is usually administered. In previously irradiated patients, in whom additional EBRT of 20 Gy to 30 Gy is feasible, the dose of IORT generally ranges between 15 Gy to 20 Gy. In patients in whom no or very limited EBRT is planned, IORT doses from 25 Gy to 30 Gy have been administered; however, doses in this range should be judiciously employed given the risk of normal tissue damage, specifically peripheral nerve injury. As discussed previously, although not clearly defined, the biological effectiveness of single-dose IORT on tumor/acute reacting tissues generally appears to be 1.5 to 2.5 times greater than that delivered by conventional fractionation (1). Therefore, the effective tumor dose (when "normalized" to fractionated EBRT doses) of a 20-Gy IORT treatment would be estimated to be 30 Gy to 50 Gy.

### Intraoperative Radiation Therapy Normal Tissue Tolerance

Late normal tissue complications are often the dose-limiting sequelae of IORT administration. IORT tolerance for intact or surgically manipulated organs or structures in animals (primarily canines) is seen in Table 8.3. Much of this information has been derived from studies performed on dogs at the National Cancer Institute (NCI) (6–11) and Colorado State University (CSU) (12–14).

Several dose-sensitive structures have been studied in humans receiving IORT, including the ureter and the peripheral nerve, discussed in the next section. However, when considering the toxicity from IORT, it is also important to consider the severe morbidity and mortality associated with locally recurrent tumors. For a more comprehensive review of normal tissue tolerance, the reader is referred to a dedicated IORT textbook (2).

### Ureter

Reports from the Mayo Clinic describe the impact of IORT on rates of ureteral obstruction in human cancer patients. In their original report, among patients with no evidence of obstruction at the time of IORT, doses of 10 Gy administered intraoperatively resulted in a 50% incidence of ureteral obstruction, increasing to 70% with doses from 15 Gy to 25 Gy (15).

In an update of this study, including 146 patients with locally advanced malignancies receiving IORT (7.5–30 Gy) to one or both ureters, these investigators reported that the risk of obstruction following IOERT is significant and increases with time and IORT dose. The rates of a clinically apparent type 1 obstruction (an obstruction from any cause) after IOERT at 2, 5, and 10 years were 47%, 63%, and 79%, respectively. The rates of a clinically apparent type 2 obstruction (obstruction occurring at least 1 month after IOERT, excluding obstruction caused by a tumor, an abscess, or patient stents) at 2, 5, and 10 years were 27%, 47%, and 70%, respectively. However, the obstruction risk for ureters not receiving IOERT was also high, which suggests an underlying risk of ureteral injury from other causes (EBRT or the surgical manipulation of ureters) (16).

### Peripheral Nerve

In the pelvis and retroperitoneum, peripheral nerve tissue is the principal dose-limiting normal tissue for IORT. Often, peripheral nerve tissue is directly adjacent to or involved with the tumor. As a result the relative surgical "immobility" of the peripheral nerve and the inability to shield the nerve from the IORT

**TABLE 8.3**  Normal tissue tolerance to intraoperative irradiation in dogs

| Tissue | Dose (Gy) | End point |
| --- | --- | --- |
| *Intact Structure* | | |
| Aorta, vena cava | 30 | Threshold for fibrosis (patency up to 50 Gy) |
| Peripheral nerve | 15 | Threshold for neuropathy, sensory-motor |
| Bladder | 30 | Ureterovesical junction stenosis |
| Ureter | 30 | Threshold for fibrosis and stenosis |
| Kidney | 15 | Threshold for tubular loss (30 Gy complete intensified fibrosis) |
| Bile duct | 20 | Threshold for fibrosis and stenosis |
| Small intestine | 20 | Ulceration, fibrosis, stenosis |
| Esophagus | | |
| Full thickness | 20 | Threshold for ulcerations and strictures |
| Partial thickness | 40 | No sequelae at this dose |
| Heart (right atrium) | 20 | Fibrosis |
| Lung | 20 | Fibrosis |
| Trachea | 30 | Submucosal fibrosis |
| *Surgically manipulated* | | |
| Aorta anastomosis | 45 | Threshold for late fistula formation (fibrosis and stenosis at 20 Gy) |
| Aortic prosthetic graft | 25 | Threshold for stenotic graft occlusion |
| Biliary-enteric anastomosis | 20 | Anastomotic breakdown |
| Small intestine (defunctionalized) | 45 | Threshold for fistula formation (fibrosis and stenosis at 20 Gy) |
| Bladder | 30 | Healing but contracture |
| Bronchial stump | 40 | Absence of air leak |

field can often lead to nerve tissue receiving the full dose of EBRT and IORT. All patients considered for IORT should complete a thorough pretreatment informed consent, including a discussion regarding neuropathy–related side effects. Peripheral nerve tolerance has been shown to depend on the volume of nerve irradiated and the total dose delivered. Reports from the Mayo Clinic on human patients describe the frequency and risk factors for neuropathy following IORT.

In an initial analysis from the Mayo Clinic, 51 patients with primary or recurrent pelvic malignancies were treated with EBRT (median 50.4 Gy), maximal resection, and an IOERT boost (10–25 Gy using 9–18 MeV electrons) (15). Sixteen (32%) patients experienced grade I through III peripheral neuropathy as manifested by pelvic/extremity pain, leg weakness, numbness, or tingling. The pain was severe (grade III) in 3 out of 51 patients (6%). A follow-up study from the Mayo Clinic evaluated 178 patients with previously unirradiated primary or locally recurrent colorectal cancer (17,18). They reported a relationship between increasing doses of IOERT and the incidence of clinically significant neuropathy. Grade 2 to 3 neuropathy was seen in 3% to 7% of patients receiving an IOERT dose of less than or 12.5 Gy and 19% to 23% of patients receiving greater than or equal to 15 Gy. Finally, a more recent Mayo Clinic analysis of 607 patients with locally recurrent colorectal cancer receiving IORT reported an incidence of grade 1 through grade 3 neuropathy of 15% (grade 1, 5%; grade 2, 7%; grade 3, 3%). A dose-related increase in grade 2 and grade 3 neuropathy was seen in patients receiving greater than or equal to 15 Gy versus less than or equal to 12.5 Gy (19).

## INTRAOPERATIVE RADIATION THERAPY RESULTS FOR SELECTED DISEASE SITES

A summary of IORT results in selected disease sites will now be presented. Much of this data is from nonrandomized studies, with few prospective, randomized studies. For a more comprehensive review, the reader is referred to dedicated chapters on each site in an IORT text (3).

### Breast Cancer
### Intraoperative Radiation Therapy Alone
Randomized trials have demonstrated equivalent disease-free survival (DFS) and overall survival (OS) in selected breast cancer patients undergoing either a mastectomy or breast-conserving surgery followed by EBRT (20). More contemporary data report a possible survival advantage to breast-conserving therapy (21). Based on the finding that local recurrences frequently occur at or adjacent to the original tumor bed following breast conserving surgery, there has been increasing interest in accelerated partial breast irradiation (APBI). Besides the appeal of a shorter radiation course, APBI also has been shown to decrease radiation exposure to critical normal structures, including the lungs and heart. A recent phase III randomized noninferiority trial showed APBI with interstitial multicatheter brachytherapy alone to be noninferior in 5-year local control compared to whole-breast radiation therapy (WBRT) with a boost in low-risk breast cancer (22). Single-fraction IORT has also been studied as a technique

to deliver APBI. Two randomized phase III trials comparing IORT to standard whole-breast EBRT in early-stage breast cancer have been reported: the electron IORT ELIOT trial and the targeted intraoperative radiotherapy TARGIT trial, which used kV-IORT. The results of these trials are reviewed next.

The Italian ELIOT trial randomized 1,305 women with early-stage breast cancer (tumors 2.5 cm or less and clinically node-negative) to 21 Gy IOERT prescribed to the 90% isodose line versus 50 Gy of whole-breast EBRT and a 10-Gy boost (23). IORT was delivered with a mobile linear accelerator using 6 MeV to 9 MeV electrons while shielding the thoracic wall with a lead plate. After a median follow-up of 5.8 years, 35 patients in the IORT group and 4 patients in the EBRT group had had an ipsilateral breast tumor recurrence (IBTR) ($P<.0001$). The 5-year event rate for IBRT was 4.4% in the IORT group and 0.4% in the EBRT group. This difference was within the prespecified equivalence margin. There was no significant difference in 5-year OS (96.8% vs. 96.9% for IORT vs. EBRT, respectively). Significantly fewer skin side effects were seen in women who received IORT compared to women who received EBRT ($P=.0002$). On subset analysis the cohort of patients identified as low risk (based on the absence of high-risk factors, including a tumor over 2 cm, four or more positive nodes, a poorly differentiated tumor, and a triple negative status) had a 1.5% 5-year IBTR rate with IORT. In contrast, the IBTR rate was 11.3% in patients with one or more risk factors. The authors acknowledge the need for longer follow-ups and improved selection of patients for IORT (23).

The TARGIT-A trial randomized 3,451 patients with early breast cancer (a tumor 3.5 cm or less, N0-1, and unifocal) to whole-breast EBRT versus kV-IORT (24). The IORT prescription was 20 Gy at the surface of the applicator, delivered using the 50-kV INTRABEAM device. If resected patients were at high risk of local recurrence in other quadrants (ie, findings of extensive intraductal components, extensive lymphovascular invasion, nodal metastases, etc) then EBRT could be delivered postoperatively. Supplemental EBRT after IORT was necessary in 15.2% of patients. With a median follow-up of 29 months, the 5-year risk for local recurrence in the conserved breast was 3.3% for IORT versus 1.3% for EBRT ($P=.042$) (noninferior). No significant difference in breast cancer mortality was found between treatment groups ($P=.56$), but there were significantly fewer non–breast cancer deaths with TARGIT (1.4% vs. 3.5%, P=.0086). The overall mortality was 3.9% for IORT versus 5.3% for EBRT ($P=.099$). Grade 3 or 4 skin complications were significantly reduced with TARGIT (4 of 1,720 vs. 13 of 1,731, P=.029). Late toxicity data available in 305 patients showed significantly less telangiectasias in the arm receiving IORT alone (25). Although longer follow-up times are needed, early results of the protocol of IORT with risk-adapted WBRT show promising outcomes in a well-selected cohort.

## Intraoperative Radiation Therapy Plus External Beam Radiation Therapy

Boost treatments to the lumpectomy bed following EBRT have been shown to reduce local recurrence rates by approximately 50% in all age groups compared to EBRT alone (26). The potential advantages of an IORT versus an EBRT boost include a more precise delivery of irradiation to the tumor bed, skin sparing so that the associated late cosmetic sequelae are avoided, and a smaller boost area with a more homogeneous dose distribution.

The largest series of patients treated with IORT as a boost prior to WBRT comes from a collaborative analysis of European International Society of Intraoperative Radiation Therapy (ISIORT) member institutions. Each institution conducted a prospective program on breast-boost IOERT. Data on over 1,200 patients were collected. Using IOERT, a median single-fraction dose of 10 Gy was applied to the 90% reference isodose. Standard fractionation WBRT (50–54 Gy) was then given at a median of 6.8 weeks following IOERT (27,28). At a median follow-up of 72.4 months, local tumor control was 99.2% with an annual in-breast recurrence rate of 0.64%, 0.34%, 0.21%, and 0.16% in patients aged less than 40 years, 40 to 49 years, 50 to 59 years, and more than or equal to 60 years, respectively (29). The authors concluded that an IOERT boost during breast conservation therapy results in an optimal dose delivery and outstanding local control rates.

The results of the TARGIT trial using kV-IORT as a boost therapy have also been reported (30). A total of 299 patients underwent a single 20-Gy IORT treatment to the tumor bed at the time of resection. Patients then received conventionally fractionated WBRT. At a median follow-up of 60.5 months, the 5-year estimate for ipsilateral recurrence was 1.73%. The authors commented that the local recurrence rate compared favorably to patients treated in the EORTC boost trial (4.3%) and the UK Standardisation of Breast Radiotherapy (UK START)-B boost trial (2.8%). The reported acute toxicity was "rare," but a comprehensive toxicity analysis was not provided.

## Pancreatic Cancer

Although patients with pancreatic cancer are at a high risk of systemic metastatic failure, many will also present with isolated or concurrent local failure or progression. The available data in patients receiving IORT following pancreaticoduodenectomy demonstrate an improvement in local control; however, a clear survival benefit has not been demonstrated (31–33). Series of patients with locally advanced pancreatic cancer suggest local control and pain relief, with select studies demonstrating an OS benefit (34–38). Although improving local control in pancreatic cancer patients may achieve modest gains in survival, the high rate of distant metastases limits significant improvements in long-term survival using IORT approaches. Further research will need to evaluate the role of IORT integrated with more effective systemic therapies.

## Retroperitoneal and Pelvic Soft Tissue Sarcomas

For patients with primary and recurrent retroperitoneal sarcomas, IORT combined with EBRT and resection offers an effective means of improving local disease control. This has been demonstrated in a small randomized trial from the NCI as well as multiple U.S. and European single-institution studies (39–47). NCI investigators conducted a randomized phase III trial in patients undergoing a surgical resection of primary retroperitoneal sarcoma (39). Thirty-five patients were randomized to receive 20 Gy of IOERT followed by 35 Gy to 40 Gy of EBRT postoperatively, versus postoperative EBRT alone to a dose of 50 Gy to 55 Gy. Patients receiving IOERT were treated with concurrent misonidazole given 15 to 30 minutes prior to treatment. The local-regional recurrence was significantly lower among those who received IOERT and EBRT (6:15) compared to EBRT alone (16:20, $P<.001$). There was no difference in survival. Patients receiving IOERT and EBRT experienced fewer episodes of radiation enteritis than patients receiving EBRT alone (2:15 vs. 10:20, $P<.05$); however, radiation-related peripheral neuropathy was more frequent in patients receiving IOERT (9:15 vs. 1:20, $P<.01$).

In the NCI trial, the rate of tumor bed relapse was high (80%) in patients treated with postoperative EBRT alone, likely due to the inability to deliver effective EBRT doses given normal tissue constraints. Because these results are similar to the reports on resection alone, the use of adjuvant EBRT without IORT following marginal resection could be questioned. A preferable approach for patients with locally advanced or locally recurrent disease would be to deliver preoperative EBRT following a confirmation of the diagnosis by thin-needle biopsy. This would be followed by resection at an institution capable of delivering IORT. A recently reported prospective phase I/II trial demonstrated good results in terms of local control and survival when patients with high-risk retroperitoneal sarcomas were managed with preoperative dose-escalated EBRT (IMRT with an integrated boost to 50–56 Gy), surgical resection, and IOERT (10–12 Gy) (48). With a median follow-up of 33 months in 27 patients, 5-year local control was 72%, and 5-year OS was 74%.

## Gynecologic Cancers

The prognosis for patients with locally advanced or locally recurrent gynecologic cancers is poor. Often in these situations, there is direct tumor extension to the pelvic sidewall, the pelvic lymph nodes, or the para-aortic nodes, and standard radiation or surgical therapy has failed. The use of radical resection and IORT with or without EBRT and/or chemotherapy may benefit patients when compared with EBRT alone. Analyses from the Mayo Clinic study described the outcomes of 148 patients with primary (23 patients) or recurrent (125 patients) gynecologic malignancies treated with IOERT-containing regimens (49–51). Preoperative or postoperative EBRT was delivered in 113 patients, and 85 patients had received prior EBRT. The 5-year OS for all patients was 27%, and the 5-year local failure rate was 40%. On subset analysis, patients with R0 or R1 resections had improved 5-year OS compared to patients with R2 resections (31% vs. 13%, $P=.01$), and patients with no prior EBRT had better OS than those with prior EBRT (35% vs. 15%, $P=.01$) (49–51). These data suggest that regimens with IORT have the potential to cure selected patients with locally advanced and recurrent gynecologic cancers.

## Colorectal Cancer

### Primary Locally Advanced Colorectal Cancers

For colorectal cancers adherent or fixed to adjoining structures, such as the sacrum or pelvic sidewall, curative resection is often not feasible. In selected patients the optimal management approach is to administer preoperative chemoradiation in an effort to "downstage" the disease and facilitate surgical resection. At the time of resection, if clinical suspicion of involved margins is high, the use of IORT may be appropriate. Multimodality treatment involving IORT has been shown in multiple single-institution studies to provide high rates of local control and improved survival.

In a series from Massachusetts General Hospital (MGH), 64 patients with locally advanced primary rectal cancer underwent preoperative irradiation (with or without 5-FU) followed by resection and IOERT (52). Patients undergoing margin-negative resection had a five-year actuarial local control and disease-specific survival (DSS) of 91% and 63%, respectively. Patients with microscopically involved margins experienced 5-year local control and DSS of 65% and 47%, respectively, and patients with gross disease experienced 5-year local control and DSS of 57% and 14%, respectively.

A Mayo Clinic report described the outcomes of 146 patients with locally unresectable primary colorectal cancers who received IOERT in addition to pre- or postoperative combined modality therapy (53). The median survival was

44 months with 5-year OS of 52%. The 5-year rates of freedom from local and distant recurrence were 86% and 51%, respectively. OS was higher in patients receiving preoperative versus postoperative combined modality treatment (5-year OS 55% vs. 38%, $P = .02$).

## Locally Recurrent Colorectal Cancer

Local recurrence following the curative resection of primary colorectal cancer is a challenging clinical situation and is often treated with palliative intent. For patients undergoing surgery alone for the pelvic recurrence of rectal cancer, the reported 5-year survival rates are 0% (54). In select patients with recurrent colorectal cancer, combined modality treatment with IORT can facilitate improved local control and potentially long-term survival. It has been possible to achieve 5-year OS rates in the range of 20% when IORT is combined with EBRT with or without chemotherapy and surgical salvage (17,54–58).

In an MGH analysis of 41 patients with locally recurrent rectosigmoid cancer undergoing IOERT, patients with gross residual disease experienced 5-year local control and DFS of 21% and 7%, respectively, versus 47% and 21%, respectively, for patients with clear or microscopically positive margins (55). A Mayo Clinic report described the outcome of 106 patients undergoing palliative resection of locally recurrent nonmetastatic rectal cancer. Forty-two patients received IOERT as a component of treatment (most 15–20 Gy), and 41 received EBRT (most $\geq$ 45 Gy). Patients with gross residual disease experienced a significantly worse outcome versus those with microscopically involved margins (5-year survival of 9% versus 33%; $P = .03$). Patients receiving IOERT had a 5-year survival rate of 19% versus 7% without IOERT ($P = .0006$). A more recent Mayo Clinic analysis of 607 patients with recurrent colorectal cancer who received IOERT as a component of treatment reported 5-year OS to be 30% (19). The 3-year cumulative incidence of central, local, and distant relapse was 12%, 23%, and 49%, respectively. Complete resection was associated with improved survival. Figure 8.6 includes photographs from an HDR-IORT procedure performed on a patient with locally recurrent rectal cancer.

## Other Sites

The data and experiences with IORT at other disease sites have been reviewed in detail in a dedicated IORT textbook (3). In brief, IORT has been used in nearly every disease site, with the intent to escalate the radiation dose to facilitate local disease control.

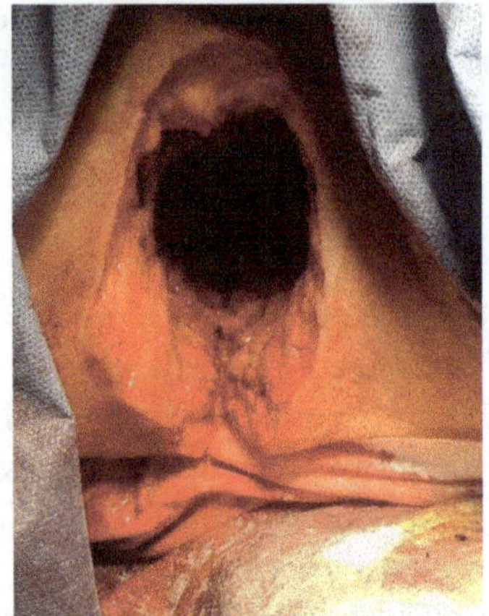

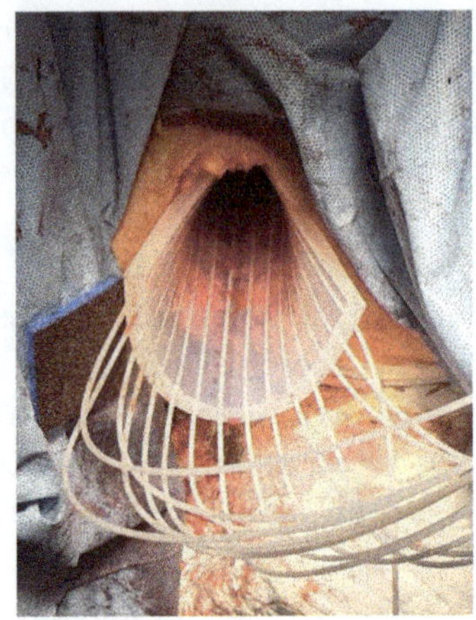

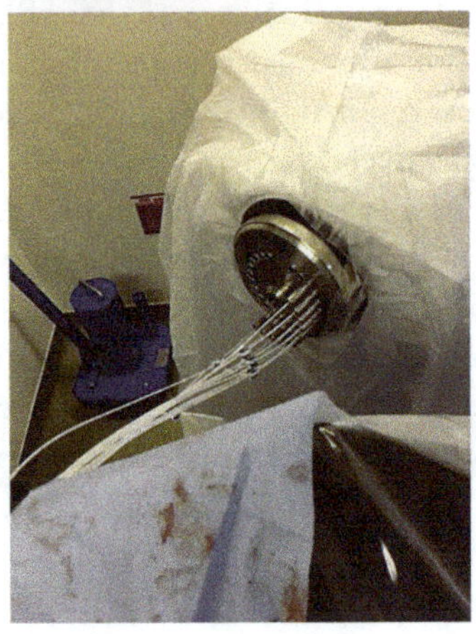

**FIGURE 8.6** HDR-IORT using the HAM applicator following abdominoperineal resection of locally recurrent rectal adenocarcinoma

*Note:* HAM, Harrison-Anderson-Mick; HDR-IORT, intraoperative high–dose rate brachytherapy.

*Source:* Courtesy of Daphna Spiegel, MD.

## CONCLUSIONS

IORT has proven to be an important component of the multidisciplinary management of many malignancies. Numerous studies support the use of IORT for dose escalation to optimize local control in locally advanced or recurrent cancer. Recent phase III trials have demonstrated the potential of IORT to replace a component of or all EBRT approaches in selected patients with breast cancer undergoing breast conservation therapy. Newer technologies, including mobile IOERT, HDR, and kV-IORT units, promise to improve the availability and efficiency of IORT while providing different means to precisely treat all disease sites. Dedicated IORT facilities have also been created at many institutions to facilitate multidisciplinary management involving IORT. Further research, including phase II/III studies, is needed to best understand how to integrate IORT into varying oncology treatment approaches.

## References


1. Okunieff P, Sundararaman S, Chen Y. Biology of large dose per fraction radiation therapy. In: Gunderson L, Willett C, Harrison L, Calvo F, eds. *Intraoperative Irradiation—Techniques and Results*. 2nd ed. New York: Humana Press; 2011:27–47.

2. Vujaskovic Z, Willett C, Tepper J, et al. Normal tissue tolerance to IOERT, EBRT, or both animal and clinical studies. In: Gunderson L, Willett C, Calvo FA, Harrison LB, eds. *Intraoperative Irradiation—Techniques and Results*. 2nd ed. New York: Humana Press; 2011.

3. Gunderson L, Willett C, Harrison L, et al. *Intraoperative Irradiation—Techniques and Results*. 2nd ed. New York: Humana Press; 2011.

4. Mills MD, Fajardo LC, Wilson DL, et al. Commissioning of a mobile electron accelerator for intraoperative radiotherapy. *J Appl Clin Med Phys*. 2001;2:121–130.

5. Nag S, Willett C, Gunderson L, et al. IORT with electron-beam, high dose rate brachytherapy or low-kV/electronic brachytherapy: methodological comparisons. In: Gunderson L, Willett C, Harrison L, Calvo F, eds. *Intraoperative Irradiation—Techniques and Results*. 2nd ed. New York: Humana Press; 2011.

6. Johnstone P, Sindelar WF, Kinsella TJ. Experimental and clinical studies of intraoperative radition. *Int J Radiat Oncol Biol Phys*. 1986;12:1687–1695.

7. Kinsella TJ, DeLuca AM, Barnes M, et al. Threshold dose for peripheral neuropathy following intraoperative radiotherapy (IORT) in a large animal model. *Int J Radiat Oncol Biol Phys*. 1991;20:697–701.

8. Kinsella TJ, Sindelar WF, DeLuca AM, et al. Tolerance of the canine bladder to intraoperative radiation therapy: an experimental study. *Int J Radiat Oncol Biol Phys*. 1988; 14:939–946.

9. Sindelar WF, Tepper J, Travis EL. Tolerance of bile duct to intraoperative irradiation. *Surgery*. 1982;92:533–540.

10. Sindelar WF, Tepper JE, Kinsella TJ, et al. Late effects of intraoperative radiation therapy on retroperitoneal tissues, intestine, and bile duct in a large animal model. *Int J Radiat Oncol Biol Phys*. 1994;29:781–788.

11. Sindelar WF, Johnstone PA, Hoekstra H, et al. *Normal Tissue Tolerance to IORT: The NCI Experimental Studies*. Totowa, NJ: Humana Press; 1999.

12. LeCouteur RA, Gillette EL, Powers BE, et al. Peripheral neuropathies following experimental intraoperative radiation therapy (IORT). *Int J Radiat Oncol Biol Phys*. 1989; 17:583–590.

13. Gillette EL, Gillette S, Vujaskovic Z, et al. *Influence of Volume on Canine Ureters and Peripheral Nerves Irradiated Intraoperatively*. Essen, Germany: Verlag Die Blaue Eule; 1993.

14. Gillette EL, Gillette S, Powers BE. *Studies at Colorado State University of Normal Tissue Tolerance of Beagles to IOERT, EBRT or a Combination*. Totowa, NJ: Humana Press; 1999.

15. Shaw EG, Gunderson LL, Martin JK, et al. Peripheral nerve and ureteral tolerance to intraoperative radiation therapy: clinical and dose-response analysis. *Radiother Oncol*. 1990;18:247–255.

16. Miller RC, Haddock MG, Petersen IA, et al. Intraoperative electron-beam radiotherapy and ureteral obstruction. *Int J Radiat Oncol Biol Phys*. 2006;64:792–798.

17. Gunderson LL, Nelson H, Martenson JA, et al. Intraoperative electron and external beam irradiation with or without 5-fluorouracil and maximum surgical resection for previously unirradiated, locally recurrent colorectal cancer. *Dis Colon Rectum*. 1996;39:1379–1395.

18. Gunderson LL, Nelson H, Martenson JA, et al. Locally advanced primary colorectal cancer: intraoperative electron and external beam irradiation +/- 5-FU. *Int J Radiat Oncol Biol Phys*. 1997;37:601–614.

19. Haddock MG, Miller RC, Nelson H, et al. Combined modality therapy including intra-operative electron irradiation for locally recurrent colorectal cancer. *Int J Radiat Oncol Biol Phys.* 2011;79:143–150.

20. Fisher B, Anderson S, Bryant J, et al. Twenty-year follow-up of a randomized trial comparing total mastectomy, lumpectomy, and lumpectomy plus irradiation for the treatment of invasive breast cancer. *N Engl J Med.* 2002;347:1233–1241.

21. van Maaren MC, de Munck L, de Bock GH, et al. 10 year survival after breast-conserving surgery plus radiotherapy compared with mastectomy in early breast cancer in the Netherlands: a population-based study. *Lancet Oncol.* 2016;17:1158–1170.

22. Strnad V, Ott OJ, Hildebrandt G, et al. 5-year results of accelerated partial breast irradiation using sole interstitial multicatheter brachytherapy versus whole-breast irradiation with boost after breast-conserving surgery for low-risk invasive and in-situ carcinoma of the female breast: a randomised, phase 3, non-inferiority trial. *Lancet.* 2016;387: 229–238.

23. Veronesi U, Orecchia R, Maisonneuve P, et al. Intraoperative radiotherapy versus external radiotherapy for early breast cancer (ELIOT): a randomised controlled equivalence trial. *Lancet Oncol.* 2013;14:1269–1277.

24. Vaidya JS, Wenz F, Bulsara M, et al. Risk-adapted targeted intraoperative radiotherapy versus whole-breast radiotherapy for breast cancer: 5-year results for local control and overall survival from the TARGIT—a randomised trial. *Lancet.* 2013;383:603–613.

25. Sperk E, Welzel G, Keller A, et al. Late radiation toxicity after intraoperative radiotherapy (IORT) for breast cancer: results from the randomized phase III trial TARGIT A. *Breast Cancer Res Treat.* 2012;135:253–260.

26. Bartelink H, Horiot JC, Poortmans PM, et al. Impact of a higher radiation dose on local control and survival in breast-conserving therapy of early breast cancer: 10-year results of the randomized boost versus no boost EORTC 22881-10882 trial. *J Clin Oncol.* 2007;25:3259–3265.

27. Sedlmayer F, Fastner G, Merz F, et al. IORT with electrons as boost strategy during breast conserving therapy in limited stage breast cancer: results of an ISIORT pooled analysis. *Strahlenther Onkol.* 2007;183(2, theme issue):32–34.

28. Sedlmayer F, Fastner G, Merz F, et al. ISIORT pooled analysis on linac-based IORT as boost strategy during breast conserving therapy. *Rev Cancer.* 2008;22:21–22.

29. Fastner G, Sedlmayer F, Merz F, et al. IORT with electrons as boost strategy during breast conserving therapy in limited stage breast cancer: long term results of an ISIORT pooled analysis. *Radiother Oncol.* 2013;108:279–286.

30. Vaidya JS, Baum M, Tobias JS, et al. Long-term results of targeted intraoperative radiotherapy (Targit) boost during breast-conserving surgery. *Int J Radiat Oncol Biol Phys.* 2011;81:1091–1097.

31. Reni M, Panucci MG, Ferreri AJ, et al. Effect on local control and survival of electron beam intraoperative irradiation for resectable pancreatic adenocarcinoma. *Int J Radiat Oncol Biol Phys.* 2001;50:651–658.

32. Ogawa K, Karasawa K, Ito Y, et al. Intraoperative radiotherapy for resected pancreatic cancer: a multi-institutional retrospective analysis of 210 patients. *Int J Radiat Oncol Biol Phys.* 2010;77:734–742.

33. Valentini V, Calvo F, Reni M, et al. Intra-operative radiotherapy (IORT) in pancreatic cancer: joint analysis of the ISIORT-Europe experience. *Radiother Oncol.* 2009;91:54–59.

34. Willett CG, Del Castillo CF, Shih HA, et al. Long-term results of intraoperative electron beam irradiation (IOERT) for patients with unresectable pancreatic cancer. *Ann Surg.* 2005;241:295–299.

35. Cai S, Hong TS, Goldberg SI, et al. Updated long-term outcomes and prognostic factors for patients with unresectable locally advanced pancreatic cancer treated with intraoperative radiotherapy at the Massachusetts General Hospital, 1978 to 2010. *Cancer*. 2013; 119:4196–4204.

36. Roldan GE, Gunderson LL, Nagorney DM, et al. External beam versus intraoperative and external beam irradiation for locally advanced pancreatic cancer. *Cancer*. 1988;61: 1110–1116.

37. Shipley WU, Wood WC, Tepper JE, et al. Intraoperative electron beam irradiation for patients with unresectable pancreatic carcinoma. *Ann Surg*. 1984;200:289–296.

38. Shibamoto Y, Manabe T, Ohshio G, et al. High-dose intraoperative radiotherapy for unresectable pancreatic cancer. *Int J Radiat Oncol Biol Phys*. 1996;34:57–63.

39. Sindelar WF, Kinsella TJ, Chen P. Intraoperative radiotherapy and retroperitoneal sarcomas final results of a prospective, randomized, clinical trial. *Arch Surg*. 1993;128:402–410.

40. Petersen IA, Haddock MG, Donohue JH, et al. Use of intraoperative electron beam radiotherapy in the management of retroperitoneal soft tissue sarcomas. *Int J Radiat Oncol Biol Phys*. 2002;52:469–475.

41. Petersen IA, Haddock M, Stafford S, et al. Use of intraoperative radiation therapy for retroperioneal sarcomas: update of the Mayo Clinic Rochester experience. *Rev Cancer*. 2008;22.

42. Gieschen HL, Spiro IJ, Suit HD, et al. Long-term results of intraoperative electron beam radiotherapy for primary and recurrent retroperitoneal soft tissue sarcoma. *Int J Radiat Oncol Biol Phys*. 2001;50:127–131.

43. Pierie JP, Betensky RA, Choudry U, et al. Outcomes in a series of 103 retroperitoneal sarcomas. *Eur J Surg Oncol*. 2006;32:1235–1241.

44. Krempien R, Roeder F, Buchler MW, et al. Intraoperative radiation therapy (IORT) for primary and recurrent retroperitoneal soft tissue sarcoma: first results of a pooled analysis. *Cancer*. ISIORT. 2008; Madrid: 56.

45. Gunderson LL, Nagorney DM, McIlrath DC, et al. External beam and intraoperative electron irradiation for locally advanced soft tissue sarcomas. *Int J Radiat Oncol Biol Phys*. 1993;25:647–656.

46. Calvo F, Azinovic I, Martinez R, et al. Intraoperative radiotherapy for the treatment of soft tissue sarcomas of central anatomic sites [abstract]. *IORT 94 5th International Symposium Abstracts*. 1994:4.

47. Dubois JB, Hay MH, Gely S, et al. Intraoperative radiation therapy (IORT) in soft tissue sarcoma [abstract]. *IORT 94 5th International Symposium Abstracts*. 1994.

48. Roeder F, Ulrich A, Habl G, et al. Clinical phase I/II trial to investigate preoperative dose-escalated intensity-modulated radiation therapy (IMRT) and intraoperative radiation therapy (IORT) in patients with retroperitoneal soft tissue sarcoma: interim analysis. *BMC Cancer*. 2014;14:617.

49. Haddock MG, Petersen IA, Webb MJ, et al. IORT for locally advanced gynecological malignancies. *Front Radiat Ther Oncol*. 1997;31:256–259.

50. Haddock M, Petersen IA, Webb MJ, et al. Intraoperative radiation therapy for locally advanced gynecological (GYN) malignancies. Paper presented at: 3rd International ISIORT Meeting; 2002; Aachen, Germany.

51. Haddock M, ed. Intraoperative radiation therapy for locally advanced gynecologic malignancies. In: *ISIORT*. 2005.

52. Willett CG, Shellito PC, Tepper JE, et al. Intraoperative electron beam radiation therapy for primary locally advanced rectal and rectosigmoid carcinoma. *J Clin Oncol*. 1991;9:843–849.

53. Mathis KL, Miller R, Nelson H, et al. Unresectable colorectal cancer can be cured with multimodality therapy. *Ann Surg.* 2008;248:592–598.

54. Suzuki K, Gunderson LL, Devine RM, et al. Intraoperative irradiation after palliative surgery for locally recurrent rectal cancer. *Cancer.* 1995;75:939–952.

55. Willett CG, Shellito PC, Tepper JE, et al. Intraoperative electron beam radiation therapy for recurrent locally advanced rectal or rectosigmoid carcinoma. *Cancer.* 1991;67:1504–1508.

56. Dresen R, Goesns M, Martijm H, et al. Radical resection after IOERT containing multimodality treatment is an important determinant for outcomes in patients treated for locally recurrent rectal cancer. *ISIORT Rev Cancer.* 2008;22:45–46.

57. Wallace HJ III, Willett CG, Shellito PC, et al. Intraoperative radiation therapy for locally advanced recurrent rectal or rectosigmoid cancer. *J Surg Oncol.* 1995;60:122–127.

58. Abuchaibe O, Calvo FA, Azinovic I, et al. Intraoperative radiotherapy in locally advanced recurrent colorectal cancer. *Int J Radiat Oncol Biol Phys.* 1993;26:859–867.

# Nanomedicines 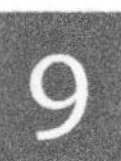

## DIAGNOSTIC AND THERAPEUTIC APPLICATIONS IN RADIATION ONCOLOGY

*Joseph M. Caster, Tian Zhang, Artish N. Patel,*
*Nichole J. Newman, and Andrew Z. Wang*



---

**List of Abbreviations**

| | |
|---|---|
| ALL | acute lymphoblastic leukemia |
| AML | acute myelogenous leukemia |
| AMR | ataxia telangiectasia mutated |
| APC | antigen-presenting cell |
| AUC | area under curve |
| CNS | central nervous system |
| CRT | chemoradiotherapy |
| CTLA-4 | cytotoxic T lymphocyte antigen 4 |
| EMA | European Medical Agency |
| EPR | enhanced permeability and retention effect |
| FDA | Food and drug Administration |
| FU | fluorouracil |
| GBM | glioblastoma multiforme |
| GCSF | granulocyte colony-stimulating factor |
| HAART | highly active antiretroviral therapy |
| HER2 | human epidermal growth factor receptor family 2 |
| IC50 | half maximal inhibitory concentration |
| KRAS | Kirstin rat sarcoma viral oncogene homologue |
| KS | Kaposi sarcoma |
| KSP | kinesin spindle protein |
| LH-RH | luteinizing hormone–releasing hormone |
| MBC | metastatic breast cancer |

| | |
|---|---|
| MMP | metalloproteinase |
| MTD | maximum tolerated dose |
| NIR | near infrared |
| NSCLC | non–small cell lung cancer |
| NP | nanoparticle |
| OI | optical imaging compound |
| ORR | overall response rate |
| OS | overall survival |
| PD-1 | Programmed cell death protein 1 |
| PFS | progression-free survival |
| pCR | complete response |
| PN | peripheral neuropathy |
| QD | quantom dot |
| RES | reticuloendothelial system |
| RRM2 | ribonucleotide reductase 2 |
| RT | radiotherapy |
| SBRT | stereotactic body radiation therapy |
| SPIONs | supraparamagnetic iron oxide NPs |
| STM | solid tumor malignancy |
| TNF | tissue necrosis factor |
| TTF | time to failure |
| TTP | time to progression |
| STM | Solid tumor malignancy |
| VEGF | vascular endothelial growth factor |

## INTRODUCTION

### Background

Broadly defined, *nanomedicine* refers to the application of nanoscale materials to health and medicine (1–2). Nanoscale medicines (ranging from a few to several hundred nanometers) are often referred to as *nanoparticles* (NPs). Specific entities referenced as NPs include liposomes, polymeric micelles, drug-polymer conjugates, drug-protein conjugates, dendrimers, quantum dots, quantum rods, bucky balls, carbon nanotubes, nanocrystals, inorganic nanostructures or emulsions, and "nano-viruses" (nanoparticle viral mimetics), among others. Figure 9.1 provides a schematic representation of different compounds classified as NPs.

NPs have been investigated for both therapeutic and diagnostic uses. The overwhelming majority of clinical experiences with NPs to date have been with therapeutic NPs. Many of the approved and experimental therapeutic NPs are

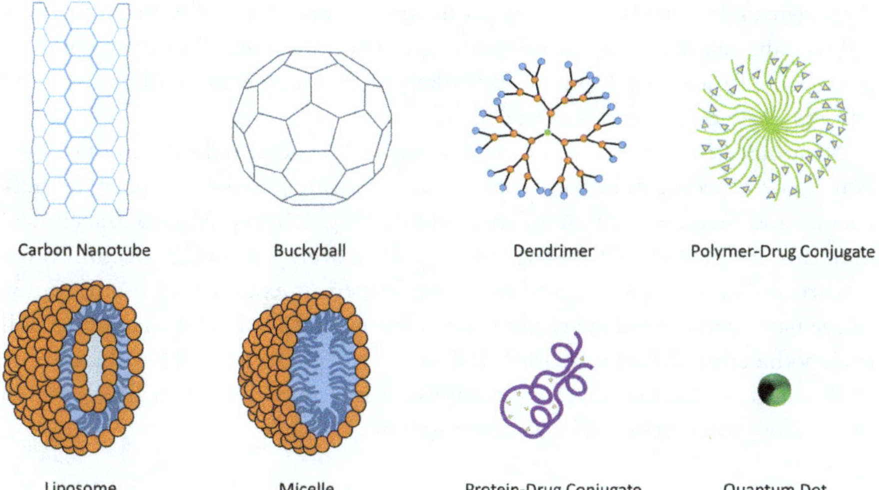


**FIGURE 9.1** Nanoparticle compounds

nanoformulations of approved drugs (3). NP formulation improves drug delivery by imparting favorable physical characteristics of the nanomaterial (polymer, protein, ion, etc) to the complex as a whole. These advantages include improved solubility; decreased renal clearance; protection against degradation; increased (or decreased) volume of distribution; increased half-life; and prolonged, sustained drug release. Many common chemotherapeutics are ideal candidates for NP drug delivery because they are hydrophobic, highly toxic, and/or unstable with short half-lives in vivo. NPs with inherent tissue specificity can also be generated to improve drug targeting. As material science continues to rapidly evolve, nanostructures can be finely tuned to maximize desired drug delivery characteristics.

NP drug formulation has been used to improve the pharmacokinetic profiles of a vast array of drug classes, including chemotherapeutics, immunomodulatory drugs, endocrine therapies, anesthetics, antibiotics, and central nervous system (CNS)-directed therapies. Clinical trials have been initiated for close to 300 nanomedicines and counting (4). Approximately one quarter of these have been developed for oncologic applications, of which almost 20 have gained regulatory approval from at least one major regulatory agency (5). Despite these achievements, the successful translation of nanomedicines still faces many challenges. The development of novel compounds is time-consuming and cost-intensive, and many of the experimental products currently in clinical trials are in direct competition with each other as well as other novel classes of therapeutics. It is likely that many promising experimental NPs will ultimately fail to gain regulatory approval. Still, given the sheer number of nanotherapeutics in clinical development, it is likely that at least some will be approved and regularly encountered in the clinic.

Nanomedicine must also continue to expand its potential roles in oncology. Nanoscale objects can be formulated with exquisite precision to provide therapeutic and diagnostic value independent of drug delivery. Most of the clinical literature is devoted to NP drug delivery. However, within the preclinical literature and early-phase clinical trials are numerous examples of useful, innovative nanomedicines that are not drug-delivery vectors. In this chapter we will review the clinical literature for NP drug delivery systems and highlight some of the most promising novel applications for nanomedicines that have entered or are close to entering clinical investigation.

## NANOMEDICINE IN ONCOLOGY

### Approved Nanotherapeutics in Oncology

NP drug delivery systems are particularly appealing for oncologic applications because they inherently provide a preferential accumulation of drugs within tumors. Normal capillaries are highly ordered structures that tightly regulate the diffusion of all but the very smallest of molecules. In contrast, tumor vasculature is abnormally leaky, with irregular gaps and pores through which nanoscale materials can readily penetrate (6). Furthermore, tumors have reduced lymphatic drainage, and once extravasated, materials are retained within extracellular tumor space. This phenomenon is referred to as *enhanced permeability and retention* (EPR) (7). It is worth noting that the clinical relevance of EPR has recently come under some scrutiny in the literature. Although EPR is easy to demonstrate in preclinical animal models, such as tumor xenografts, some authors have argued that spontaneous patient tumors are physiologically different from animal tumor models and may be less susceptible to EPR (8). Clinical experience has thus far demonstrated that NPs do preferentially accumulate in spontaneous human tumors, albeit less than animal models have predicted (9). Some NPs have been developed that incorporate specific molecular tags to improve tumor targeting (10). Preclinically, molecular targeting improves particle uptake and drug accumulation within tumors. However, clinical experience with targeted NPs is limited, and it remains to be seen if particle targeting provides any clinically meaningful advantages in patients.

Clinical experience with NP chemotherapeutics continues to expand rapidly. Approximately 20 Food and Drug Administration (FDA) or European Medical Agency (EMA) nanoformulations of drugs have been approved for use in clinical oncology, with many more in clinical trials. Several approved formulations are regularly encountered in the clinic. Some, such as Neulasta (a pegylated form of granulocyte colony-stimulating factor [GCSF]), are not regularly marketed as nanomedicines, and many clinicians may be unaware that they have been prescribing NP therapeutics for some time (11). Others have been aggressively highlighted as nanomedicines to distinguish them from existing formulations. Table 9.1 provides an overview of currently approved NP chemotherapeutics.

The overall clinical benefits of NP chemotherapeutics have been relatively consistent. We will review the clinical experiences of two such compounds, Doxil and Abraxane, to highlight the generalizable results of clinical nanomedicines in oncology. Doxil is a pegylated liposomal formulation of doxorubicin and was one of the seminal NP chemotherapeutics (12). Doxil was initially tested in patients with AIDS-related Kaposi sarcoma (KS). Doxil received accelerated approval for KS by the FDA following several phase II studies that showed promising response rates (a 70%–80% overall response rate [ORR]) with lower than expected rates of cardiotoxicity compared to traditional anthracycline regimens (13,14). The drug never gained full approval for KS, largely as a result of treatment being supplanted by highly active antiretroviral therapy (HAART) (15). However, following the accelerated approval, Doxil was also tested in patients with advanced multiple myeloma, as well as refractory breast and ovarian cancers. Doxil was given accelerated approval for the treatment of refractory ovarian cancer based on several phase II studies and the long-term follow-up of a noninferiority phase III trial of Doxil versus topotecan (16,17). This trial included 481 patients with metastatic ovarian cancer and did not meet the primary end point of improved time to progression (TTP). However, longer follow-up indicated an approximately 5% overall survival (OS) benefit in the Doxil group starting at about 18 months and maintained through follow-up (5 years). Doxil was never compared to standard doxorubicin in a randomized trial for ovarian cancer. However, the two were compared head-to-head in patients with metastatic breast cancer (MBC). A phase III noninferiority trial randomized 509 patients with MBC to 50 mg/m$^2$ of Doxil every 4 weeks or 60 mg/m$^2$ of doxorubicin every 3 weeks (18). The primary end points were progression-free survival (PFS) and cardiotoxicity. Doxil was no more efficacious than the free drug, and there were no differences in PFS or OS. However, the nanoformulation of Doxil did appreciably reduce the incidence of clinically significant cardiac events. The EMA approved Doxil for use with MBC patients at increased risk of cardiac events, but the drug never gained full FDA approval for this indication. Randomized trials with Myocet (a nonpegylated liposomal formulation of doxorubicin) yielded very similar results

**TABLE 9.1**  Approved nanomedicines in oncology

| Drug | Active drug | Nanoformulation | Indication | Manufacturer | Year approved |
| --- | --- | --- | --- | --- | --- |
| DOXIL | Doxorubicin | Pegylated liposomal | HIV-related KS, MBC, metastatic ovarian cancer, advanced multiple myeloma | Janssen | 1995 |
| Caelyx[1] | Doxorubicin | Pegylated liposomal | HIV-related KS, MBC, metastatic ovarian cancer, advanced multiple myeloma | Janssen | 1996 |
| Lipodox | Daunorubicin | Pegylated liposomal | HIV-related KS, metastatic ovarian cancer | Sun Pharma | 2013 |
| Daunoxome | Daunorubicin | Liposomal | HIV-related KS | Galen Limited | 1996 |
| DepoCyt(e) | Cytarabine | Liposomal | Lymphomatous Meningitis | Sigma-Tau | 2007 |
| Marqibo | Vincristine | Liposomal | Adult AML | Spectrum Pharma | 2012 |
| Myocet[1] | Doxorubicin | Liposomal | MBC | Enzon | 2000 |
| Abraxane | Paclitaxel | Albumin-bound | MBC, metastatic adenocarcinoma of the pancreas | Celgene | 2005 |
| Genexol-PM[2] | Paclitaxel | Polymeric micelle | MBC, advanced NSCLC | Sorrento | 2007 |
| Oncaspar | Pegaspargase | Pegylated asparaginase | ALL | Sigma-Tau | 1994 |
| Ontak | Denileukin Diftitox | Immunotoxin (fusion protein) | Cutaneous T cell lymphoma | Eisai | 2008 |
| Onivyde | Irinotecan | Liposomal | Metastatic pancreatic cancer | Merrimack Pharma | 2015 |

*Note:* ALL, acute lymphoblastic leukemia; AML, acute myelogenous leukemia; KS, Kaposi sarcoma; MBC, metastatic breast cancer; NSCLC, non–small cell lung cancer.

1. Approved in Europe.

2. Approved in South Korea.

in patients with MBC: decreased cardiotoxicity but no improvements in PFS or OS compared to free doxorubicin (19).

Abraxane (AB-007) is a formulation of paclitaxel conjugated to albumin (20). Although paclitaxel (Taxol) is a potent anticancer drug, it is plagued by poor solubility and the need for toxic solvents (cremophor) for in vivo administration (21). Cremophor-based Taxol is associated with clinically significant hypersensitivity reactions in 20% to 40% of patients and requires aggressive hydration and premedication (20). Albumin-bound paclitaxel (Abraxane) is a soluble, cremophor-free solution that demonstrated improved efficacy and decreased toxicity compared to solvent-based paclitaxel in preclinical tumor models (22). The FDA initially approved Abraxane for the treatment of MBC in 2005 following the results of a randomized controlled trial that randomized 460 patients with MBC to Abraxane (260 mg/m$^2$) or paclitaxel (175 mg/m$^2$) (23). There were modest improvements in clinical end points with Abraxane, including ORR (33% vs. 19%), median OS (56.4 weeks vs. 46.7 weeks), and TTP (24 weeks vs. 19.7 weeks). Grade IV neutropenia was less common with Abraxane (9% vs. 22%), but rates of grade II peripheral neuropathy were increased (10% vs. 2%).

Abraxane was next approved for the treatment of advanced (stage IIIB or IV) non–small cell lung cancer (NSCLC). This approval was largely based on the results of a trial that randomized 1,052 patients to either combination weekly Abraxane (100 mg/m$^2$) with carboplatin (area under the curve [AUC] = 6) or Taxol (200 mg/m$^2$) every 3 weeks with carboplatin (AUC = 6). The results of this study showed improved radiographic ORR (33% vs. 25%), median PFS (6.3 months vs. 5.8 months), and median OS (12.1 months vs 11.2 months) with Abraxane compared to solvent-based Taxol (24). Peripheral neuropathy and neutropenia were both less common with Abraxane than Taxol. Abraxane has also been approved in combination therapy with gemcitabine for the treatment of metastatic adenocarcinoma of the pancreas (25).

As a whole, the collective experiences with NP chemotherapeutics have produced remarkably similar results. Table 9.2 highlights the results of phase III trials that supported the approval of several nanomedicines. The most consistently achieved clinical benefits are reductions in dose–limiting toxicities. It is worth noting that not all toxicities are decreased with nanoformulation. Because NPs have higher MTDs, patients are often treated with much higher equivalent drug doses. As a result, certain toxicities, such as peripheral neuropathy (taxanes), are occasionally more common in the NP treatment arms. In addition to decreased toxicity, the majority of NPs have also demonstrated some improvements in clinical efficacy compared to free drugs. Although these improvements may be modest, they are comparable to the historical benefits obtained with novel compounds tested in patients with treatment refractory

**TABLE 9.2**  Phase III trials comparing NP and free drug formulations

| Drug | Trial | # Patients | Disease | Treatment | Outcomes |
|---|---|---|---|---|---|
| Abraxane | Socinski et al | 1052 | Advanced NSCLC | Abraxane + carboplatin vs. Taxol + carboplatin | PFS: 6.3 vs. 5.8 months OS: 12.1 vs. 11.2 months Gr III/IV PN: 3% vs. 12% Gr III/IV NP: 47% vs. 56% |
| | Gradisher et al | 460 | MBC | Abraxane vs. Cremophor EL–based | TTP: 23 vs. 16.9 weeks OS: 56.4 vs. 46.7 weeks Gr IV NP: 9% vs. 22% |
| Myocet | Chan et al | 160 | MBC | Myocet vs. epirubicin | TTF: 5.7 vs. 4.4 months TTP: 7.7 vs. 5.6 months OS: 18.3 vs. 16 months |
| DOXIL | O'Brien et al | 509 | MBC | Doxil vs. free doxorubicin | PFS: 7.8 vs. 6.9 months OS: 22 vs. 21 months NP: 4% vs. 10% |
| Daunoxome | Gill et al | 232 | AIDS-related Kaposi sarcoma | Daunoxome vs. ABV | Gr IV NP: 5% vs. 15% MS: 369 vs. 342 days |

*Note:* MBC, metastatic breast cancer; MS, median survival; NP, neutropenia; NSCLC, non–small cell lung cancer; OS, overall survival; PFS, progression-free survival; PN, peripheral neuropathy; TTF, time to treatment failure; TTP, time to progression.

metastatic tumors. Thus, clinical experience with nanomedicines has correlated well with preclinical studies, demonstrating an improvement in the therapeutic index.

### Investigational Nanotherapeutics in Oncology

A diverse array of nanomedicines is currently under clinical development in the field of oncology. Table 9.3 lists all the chemotherapeutic nanomedicines currently in clinical trials. The clinical status of all these compounds has been reviewed in detail elsewhere (3). With advances in the material sciences, novel NPs can be carefully and rapidly fine-tuned for specific applications. Several experimental particles have characteristics that articulately highlight the novel

**TABLE 9.3**  Nanochemotherapeutics currently in clinical development

| Drug | Active drug | Nanoformulation | Investigational use | Company | Clinical phase |
|---|---|---|---|---|---|
| Onco TCS | Vincristine | Liposome | Hodgkin lymphoma | INEX | III |
| Thermodox | Doxorubicin | Liposome | Metastatic malignant melanoma, liver cancer | Celsion Corp. | III |
| Xyotax/ Opaxio | Paclitaxel | Poliglumex | Lung cancer, ovarian cancer | CTI BioPharma | III |
| Livatag | Doxorubicin | Transdrug™ | Hepatocellular carcinoma | Onxeo | III |
| Promitil | Mitomycin-C | Liposomal | Advanced STMs | Lipomedix | I |
| Cynviloq | Paclitaxel | Polymeric micelle | MBC, advanced NSCLC | NantWorks | III |
| NK105 | Paclitaxel | Polymeric micelle | Various cancers | Nippon Kayaku Co., Ltd. | III |
| CRLX-101 | Camptothecin | Cyclodextran conjugated | Advanced STMs, rectal cancer | Cerulean Pharma | II |
| LE-SN38 | SN38 | Liposomal | Colorectal cancer | NeoPharm | II |
| MM-302 | Doxorubicin | Liposomal | MBC | Merrimack | II |
| IHL-305 | Irinotecan | Liposomal | Advanced STMs | Yakult Honsha | I |
| Nanoplatin (NC-6004) | Cisplatin | Polymeric micelle | Advanced STMs | Orient Europharma | II/III |
| DTX-SPL8783 | Docetaxel | Dendrimer conjugated | Advanced STMs | Starpharma | I |
| CRLX-301 | Docetaxel | Polymer conjugated | Refractory tumors | Cerulean | I/II |
| NC-4016 | Oxaliplatin | Polymeric micelle | Advanced STMs | NanoCarrier | I |

*Note:* GBM, glioblastoma multiforme; MBC, metastatic breast cancer; STM, solid tumor malignancy; NSCLC, non–small cell lung cancer.

potential of emerging nanomedicines. Here, we will review several clinically relevant compounds that demonstrate unique characteristics to exploit with nanomedicine.

One way to improve the target specificity of drugs is to utilize prodrugs, which are inactive until converted to an active form within tumors. Therapeutic prodrugs have been utilized for many years. However, with traditional drug delivery, only a small portion of the total drug administered makes it to the intended location. The excess drug is either wasted or partially activated at nonspecific sites, which increases treatment toxicity. Promitil is a pegylated-liposomal particle conjugated to a mitomycin C prodrug via a cleavable disulfide linker (26). The active drug is only released once the linker is cleaved by reducing substances such as glutathione, which are found in substantially higher concentrations within tumors than normal tissues. NPs such as Promitil can maximize tumor specificity by utilizing both passive tumor targeting (via EPR) and drug activation within the tumor microenvironment. Inducible drugs such as Promitil offer another intriguing therapeutic potential. Tumors release high concentrations of reducing agents in response to targeted therapies, such as conformal radiation. Therefore, it may be possible to engineer particles that enable a treatment-stimulated drug release to further enhance the synergy of combined modalities and decrease off-target effects.

Monoagent chemotherapy is virtually never used alone in the definitive setting. Chemotherapies are generally used in combination with other agents that have synergistic mechanisms of action. Optimal treatment conditions, including specific molar ratios and sequences of drug exposure, can be identified in vitro. Unfortunately, with traditional drug-delivery methods, it is difficult to maintain such specific delivery characteristics on a tissue or cellular level. With nanomedicines, it is possible to coencapsulate multiple drugs within a single carrier at fixed ratios with finely tuned release rates. This method ensures that tissues and cells exposed to one drug are also exposed to the other under the prespecified conditions. Preclinically, coencapsulation provides superior tumor control compared to the administration of free drugs or the concurrent administration of single-drug NPs. CPX-351 is a liposomal formulation that delivers cytarabine and daunorubicin in a 5:1 fixed molar ratio for the treatment of acute myelogenous leukemia (AML) (27). Several phase II studies have been completed, and response rates appear significantly higher than historic controls using standard cytarabine and daunorubicin, particularly in high-risk patients (28). A phase III trial is currently accruing patients (29).

Nanomedicines are also being developed to deliver biological agents. Tissue necrosis factor (TNF) alpha is a very potent cytotoxin that, as its name implies, mediates cell death signaling pathways (30). TNFα has almost no clinical utility because it causes profound systemic toxicities. Its current clinical utility is restricted to single-limb perfusion to reduce systemic exposure (31). Several gold NP TNF conjugates have been generated. Aurimune (CYT-6091) is a pegylated gold NP conjugate of TNFα that has progressed to early-phase trials. Pegylation is necessary to avoid rapid clearance by the reticuloendothelial system (RES). A phase I trial of patients with advanced tumors showed no clinically significant infusion reactions (32). Only two patients developed diastolic blood pressure readings that were outside the normal limits for the study. Phase II trials are currently accruing patients to assess Aurimune's therapeutic efficacy.

Another emerging technique is the generation of NPs composed of therapeutically active subunits that do not require any payload. Particles composed of high Z materials, including gold and hafnium oxide, are potent radiosensitizers that release substantial amounts of energy (heat) when exposed to high-energy ionizing radiation (33). NBTXR3 is a hafnium oxide NP given as a direct intratumoral injection to enhance tumor radiosensitivity. It is being tested in phase I trials of patients with head and neck cancers (34). Although they are not oncologic, particles composed of potent antimicrobial subunits, including the dendrimer-based Vivagel and the highly charged quaternary ammonium polyethyleneimine-based polymers, have been used in clinical settings (35,36). Utilizing active subunit particles simultaneously as drug carriers and active agents can further enhance their efficacy.

## Diagnostic Nanomedicines

Diagnostic NPs are not regularly encountered in the clinic. However, a strong need exists for novel imaging modalities with improved sensitivity in order to better stage patients and to more accurately evaluate treatment responses. Addressing these diagnostic shortcomings is essential to improving treatment recommendations, such as the use of adjuvant therapies or the omission of intense local therapies in metastatic patients. NPs are appealing as imaging agents because they can be finely tuned to incorporate targeting and imagable moieties in stable platforms (37). Several experimental compounds appear promising and have enabled the reproducible visualization of submillimeter tumors, which is not possible with modern imaging modalities (PET–CT or MRI).

The earliest diagnostic NPs were high Z elements, such as iron oxide (referred to as *supraparamagnetic iron oxide NPs* [SPIONs]), largely developed for use as contrast agents in the 1990s (38). Several specific compounds were thoroughly studied, but ultimately only a few gained regulatory approval because they were not clearly superior to other contrast modalities (39,40). One limitation to bare SPIONs is that they are only poorly taken up by tumor cells. Several groups have demonstrated that the conjugation of specific tags that target cell surface receptors (human epidermal growth factor receptor family 2 [HER2], luteinizing hormone–releasing hormone [LH–RH], folate, glial markers, etc) markedly enhances SPION intracellular uptake and improves the sensitivity of in vivo tumor imaging. Gold-based NPs and gadolinium-conjugated dendrimeric NPs are also being extensively investigated as metallic imaging agents.

Optimal imaging compounds (OIs) represent the other major class of imaging agents. These compounds utilize fluorescent or bioluminescent properties to enable in vivo imaging. Molecular imaging, the incorporation of OIs with specific molecular probes, has been an area of intense research interest for many years. The translation of OIs has largely been inhibited by issues with in vivo delivery. The majority of OIs have very short half-lives and are poorly taken up by target cells, which limits their exposure to intracellular targets. NP-based OIs are promising because they have long half-lives and can incorporate additional signals to facilitate intracellular delivery. The quantum dot (QD) is one popular NP OI system (41). These particles are composed of semiconducting nanocrystals with broad fluorescent spectra. QDs are frequently coated with polymeric or lipid (lipodots) shells to prevent enzymatic degradation and improve in vivo half-life. Preclinical models have incorporated various tags to QDs and have enabled the sensitive imaging of breast, ovarian, pancreatic, lung, and prostate cancers with virtually no measurable toxicity and favorable pharmacokinetic profiles (42).

Near-infrared (NIR) polymeric NPs have also received attention as OIs (43). Tumor-targeting polymeric NP OIs have promising sensitivities in preclinical models. In one instance a Cy5-labeled dendrimer detected micrometastatic deposits down to 200 microns (0.2 mm) in diameter. Functional polymeric OIs are also being developed to identify cell lineage or assess the levels of specific cell signaling pathways in vivo. Probes can be designed so that specific intracellular enzymes, such as metalloproteinases (MMPs) or caspases, can quench or activate them.

## CHALLENGES AND OPPORTUNITIES

In many respects, NP drug delivery has been a success story. A number of compounds have received approval and are frequently encountered in the clinic. Many more are currently undergoing clinical development. Despite these achievements, enthusiasm for NP chemotherapeutics has waned somewhat in recent years. One of the major criticisms of NP chemotherapeutics is that they have not yet been "game changers." Most of the clinical benefits achieved to date have been reductions in toxicity as opposed to improvements in efficacy. Many clinicians have expressed disappointment that NPs have failed to significantly change the overall clinical course of patients with advanced cancers. Viewed in the appropriate context, the collective clinical experiences with NPs are not at all surprising, and disappointment can be tempered by opportunity.

Chemotherapy alone is rarely curative for macroscopic solid tumors. Dose reductions for toxicity can limit the efficacy of chemotherapy. However, inadequate drug dosing is not the primary reason chemotherapeutics ultimately fail to control solid tumors. A number of well- characterized mechanisms cause tumors to resist chemotherapy, including the loss of molecular targets, the upregulation of alternate signaling pathways, the expression of drug efflux pumps, et cetera. Simply increasing the dose or duration of drug exposure is unlikely to overcome many of these resistance mechanisms. Even in the simplest in vitro model systems, it is difficult to achieve greater than two to three logs of tumor cell kills using chemotherapy alone without large increases in drug doses (generally orders of magnitude above the half maximal inhibitory concentration [$IC_{50}$]). It is simply not realistic to assume that improvements in drug delivery will result in sufficient amounts of cell killing in vivo to produce higher cure rates in patients with advanced cancer treated with chemotherapy alone. Accordingly, the pivotal trials for successful NPs, such as Abraxane and Doxil, were primarily designed to show equivalent efficacy (noninferiority) or modest improvements in PFS. The principal hypothesis was that nanoformulations would be *at least* as effective as small molecule drugs but less toxic. These drugs were not expected to dramatically alter the course of metastatic disease. The goal of these early trials was to show some measurable clinical benefit to gain regulatory approval. The long-term clinical benefits of NPs, as with virtually all chemotherapeutics, will most likely be realized when utilized in potentially curable patients in whom modest improvements in tumor cell killing could directly translate into improved cure rates or long-term tumor control.

The continued development of nanoformulations of approved chemotherapeutics is likely of limited value. The majority of ideal candidates for nanoformulation (poorly soluble and highly toxic) have already been tried, often in multiple platforms. "Improved" formulations of drugs such as paclitaxel and doxorubicin will face a more rigorous approval process. Whereas early NPs, such as Abraxane and Doxil, could gain approval by demonstrating improvements compared to small molecule equivalents, newer formulations will need to exhibit some meaningful benefits above those obtained with existing NPs. A more fruitful approach for NP drug delivery may be the up-front nanoformulation of novel chemotherapeutics.

Perhaps the most promising strategy for nanomedicine as a field is to move beyond simple drug delivery. Nanomedicine has many opportunities to help translate potentially paradigm-shifting experimental therapies. Nucleic acid–based therapies are one such class of technology. The ability to alter gene expression using methods such as siRNA, RNAi, and mRNA delivery has been experimentally possible for well over a decade. However, barriers to in vivo delivery have proven difficult to overcome. Nucleic acids must be protected from degradation, targeted to the appropriate cell types, and taken up by the target cell without destroying the cargo in the process. NPs can be finely tuned to accomplish many of these goals, and clinical experience with NP–based nucleic acid therapies is rapidly expanding. Early experiences were trying, and the development of several compounds, including CALAA-01 (an RRM2-targeting therapy), was terminated because signal alteration was both limited and transient

**TABLE 9.4**  Nucleic acid–based nanomedicines for oncology in clinical trials

| Compound | Gene target | Disease treated | Current trial phase | Clinical identifier |
|---|---|---|---|---|
| SGT-53 | P53 | Adult, pediatric tumors | Phase II | NCT02340156 |
| siG12D-LODER | KRAS | Pancreatic cancer | Phase II | NCT01676259 |
| ALN-VSP | KSP and VEGF | Solid tumor malignancies | Phase I (extension trial recently completed) | NCT01158079 |
| CALAA-01 | RRM2 | Solid tumor malignancies | Phase 1 (terminated) | NCT00689065 |
| EphA2-DOPC | EphAS | Recurrent solid tumors | Phase I | NCT01591356 |
| miR-RX34 | RX34 microRNA | Solid tumor malignancies | Phase I | NCT01829971 |
| DOTAP-Chol-Fus1 | Fus1 gene (insertion) | NSCLC | Phase I | NCT00059605 |
| DC-Chol-EGFR | EGFR | Oral squamous cell carcinoma | Phase I | NCT00009841 |
| LErafAON | cRaf | Solid tumor malignancies | Phase I | NCT00024648 |
| siRNA-EphA2-DOPC | EphA2 | Advanced cancers | Phase I | NCT01591356 |
| Atu027 | PKN3 | Solid tumors | Phase I | NCT00938574 |
| TKM-080301 | PLK1 | Cancer | Phase I | NCT01262235 |

*Note:* KRAS, Kirstin rat sarcoma viral oncogene homologue; KSP, kinesin spindle protein; RRM2, ribonucleotide reductase 2; VEGF, vascular endothelial growth factor.

(44). However, the community has built on early experiences, and several promising compounds have achieved potent, long-lasting target knock down, progressing to late-stage clinical trials (45). Table 9.4 describes the many nucleic acid–based nanomedicines currently in clinical development.

Immune-modulating therapies are currently viewed by many as the future of advanced cancer therapies. Checkpoint inhibitors, including the specific inhibitors of cytotoxic T lymphocyte antigen 4 (CTLA-4) and programmed cell death protein 1 (PD-1), have demonstrated curative potential in patients with metastatic "immunologically responsive" cancers, including melanoma and NSCLC (46,47). Excitement about these breakthrough treatments is warranted, as very few therapies have ever shown curative potential in patients with widely metastatic disease (48). Unfortunately, long-term cures remain the exception and are rarely achieved in more than 10% to 20% of patients. Successfully mounting an immunologic response to a specific stimulus is a tightly regulated process that requires multiple signals and that can be modulated by host and target factors at almost every step. Maximizing this process will require coordinated signaling events at specified intervals. Nanocarriers have the potential to maintain the spatial and temporal arrangement of multiple targeted signals. Rationally designed compounds may be able to more reproducibly harness the full potential of immunologically based cancer therapies (49).

## NANOMEDICINE AND RADIATION ONCOLOGY

The futures of nanomedicine and radiation oncology may be closely linked in various ways. Many of the potential benefits of nanomedicines are complimentary to the needs of radiation oncology. The incorporation of NP chemotherapeutics into definitive chemoradiotherapy (CRT) paradigms could renew interest in NP drug delivery (50). Intense research efforts are currently identifying novel ways to improve the therapeutic index of CRT. Advances in radiation delivery methods, such as IMRT, have been helpful in reducing the toxicity associated with CRT. However, there is still a need for further improvement, and NP drug delivery may be ideally suited to this task. By preferentially accumulating in tumors, the NP formulations of radiosensitizers can preferentially sensitize tumors, instead of normal tissues, to radiotherapy (RT). Multiple preclinical models and early-phase clinical trials have demonstrated markedly reduced in-field normal tissue toxicity with nanoformulations. The combination of precise radiotherapy (such as with IMRT) and NP drug delivery represents a viable method to maximize the differences between tumor and normal tissue sensitivity to CRT.

Potently sensitizing NPs could be incorporated into CRT as a means to intensify treatment for tumors that are difficult to control locally. Many potent and toxic radiosensitizers have been developed, including specific inhibitors of key DNA repair proteins, such as ataxia telangiectasia mutated (ATM), ATM and Rad3 related (ATR), and DNApk. Appropriate concerns over normal tissue toxicity have limited the clinical utility of these promising agents in CRT. NP formulations of these potent radiosensitizers may provide better tumor control than reduced-dose regimens of traditional chemotherapeutics like cisplatin (51). In addition to use as single agents, there is strong interest in adding NP radiosensitizers to traditional free drug CRT protocols in an effort to maximize therapeutic efficacy. As an example, there is an ongoing clinical phase I/II trial incorporating CRLX101 (a drug-polymer conjugate of camptothecin) into

5-fluorouracil (FU)–based preoperative CRT for the treatment of locally advanced rectal cancer with a primary end point of pathologic complete response (pCR) at the time of surgical resection.

In contrast to chemotherapy alone, the clinical benefits of nanoformulation may not be limited to decreased toxicity. Preclinical experimental models suggest that nanoformulation could significantly increase the efficacy of CRT and improve clinical outcomes for patients with locally advanced diseases (52,53). In classical radiobiologic assays, small changes in drug concentration can markedly enhance radiation–induced cell killing on the order of two to three logs. It is relatively easy to achieve more than six logs of cell killing with modest doses of radiation and radiosensitizers in vitro. These observations suggest that under ideal conditions, improvements in drug delivery with nanoformulation could produce robust increases in tumor control in vivo. A large preclinical literature, which consistently demonstrates significantly improved therapeutic efficacy with NP CRT, supports this hypothesis. Clinical experiences with NP CRT are currently limited, and it remains to be seen if positive preclinical results will translate into clinically meaningful gains in patients.

Another potentially interesting role of nanomedicine in radiation oncology is in the use of theranostic NPs. Theranostic agents are both diagnostically and therapeutically useful. To date there are very few clinically useful theranostic devices. A number of groups are attempting to generate therapeutic NPs that can also be visualized on CT or MRI. This is frequently accomplished by utilizing inorganic particle scaffolds encapsulating chemotherapeutics (54,55). This strategy could be particularly fruitful in CRT. Inorganic NPs are generally formulated with high Z materials, such as iron, gold, and hafnium. High Z elements are potent radiosensitizers because they release a substantial amount of energy when exposed to high-frequency or ionizing radiation. In addition to being therapeutically useful, enhancing the visualization of tumors with theranostic NPs could also aid in assessing tumor responses and utilizing adaptive treatment planning during the course of radiation. The majority of theranostic NPs are currently still in preclinical development, and it will likely be quite some time before the clinical potential of these compounds is rigorously tested in humans (56).

Combined modality treatment will also be important to the successful use of nucleic acid–based therapy. The most effective formulations to date provide signal interference on the order of 4 to 6 weeks. The indefinite suppression of signaling would require the repeated administration of NPs. The lifetime limits of particle administration is currently unknown but would likely restrict this approach. Further, tumor resistance to treatment via alternative signaling pathways is almost guaranteed over time. A better approach may be to target specific pathways that transiently render tumors phenotypically more responsive to chemotherapy and radiation. Many naturally occurring phenotypes with favorable responses to therapy have been identified in subsets of patients, and it may be possible to convert wild-type tumors to the more favorable subtype with transient nucleic acid therapy. This approach could obviate the need for prolonged signal modulation and may circumvent tumor resistance mechanisms.

Nanomedicine also has the potential to improve the systemic efficacy of radiotherapy. The combined use of focused radiation (stereotactic body radiation therapy, or SBRT) with immune checkpoint inhibitors (including anti-CTLA-4 or anti-PD-1 therapies) has renewed interest in trying to clinically utilize the abscopal effect. This phenomenon was first observed almost 50 years ago. In very rare cases, focused radiation to a single site of disease is followed by the regression of distant disease that was not in the primary radiation field. For many years it was speculated that this resulted from the generation of a tumor-specific immune response stimulated by radiation therapy. A landmark case report of a patient with widely metastatic melanoma who developed tumor-specific antibodies and subsequent disease regression following palliative RT for a rib metastasis while on ipilimumab supported this hypothesis (57). Since that time, there has been an explosion of research focused on combining radiation and immunologic therapies to stimulate tumor-specific immune responses. The preclinical literature supports this as a feasible approach. Unfortunately, this phenomenon is difficult to trigger in patients, and the long-term safety of combining immune-modulating therapies with hypofractionated RT is almost completely unknown (58). As already discussed, the stimulation of a tumor-specific immune response requires robust antigen presentation and coordinated signaling events. NPs have the potential to improve the method of antigen capture and presentation to antigen-presenting cells (APCs) and coordinate T cell processes in a carefully designed manner.

## CONCLUSIONS

Nanomedicine has come a long way over its short history. Several NP drug carriers have gained regulatory approval, and many more are in clinical development. Although nanotherapeutics have yet to be game changers in oncology, they remain by and large untested in the definitive setting, and their full potential is thus unexplored. Therapeutic nanomedicines may be particularly useful when combined with other treatment modalities, including radiation therapy. Importantly, nanomedicines are poised to aid in the translation of novel therapies that may drastically alter the clinical course of patients with advanced or difficult-to-control cancers.

## References

1. Wagner V, Dullaart A, Bock AK, et al. The emerging nanomedicine landscape. *Nat Biotechnol.* 2006;24(10):1211–1217.

2. Webster TJ. Nanomedicine: what's in a definition? *Int J Nanomedicine.* 2006;1(2): 115–6.

3. Min Y, Caster JM, Eblan MJ, et al. Clinical Translation of Nanomedicine. *Chem Rev.* 2015;115(19):11147–11190.

4. Etheridge ML, Campbell SA, Erdman AG, et al. The big picture on nanomedicine: the state of investigational and approved nanomedicine products. *Nanomedicine.* 2013;9(1): 1–14.

5. Caster JM, Patel AN, Zhang T, et al. Investigational nanomedicines in 2016: a review of nanotherapeutics currently undergoing clinical trials. *Wiley Interdiscip Rev Nanomed Nanobiotechnol.* 2017;9(1). doi: 10.1002/wnan.1416. .

6. Jain RK, Safabakhsh N, Sckell A, et al. Endothelial cell death, angiogenesis, and microvascular function after castration in an androgen-dependent tumor: role of vascular endothelial growth factor. *Proc Natl Acad Sci U S A.* 1998;95(18):10820–10825.

7. Maeda H. Vascular permeability in cancer and infection as related to macromolecular drug delivery, with emphasis on the EPR effect for tumor-selective drug targeting. *Proc Jpn Acad Ser B Phys Biol Sci.* 2012;88(3):53–71.

8. Maeda H. Toward a full understanding of the EPR effect in primary and metastatic tumors as well as issues related to its heterogeneity. *Adv Drug Deliv Rev.* 2015;91(30):3–6.

9. Gabizon A, Catane R, Uziely B, et al. Prolonged circulation time and enhanced accumulation in malignant exudates of doxorubicin encapsulated in polyethylene-glycol coated liposomes. *Cancer Res.* 1994;54(4):987–992.

10. Salata O. Applications of nanoparticles in biology and medicine. *J Nanobiotechnology.* 2004;2(1):3.

11. Renwick W, Pettengell R, Green M. Use of filgrastim and pegfilgrastim to support delivery of chemotherapy: twenty years of clinical experience. *BioDrugs.* 2009;23(3):175–186.

12. Allen TM, Cullis PR. Liposomal drug delivery systems: from concept to clinical applications. *Adv Drug Deliv Rev.* 2013;65(1):36–48.

13. Barenholz Y. Doxil(R)--the first FDA-approved nano-drug: lessons learned. *J Control Release.* 2012;160(2):117–134.

14. Batist G, Ramakrishnan G, Rao CS, et al. Reduced cardiotoxicity and preserved antitumor efficacy of liposome-encapsulated doxorubicin and cyclophosphamide compared with conventional doxorubicin and cyclophosphamide in a randomized, multicenter trial of metastatic breast cancer. *J Clin Oncol.* 2001;19(5):1444–1454.

15. Martin-Carbonero L, Barrios A, Saballs P, et al. Pegylated liposomal doxorubicin plus highly active antiretroviral therapy versus highly active antiretroviral therapy alone in HIV patients with Kaposi's sarcoma. *AIDS.* 2004;18(12):1737–1740.

16. Gordon AN, Fleagle JT, Guthrie D, et al. Recurrent epithelial ovarian carcinoma: a randomized phase III study of pegylated liposomal doxorubicin versus topotecan. *J Clin Oncol.* 2001;19(14):3312–3322.

17. Gordon AN, Tonda M, Sun S, et al. Doxil Study I. Long-term survival advantage for women treated with pegylated liposomal doxorubicin compared with topotecan in a phase 3 randomized study of recurrent and refractory epithelial ovarian cancer. *Gynecol Oncol.* 2004;95(1):1–8.

18. O'Brien ME, Wigler N, Inbar M, et al. Reduced cardiotoxicity and comparable efficacy in a phase III trial of pegylated liposomal doxorubicin HCl (CAELYX/Doxil) versus con-

ventional doxorubicin for first-line treatment of metastatic breast cancer. *Ann Oncol.* 2004;15(3):440–449.

19. Chang HI, Yeh MK. Clinical development of liposome-based drugs: formulation, characterization, and therapeutic efficacy. *Int J Nanomedicine.* 2012;7:49–60.

20. Kundranda MN, Niu J. Albumin-bound paclitaxel in solid tumors: clinical development and future directions. *Drug Des Devel Ther.* 2015;9:3767–3777.

21. Wani MC, Taylor HL, Wall ME, et al. Plant antitumor agents. VI. The isolation and structure of taxol, a novel antileukemic and antitumor agent from Taxus brevifolia. *J Am Chem Soc.* 1971;93(9):2325–2327.

22. Desai N, Trieu V, Yao Z, et al. Increased antitumor activity, intratumor paclitaxel concentrations, and endothelial cell transport of cremophor-free, albumin-bound paclitaxel, ABI-007, compared with cremophor-based paclitaxel. *Clin Cancer Res.* 2006;12(4):1317–1324.

23. Gradishar WJ, Tjulandin S, Davidson N, et al. Phase III trial of nanoparticle albumin-bound paclitaxel compared with polyethylated castor oil-based paclitaxel in women with breast cancer. *J Clin Oncol.* 2005;23(31):7794–7803.

24. Socinski MA, Bondarenko I, Karaseva NA, et al. Weekly nab-paclitaxel in combination with carboplatin versus solvent-based paclitaxel plus carboplatin as first-line therapy in patients with advanced non-small-cell lung cancer: final results of a phase III trial. *J Clin Oncol.* 2012;30(17):2055–2062.

25. Heinemann V, Boeck S, Hinke A, et al. Meta-analysis of randomized trials: evaluation of benefit from gemcitabine-based combination chemotherapy applied in advanced pancreatic cancer. *BMC Cancer.* 2008;8:82.

26. Gabizon A, Amitay Y, Tzemach D, et al. Therapeutic efficacy of a lipid-based prodrug of mitomycin C in pegylated liposomes: studies with human gastro-entero-pancreatic ectopic tumor models. *J Control Release.* 2012;160(2):245–253.

27. Tardi P, Johnstone S, Harasym N, et al. In vivo maintenance of synergistic cytarabine:daunorubicin ratios greatly enhances therapeutic efficacy. *Leuk Res.* 2009; 33(1):129–139.

28. Lancet JE, Cortes JE, Hogge DE, et al. Phase 2 trial of CPX-351, a fixed 5:1 molar ratio of cytarabine/daunorubicin, vs cytarabine/daunorubicin in older adults with untreated AML. *Blood.* 2014;123(21):3239–3246.

29. Carol H, Fan MM, Harasym TO, et al. Efficacy of CPX-351, (cytarabine:daunorubicin) liposome injection, against acute lymphoblastic leukemia (ALL) xenograft models of the Pediatric Preclinical Testing Program. *Pediatr Blood Cancer.* 2015;62(1):65–71.

30. Watanabe N, Niitsu Y, Umeno H, et al. Toxic effect of tumor necrosis factor on tumor vasculature in mice. *Cancer Res.* 1988;48(8):2179–2183.

31. Verhoef C, de Wilt JH, Grunhagen DJ, et al. Isolated limb perfusion with melphalan and TNF-alpha in the treatment of extremity sarcoma. *Curr Treat Options Oncol.* 2007;8(6):417–427.

32. Libutti SK, Paciotti GF, Byrnes AA, et al. Phase I and pharmacokinetic studies of CYT-6091, a novel PEGylated colloidal gold-rhTNF nanomedicine. *Clin Cancer Res.* 2010; 16(24):6139–6149.

33. Dreaden EC, Mackey MA, Huang X, et al. Beating cancer in multiple ways using nano-gold. *Chem Soc Rev.* 2011;40(7):3391–3404.

34. Maggiorella L, Barouch G, Devaux C, et al. Nanoscale radiotherapy with hafnium oxide nanoparticles. *Future Oncol.* 2012;8(9):1167–1181.

35. McCarthy TD, Karellas P, Henderson SA, et al. Dendrimers as drugs: discovery and preclinical and clinical development of dendrimer-based microbicides for HIV and STI prevention. *Mol Pharm.* 2005;2(4):312–318.

36. Pietrokovski Y, Nisimov I, Kesler-Shvero D, et al. Antibacterial effect of composite resin foundation material incorporating quaternary ammonium polyethyleneimine nanoparticles. *J Prosthet Dent.* 2016;116(4):603–609.

37. Esposito C, Crema A, Ponzetto A, et al. Multifunctional anti-cancer nano-platforms are moving to clinical trials. *Curr Drug Metab.* 2013;14(5):583–604.

38. Reddy LH, Arias JL, Nicolas J, et al. Magnetic nanoparticles: design and characterization, toxicity and biocompatibility, pharmaceutical and biomedical applications. *Chem Rev.* 2012;112(11):5818–5878.

39. McLachlan SJ, Morris MR, Lucas MA, et al. Phase I clinical evaluation of a new iron oxide MR contrast agent. *J Magn Reson Imaging.* 1994;4(3):301–307.

40. Bellin MF, Roy C, Kinkel K, et al. Lymph node metastases: safety and effectiveness of MR imaging with ultrasmall superparamagnetic iron oxide particles—initial clinical experience. *Radiology.* 1998;207(3):799–808.

41. Zhu Y, Hong H, Xu ZP, et al. Quantum dot-based nanoprobes for in vivo targeted imaging. *Curr Mol Med.* 2013;13(10):1549–1567.

42. Chen C, Peng J, Sun SR, et al. Tapping the potential of quantum dots for personalized oncology: current status and future perspectives. *Nanomedicine (Lond).* 2012;7(3):411–428.

43. Shan L. Gold/Silica Nanoparticles With a Near-Infrared Fluorescent and Pegylated Paramagnetic Lipid Coating. Bethesda, MD: Molecular Imaging and Contrast Agent Database (MICAD); 2004.

44. Davis ME. The first targeted delivery of siRNA in humans via a self-assembling, cyclodextrin polymer-based nanoparticle: from concept to clinic. *Mol Pharm.* 2009;6(3):659–668.

45. Pan DW, Davis ME. Cationic Mucic Acid Polymer-Based siRNA Delivery Systems. *Bioconjug Chem.* 2015;26(8):1791–1803.

46. Azijli K, Stelloo E, Peters GJ, et al. New developments in the treatment of metastatic melanoma: immune checkpoint inhibitors and targeted therapies. *Anticancer Res.* 2014;34(4):1493–1505.

47. Forde PM, Reiss KA, Zeidan AM, et al. What lies within: novel strategies in immunotherapy for non-small cell lung cancer. *Oncologist.* 2013;18(11):1203–1213.

48. Yang Y. Cancer immunotherapy: harnessing the immune system to battle cancer. *J Clin Invest.* 2015;125(9):3335–3337.

49. Shao K, Singha S, Clemente-Casares X, et al. Nanoparticle-based immunotherapy for cancer. *ACS Nano.* 2015;9(1):16–30.

50. Eblan MJ, Wang AZ. Improving chemoradiotherapy with nanoparticle therapeutics. *Transl Cancer Res.* 2013;2(4):320–329.

51. Tian X, Lara H, Wagner KT, et al. Improving DNA double-strand repair inhibitor KU55933 therapeutic index in cancer radiotherapy using nanoparticle drug delivery. *Nanoscale.* 2015;7(47):20211–20219.

52. Caster JM, Sethi M, Kowalczyk S, et al. Nanoparticle delivery of chemosensitizers improve chemotherapy efficacy without incurring additional toxicity. *Nanoscale.* 2015;7(6):2805–2811.

53. Sethi M, Sukumar R, Karve S, et al. Effect of drug release kinetics on nanoparticle therapeutic efficacy and toxicity. *Nanoscale.* 2014;6(4):2321–2327.

54. Sivakumar B, Aswathy RG, Nagaoka Y, et al. Multifunctional carboxymethyl cellulose-based magnetic nanovector as a theragnostic system for folate receptor targeted chemotherapy, imaging, and hyperthermia against cancer. *Langmuir.* 2013;29(10):3453–3466.

55. Gautier J, Allard-Vannier E, Herve-Aubert K, et al. Design strategies of hybrid metallic nanoparticles for theragnostic applications. *Nanotechnology.* 2013;24(43):432002.

56. Liu Y, Yin T, Feng Y, et al. Mammalian models of chemically induced primary malignancies exploitable for imaging-based preclinical theragnostic research. *Quant Imaging Med Surg.* 2015;5(5):708–729.
57. Postow MA, Callahan MK, Barker CA, et al. Immunologic correlates of the abscopal effect in a patient with melanoma. *N Engl J Med.* 2012;366(10):925–931.
58. Kaminski JM, Shinohara E, Summers JB, et al. The controversial abscopal effect. *Cancer Treat Rev.* 2005;31(3):159–172.

# Radiolabeled Spheres  10

*John Byun, John L. Nosher, and Salma K. Jabbour*

## INTRODUCTION

The use of infused and directed radiation sources has been well demonstrated historically. In 1947 Muller and Rossier treated lung metastases from renal cell carcinoma with zinc 63 and gold 198 in a patient with previous lung irradiation (1). This method utilized radioactive *microspheres*, inert carbon beads without specific antigen targeting that were conjugated to unsealed sources to enhance the local control of bronchial tumors (1). The interest in infusion-based, targeted radiation therapy has increased in the last few decades and has given rise to therapies such as radioembolization, which is frequently referred to as *selective internal radiation therapy* (SIRT).

Radioembolization offers unique advantages compared to external beam radiation, especially in the context of liver-dominant cancers. Although surgical resection offers the best chance for survival, only 20% of patients are candidates. External beam radiation may not be appropriate due to the volume, the number, or the location of liver cancers. Radioembolization provides a means to target liver cancer while relatively sparing normal liver tissue and addressing an otherwise unmet need.

## YTTRIUM 90 RADIOEMBOLIZATION AGENTS

Two major types of yttrium 90 (Y90) microspheres are available commercially, TheraSpheres (MDS Nordion, Ottawa, Canada) and SIR-Spheres® (SIRTeX Medical, Lake Forest, IL). TheraSpheres are glass microspheres approximately 20 to 30 microns in diameter with an activity of 2500 Bq, while SIR-Spheres similarly measure $32 \pm 10$ μm and have an activity of 50 Bq. The energy of the emitted beta particles is 2.27 MeV, with a mean of .937 MeV without primary gamma emission. The half-life of yttrium 90 is 64.1 hours, and approximately 94% of the tumoricidal radiation is delivered within 11 days as it decays to zirconium 90. TheraSpheres are low in particle number but high in activity and may primarily be considered a radiation source. In contrast, SIR-Spheres, with a high particle number and low activity per particle, combine radiation with embolization.

The principle behind radioembolization is that although the normal liver receives 80% of its blood supply from the portal vein and 20% from the hepatic artery, the reverse is true for cancers of the liver. Liver cancers receive their dominant supply (80%) from the hepatic artery. Therefore, agents delivered through the hepatic artery target the cancer while relatively sparing normal liver tissue. For this reason tumoricidal radiation doses of 300 Gy or more may be delivered with relative safety to a normal liver (2).

## METHOD OF DELIVERY

Baseline imaging studies, including CT, MRI, and PET, scan and assess the extent and location of disease in the liver as well as the extent of extrahepatic disease. These staging studies are important to select patients with liver-dominant disease for whom radioembolization is appropriate. A treatment-planning arteriogram is performed first, at which time any extrahepatic supply from the common hepatic artery is occluded to prevent radiation injury to the bowel (3). Technetium macroaggregated albumin (often referred to [99m]Tc-MAA scans) is similar in particle size to the Y90 particles and will mimic their distribution. Therefore, [99m]Tc-MAA is introduced into the common hepatic artery to assess extrahepatic distribution to the bowel and determine the lung shunt fraction from a single-photon emission CT (SPECT) nuclear medicine scan (4).

Lobar treatment is generally delivered so the initial treatment targets the most involved lobe before focusing on the second lobe a month later if indicated. This allows for the assessment of any liver dysfunction following the first treatment. Sequential lobar treatment has been shown to produce fewer complications than whole-liver treatment in a single administration of Y90 (5). Y90 mixed with contrast during delivery is used to monitor delivery, detect any premature occlusion of the target artery, and prevent an undesired reflux of the yttrium into nontarget vessels. Bremsstrahlung imaging with SPECT nuclear imaging or time of flight PET-CT is performed following delivery of the Y90 to assess its distribution (6). The patient may be discharged 4 to 6 hours after treatment, with both a steroid dose pack to reduce postembolization symptoms and a proton pump inhibitor to provide ulcer prophylaxis. The follow-up evaluation includes clinical and lab assessments (liver function tests) at 1 to 2 weeks posttreatment and follow-up imaging 4 to 8 weeks thereafter (7).

## DOSIMETRY

Manufacturer guidelines indicate a dose reduction in cases of more than 10% arterial shunting to the lung. As gauged by the [99m]Tc-MAA scintigraphy, shunting of 10% to 15% warrants a 20% administered activity dose reduction, while shunting from 16% to 20% warrants a 40% reduction. Early histological studies and serial liver function tests have demonstrated a high normal liver tolerance to yttrium 90 radiation dosages from both external and internal sources. Clinical studies have suggested a possible induction of radiation hepatitis with whole-liver external beam doses of greater than 30 Gy. In a study by Gray et al, four patients with metastatic colon adenocarcinoma demonstrated minimal changes to the normal liver parenchyma from SIRT, in which lobe mean doses ranged from approximately 40 Gy to 80 Gy (8).

Dosage calculations vary according to the individual Y90 product. Two primary methods are used to calculate the dose to deliver the empiric and partition model. For SIR-Spheres, the empiric recommended activities range based on the percentage of the liver involved; involvement of greater than 50% should receive 3 GBq; 25% to 50%, 2.5 GBq; and less than 25%, 2 GBq. As an approximate rule of thumb, 1 GBq of Y90/kg of tissue receives approximately 50 Gy. The empiric method is not favored, and the body surface area method (BSA) is preferred instead (9).

The BSA method involves a consideration of height and weight, as well as tumor and total liver volume. Activity in GBq = BSA − .2 + [(tumor volume )/total liver volume)], where BSA (in meters squared) = .20247 * height (meters) ^ .725 × weight (kilograms) ^ .425. For patients with very large BSA, there may be increased activity above 3 GBq, for which the American Association of Physicists in Medicine (AAPM) suggests caution (4).

## MECHANISM OF ACTION

As previously mentioned, liver cancers receive their primary blood supply (approximately 80%) from the hepatic artery, whereas normal liver tissue receives its primary supply from the portal vein. Therefore, hepatic arterial delivery proportionately targets the liver cancer. Arterial ratios of tumor tissue to normal liver tissue are estimated at 3:1 (10). In practice, individual cancers—even of the same type—vary in vascularity, and this ratio is cancer type- and patient-specific. For instance, neuroendocrine cancers and hepatocellular carcinomas tend to be highly vascular, while colorectal carcinoma (CRC) is less so. Radioembolization may achieve tumoricidal doses exceeding 100 Gy, depending on the relative vascularity of the cancer. Additionally, it is hypothesized that the tumor periphery experiences hyperoxygenation, for which the delivered radiation may allow for potentiated and increased tumoricidal activity.

Pathologic studies in postmortem samples demonstrated preferential tumor necrosis in the tumor nodules targeted. Four livers treated with glass microspheres, two each with hepatocellular carcinoma (HCC) and CRC, were dosimetrically mapped and examined histopathologically, revealing an estimated 50% tumor necrosis in a patient who did not respond well to treatment, while the other responders were noted to have 85%, 90%, and 90% tumor necrosis. With reconstructed spatial dosimetry using standardized Monte Carlo dose deposition kernels, three-dimensional analyses showed 300-Gy dose clouds with a rapid falloff to 100 Gy within a 4 mm range. This study also noted an absence of venoocclusive disease, radiation hepatitis, or cirrhosis (in patients without known cirrhosis) outside the tumor targeted. In a careful review of the gallbladder, cholecystitis was noted in two patients—one with and one without microspheres within the parenchyma (10).

## COMPLICATIONS

Given the highly targeted nature of the procedure, it is typically well tolerated, with mild to moderate side effects. Many patients develop fever immediately posttreatment, with reports of "several weeks" in duration (11). Generalized complaints may include fatigue, abdominal discomfort, and pain. Isolated lab abnormalities, including asymptomatic transaminitis, are also to be expected. Local complications due to the catheter-based access include local superficial wounds, superimposed infections, and possible hematomas.

Patients commonly experience tolerable gastrointestinal toxicities. The formation of ascites is one of the most common complications reported with SIRT. A case series by Goin et al has reported its occurrence as a sequelae after approximately 13% of treatments and liver failure to occur after approximately 3% of treatments (12). Gastrointestinal ulceration is reported in 3% to 8% of patients (13). Cholecystitis has also been a reported side effect, with widely varying pathologic and clinical presentations (14).

Radiation-induced liver disease (RILD) is reported in 3% to 20% of patients, occurring 2 weeks to 4 months following treatment. It presents clinically with weight gain, increased abdominal girth, and occasionally right upper quadrant pain with ascites and hepatomegaly, with or without jaundice. A diagnosis based on the characteristic pathology found on biopsy of fibrin deposition in central veins, venoocclusive disease, and hepatocyte atrophy, RILD risk increases with the increased exposure of normal liver tissue to radiation (15). Interestingly, data have suggested the possibility of a distinct clinical syndrome, known as *radioembolization-induced liver disease*, in which combined modality-induced liver disease causes jaundice, weight gain, ascites, and marked elevations in bilirubin. A recent study further suggests a possible common pathophysiologic pathway of hepatic sinusoidal obstruction (16).

## COLORECTAL CARCINOMA

Approximately 35% to 55% of patients with colorectal cancer will develop hepatic metastases during the course of their disease (17). Patients with metastatic disease commonly undergo systemic therapy for overall control, as liver metastases are a principle source of complications and death. Metastatic lesions that do not respond to chemotherapy portend poor outcomes and prognoses, as reported median survival rates are as low as 6 months (17). Accordingly, radioembolization has been studied and demonstrated to provide value in the local control of liver cancer.

Initial studies of combined modality therapy, integrating systemic chemotherapy with liver-directed SIRT, showed significant improvements in overall survival. An early Australian phase II trial of 21 patients with nonresectable liver metastases compared treatment using resin-based spheres and fluorouracil-based chemotherapy to fluorouracil-based chemotherapy alone. Radioembolization was administered on the third or fourth day of the second cycle of 5-fluorouracil chemotherapy. The time to progressive disease in the chemotherapy arm versus the chemotherapy and SIRT arm was 3.6 months versus 18.6 months, with a median survival of 12.8 months as opposed to 29.4 months. At the time of analysis, the chemotherapy dose intensity was noted to be 92% in the chemotherapy arm versus 85.4% in the SIRT arm, and quality-of-life measures were nonstatistically different for both arms when measured by patients or physicians (18).

Additional studies have included various systemic therapies combined with SIRT, including first-line regimens with oxaliplatin and irinotecan. Irinotecan inhibits DNA topoisomerase I and has been suggested to synergize with radiation. A small phase I irinotecan dose-escalation trial by van Hazel et al (19) utilized combined modality therapy with radioembolization at planned dosages of 2 GBq for patients who had previously failed fluorouracil-based systemic chemotherapy. Median overall survival was 12.2 months (2.8 months to ≥60 months), and median liver progression-free survival (PFS) was 9.2 months (range: 1.6–25.8 months). Median PFS was 6.0 months (range: 1.6–25.8 months). It was noted that with this therapy, one long-term survivor remained alive 5 years after the protocol initiation (19).

Radioembolization has been studied in conjunction with chemotherapy delivered through hepatic artery infusion pumps. A phase III trial of 74 patients with nonresectable liver metastases randomized patients to hepatic artery chemotherapy (HAC) with fluorouracil or floxuridine or hepatic artery chemotherapy plus SIR-Spheres. An advantage was seen in patients receiving Y90. Radiographic response rates were 17.6% versus 44%, and the time to progression was 9.7 months compared to 15.9 months in favor of radioembolization. Overall survival times favored the HAC plus SIRT patients: 1 year, 68% versus 72%; 2 years, 29% versus 39%; 3 years, 6.5% versus 39%; and 5 years, 0% versus 3.5%. No differences in grade 3 or 4 treatment toxicities were found between the two arms. The results of this phase III trial encouraged further trial designs (20).

The recent phase III randomized controlled SIRFLOX trial reported a benefit for SIRT in combination with modified fluorouracil, leucovorin, and oxaliplatin-based chemotherapy (mFOLFOX6) versus mFOLFOX6 alone. In this trial, 530 chemotherapy-naïve patients with stage IV colorectal cancer liver metastases were randomized to mFOLFOX6 with possible bevacizumab versus mFOLFOX6 with SIR-Spheres (at a median dose of 1.4 GBq, delivered at a median of 20 days after randomization and at 92.3% to both lobes of the liver). A significant benefit was observed in the radioembolization arm in a median liver PFS time of 20.5 months compared to 12.6 months (hazard ratio, 0.69; 95% CI [0.55–0.90]; $P = .002$) and an overall response rate of 78.7% versus 68.6% ($P = .042$). Although control of liver disease improved, no difference in overall time to progression was seen. Overall survival in this study has not yet been reported (21).

For heavily pretreated patients, SIRT has demonstrated a significant role in metastatic colorectal carcinoma patients with disease refractory to hepatic artery pump and systemic chemotherapy. A phase I trial conducted at Memorial Sloan Kettering recruited 19 patients who had received a mean of 2.9 previous lines of systemic chemotherapy and at least 1 line of hepatic artery chemotherapy. Median overall survival in these heavily pretreated patients was 14.9 months, while liver PFS was 5.2 months; PFS was 2.0 months. Adverse events and toxicities included up to 10% of patients, with grade 3 pain, ulcer, nausea, vomiting, hyperbilirubinemia, and ascites reported, but no patients experienced RILD (22).

Patients who require palliative therapy may also benefit from the fact that radioembolization compares well to chemoembolization. A single-institution retrospective review at Johns Hopkins included 36 metastatic colorectal cancer patients with liver metastases in which 21 consecutive patients treated with transarterial chemoembolization (TACE) were matched to 15 consecutive patients treated with SIRT. No significant difference was seen in median survival (7.7 months vs. 6.9 months, respectively), with similar overall survival at 1, 2, and 5 years. These results compare favorably to previously reported TACE results, which ranged from 7 months to 23 months, depending on patient selection criteria (23).

In summary, radioembolization has demonstrated efficacy in the setting of metastatic colorectal carcinoma. Radioembolization has been well studied in the context of combined modality therapy in conjunction with 5-fluorouracil (5-FU), oxaliplatin, and their respective combinations; heavily pretreated patients; and the palliation of liver metastases. We have included a summary of these retrospective series in Table 10.1 (see page 216-219).

## HEPATOCELLULAR CARCINOMA

Hepatocellular carcinoma (HCC) is the most common liver neoplasm and ranks as the fifth most common cancer worldwide, largely due to hepatitis C and B virus infections as well as chronic cirrhosis (24). After tissue or radiographic diagnosis, the patient is staged using the Barcelona Clinic Liver Cancer (BCLC) system, which incorporates the Eastern Oncology Cooperative Group (ECOG) performance status, the Child-Pugh score, and the size and number of liver lesions (25). For early-stage HCC lesions, curative treatments include surgical resection, ablation, or transplantation, which demonstrate overall survival rates of 90% at 1 year, 76% at 3 years, and 70% at 5 years and disease-free survival rates of 74%, 50%, and 36%, respectively (26). However, for intermediate and advanced disease, chemoembolization, "bland embolization" (in which no chemotherapy is given), sorafenib chemotherapy, and radioembolization offer durable local control rates.

TACE demonstrated a significant survival benefit for patients with HCC in two randomized controlled trials. In one of these trials, 80 patients with unresectable HCC Lo reported the following improved actuarial survival for patients treated with cisplatin-based TACE using gelatin sponge particles compared to supportive care: at 1 year, 57% versus 32%; at 2 years, 31% versus 11%; and at 3 years, 26% versus 3% (27).

A randomized trial by Llovet et al compared doxorubicin-based TACE, bland embolization, or supportive care for patients with multinodular disease who were less than 75 years old; possessed a good performance status; and had Child-Pugh class A or B liver function without encephalopathy, vascular invasion, ascites, extrahepatic spread, or a portosystemic shunt. To be eligible for this study, lesions were limited by size: single lesions less than 5 cm or three nodules measuring less than 3 cm. At an interim analysis at 2 years, survival rates between the TACE and the control arms were calculated as 1-year overall survival, 82% versus 63% and 2-year overall survival, 63% versus 27%, respectively. Subsequently, this trial was stopped early due to statistically significant survival improvements in the TACE arm compared to the supportive care arm (28).

Radioembolization offers an alternative liver-directed therapy for HCC. A large single-center, prospective longitudinal cohort study in 2010 reported radioembolization in 291 patients with Child-Pugh class A and B disease (29). Among the patients without extrahepatic disease were 113 with Child-Pugh class A and 114 with Child-Pugh class B disease. Overall median survival was 17.2 months and 8.2 months, respectively, with an overall response rate of 42% (29).

In the context of BCLC class B or C patients, a retrospective study compared the role of systemic sorafenib, an oral multikinase inhibitor of vascular endothelial growth factor receptor (VEGFR), to SIRT and found no significant difference in survival. Sorafenib was found in a multicenter phase III randomized controlled trial to increase survival in patients with metastatic HCC (30). When sorafenib alone was compared to SIRT in a single-institute propensity-matched control study, 137 patients (74 treated with sorafenib and 63 with SIRT) demonstrated nonstatistically different median survival times of 13.1 months versus 11.2 months. The inclusion criteria included unresectable lesions, Child-Pugh class A or B cirrhosis, and an ECOG performance status of 0 or 1 (31).

Comparisons between SIRT and TACE have demonstrated favorable findings for radioembolization. A comparative effectiveness study of 245 patients reported a significantly longer time to progression of 13.3 versus 8.4 months in SIRT versus TACE patients. The difference in survival was not significant, at 20.5 months versus 17.4 months (32). SIRTACE, a recent randomized controlled pilot open-label, multicenter study, prospectively compared SIRT and TACE in the setting of unresectable HCC with the primary end points of health-related quality of life and safety and a minimum follow-up of 12 months. Patients were randomized to receive single-session SIRT or multiple sessions of TACE until radiographic evidence of progression or stabilization. There were no significant differences in median PFS (3.6 months versus 3.7 months) for SIRT and TACE, respectively. Partial response rates were 13.3% for TACE and 30.8% for SIRT with disease control rates of 73.3% and 76.9% for TACE and SIRT, respectively. There was no difference in the frequency of all adverse events between the two groups (33). It appears that both SIRT and TACE achieve similar outcomes in patients with intermediate-stage HCC.

Radioembolization also offers the potential to downstage lesions or serve as a bridge for liver transplantation (34). A retrospective review at Northwestern University showed that for HCC patients who were not candidates for liver transplantation (UNOS T3) at the time of diagnosis, there was a statistically significant, higher rate of downstaging for those treated with radioembolization, at 58%, compared to those treated with chemoembolization, at 31% (*P*= .023). Similar rates of transplant (21% and 26%, respectively) were ultimately achieved. (35) An additional retrospective review in Italy demonstrated downstaging in approximately 20.3% of patients who received radioembolization (in abstract form) (36).

## NEUROENDOCRINE CANCERS

Neuroendocrine cancers are being diagnosed with increasing frequency, with an estimated incidence of one to three cases per 100,000 people yearly. Surgery and ablative therapy offer the best chance of a cure (37). For patients who are not surgical candidates, targeted biologic therapies, including sunitinib and everolimus, well as surgical resection or transplantation, demonstrate an improved PFS (38); these therapies have varying response rates from 36% to 80%. Peptide receptor radionuclide therapy, such as 177 Lu-DOTATATE, provides additional targeted treatment for metastatic neuroendocrine cancer (39). Liver-directed therapies, including bland embolization, chemoembolization, and radioembolization, have each demonstrated effectiveness in treating metastatic disease in the liver. Unfortunately, few randomized clinical trials are available to select on the optimal treatment regimens. However, radioembolization has been advocated as a possible means for targeted ablative and palliative therapy.

A prospective study of 42 patients with liver metastases from neuroendocrine cancer and good performance status; adequate renal, liver, and granulocyte values; andunresectable disease without extrahepatic disease reported a European Association for the Study of the Liver (EASL) complete response of 20.5% and a partial response of 43.4% after SIRT. Overall survival rates for 1, 2, and 3 years were 72.5%, 62.5%, and 45%, respectively, with a median survival of 34.4 months (40). A prospective study of 48 patients suggested that prognostic factors associated with improved survival included a complete/partial response, a low tumor burden, a gender of female, a well-differentiated histology, and the absence of extrahepatic metastases. In this group of patients, median survival was 35 months (41). A retrospective multi-institutional review of 148 patients with neuroendocrine cancer metastasized to the liver and treated with SIRT demonstrated a complete response in 2.7% of patients, a partial response in 60.5%, and stable disease in 22.7%. The median survival was 70 months (37).

## CONTRAINDICATIONS

SIRT is indicated in patients with liver-dominant metastatic disease. Several conditions may prevent the use of SIRT. SIRT requires an interventional procedure for access and microsphere delivery and has been demonstrated to induce significant toxicity in those patients with severe coagulopathy, hepatic dysfunction, or poor performance status. It requires a coordinated multidisciplinary team approach, including medical, radiation, surgical, and interventional oncologists.

Careful patient consideration includes a knowledge of the contraindications prior to treatment. Laboratory abnormalities also preclude treatment, based on manufacturer specifications. These labs include: aspartate transaminase (AST) or alanine transaminase (ALT) greater than five times the upper limit of normal, bilirubin greater than 2 mg/dL, and albumin less than 3 g/dL when tumor volume is greater than 50% of the noninvolved liver. Significant renal dysfunction may preclude the use of contrast agents, which are necessary for visualizing vessels during mapping and therapeutic approaches. Additionally, patients with coagulopathies or pulmonary insufficiency may be prohibited from interventional procedures. Microsphere delivery may cause dose deposition in critical organ areas for patients in whom arterial perfusion scintigraphy and mapping reveals shunting in the gastrointestinal tract outside the liver or the pulmonary system.

There is disagreement regarding occlusion of the main portal vein and its role in adverse events from treatment. Despite this, a 2015 prospective, single-institution study of 45 patients with unresectable HCC and radiographic evidence of portal vein thrombosis were treated with SIRT. Patients with Child-Pugh class A or B liver function, an ECOG performance status of 0 or 1, and a total tumor burden of less than 75% had a median overall survival of 13 months and a time to progression of 9 months. The thrombosed veins involved were the main portal vein (20%) and the branch (80%); occlusion was present in 77% of patients (42). Furthermore, a recent retrospective study demonstrated an overall survival benefit for patients with unresectable HCC and portal vein thrombosis treated with SIRT when compared to sorafenib alone. For these patients with radiographically or histologically confirmed HCC with tumoral portal vein thrombosis without extrahepatic spread, a World Health Organization

**TABLE 10.1** Metastatic colorectal cancer

| Author | Year | # pts | Treatment | Activity or dose | Outcome | Toxicity |
| --- | --- | --- | --- | --- | --- | --- |
| Gray et al (46) | 1992 | 29 | Y90 | 0.7–4.2 GBq | 88% patients with 50% CEA reduction, 48% patients with >50% volume reduction | Not recorded |
| Anderson et al (47) | 1992 | 7 | Y90 | 100–150 Gy | 85% SD | Not recorded |
| Andrews et al (48) | 1994 | 23 (17 MCRC) | Y90 | 50–150 Gy | CT response: 29% PR, 6% minimal, 24% SD | Gastritis/ulcer |
| Stubbs et al (49) | 2001 | 50 | Y90 +/− HAC 5-FU | 2–3 GBq | 72% overall CT response 3 months, MS=9.8 months | Duodenal ulcers, GI bleeds |
| Gray et al (50) | 2001 | 74 | HAC FUDR +/− Y-90 | 2–3 GBq | 72% overall response versus 47%, PD: 15.7 versus 9.7 months | Liver abscess, gastritis |
| Wong et al (51) | 2002 | 8 | Y90 | 135–160 Gy | 75% CEA response, 63% PET response, 25% CT response | Not recorded |
| Herba and Thirlwell (52) | 2002 | 33 | Y90 | 50–150 Gy | 41% imaging response | Ulcer, GI bleed |
| Van Hazel et al (53) | 2004 | 11 | 5-FU/LV +/− Y90 | 2.5 GBq | PD 18.6 versus 3.6 months, MS=29.4 versus 12.8 months | RILD |
| Goin et al (54) | 2005 | 43 | Y90 | Variable | 81% SD or better by CT, 19% PR, 5% CR, MS=408 days (range: 316–565 days) | Ulcers, fatigue/fever |
| Lim et al (55) | 2005 | 32 | Y90 with var SC | N/A | CT: 31% PR, 28% SD | Ulcers, RILD |
| Lewandowski et al (56) | 2005 | 27 | Y90 with var SC | 135–150 Gy | 88% PET response versus 35% CT, surv better <25% inv | Ulcer |
| Murthy et al (57) | 2005 | 12 | Y90 with var SC | 1.4 GBq median | 57% CEA response, 55% SD or better by CT | Ulcer |

**TABLE 10.1**  (*Continued*)

| Author | Year | # pts | Treatment | Activity or dose | Outcome | Toxicity |
| --- | --- | --- | --- | --- | --- | --- |
| Popperl et al (58) | 2005 | 12 | Y90 with var SC | 1.2–2.5 GBq | 75% PET response, CEA response, and SD or better by CT | Pancreatitis, ulcer |
| Kennedy et al (59) | 2006 | 208 | Y90 with var SC | 1.7+0.5 GBq | 70% CEA reduction, 91% PET response, 35% PR by CT | Ulcers |
| Mancini et al (60) | 2006 | 48 | Y90 | 1.7 GBq median | 12.5% partial response, 75% stable disease, 12.5% progression | Fever, pain, leukocytosis, chronic pain, jaundice, nausea |
| Stubbs et al (61) | 2006 | 100 | Y90+HAC FUDR | 2–3 GBq | 6.25% progressed by CT, median CEA decreased by 72% | Ulcers (2 fatal) |
| Sharma et al (62) | 2007 | 20 | Y90+FOLFOX4 dose esc | 1.7 GBq median | 90% PR by CT, 10% SD | Neutropenia, ulcers |
| Jakobs et al (63) | 2007 | 18 | Y90 | 2.13 GBq median | 76% response or stable by CT | Fever, loss of appetite, lethargy, fatigue. |
| Sato et al (64) | 2008 | 137 | Y90 | 1.83 GBq median | MS=457 days | Fatigue, abdominal pain, nausea |
| Cianni et al (65) | 2009 | 41 | Y90 | 1.82 GBq median | MS=354 days | Abdominal pain, nausea, cholecystitis, gastritis, hepatic failure |
| Mulcahy et al (66) | 2009 | 72 | Y90 | 118 Gy median | MS=14.5 mo | Fatigue, abdominal pain, nausea, fever, anoerxia, diarrhea, ulcer, hyperbilirubinemia, transaminitis |

**TABLE 10.1**  (*Continued*)

| Author | Year | # pts | Treatment | Activity or dose | Outcome | Toxicity |
|---|---|---|---|---|---|---|
| Van Hazel et al (67) | 2009 | 25 | Y90+irinotecan | 2 GBq median | MS=12.2 mo; median PFS 6.0 months. | Jaundice, DVT, leukopenia, constipation, hyperbilirubinemia |
| Cosimelli et al (68) | 2010 | 50 | Y90 | 1.7 GBq median | MS=12.6 mo. 2Y OS=19.6% | Death (2, possibly treatment related from kidney failure and liver failure), fever, pain, gastric ulcer, pain, jaundice, fatigue, leukocytosis |
| Evans et al (69) | 2010 | 249 | Y90 | 1.85 GBq median | MS=8.3 mo | Ulcer, RILD, cholecystitis |
| Hendlisz et al (70) | 2010 | 44 | FU+/−Y90 | 1.79 GBq median | Median TTP, 2.1 vs. 5.5 mo (SIRT); MS 7.3 vs 10.0mo | Fatigue, fever, stomatitis, nausea, vomiting, anorexia, gastrointestinal pain, cognitive disturbance, neurosensorial, thrombocytopenia, ulcer and ascites |
| Kosmider et al (71) | 2011 | 19 | Y90+FOLFOX/5FU or leucovorin | 1.96 Gbq median | MS=29.4 mo, median PFS 10.4 mo | Abdominal pain, feer, neutropenia, ulcers, hepatic failure (1 death) |
| Nace et al (72) | 2011 | 51 | Y90 | 1.10 GBq median | MS=10.2 mo | Fatigue, abdominal pain, nausea, ulcer |
| Bester et al (73) | 2012 | 339 | Y90 | 1.8 GBq median | MS=12.0 mo | Abdominal pain, lethargy, ulcer, RILD, cholecystitis |
| Martin et al (74) | 2012 | 24 | Y90 | 46.5 mCi median | Median PFS 3.8 mo, MS=8.9 mo. 0% CT response | Gastric ulcers |

**TABLE 10.1**  (*Continued*)

| Author | Year | # pts | Treatment | Activity or dose | Outcome | Toxicity |
|---|---|---|---|---|---|---|
| Turkmen et al (75) | 2013 | 23 | Y90 | 2 GBq median | MS=14.0 mo | Fatigue, abdominal pain, nausea, vomiting, fever, hyperbilirubinemia. |
| Lewandowski et al (76) | 2014 | 214 | Y90 | 2.35 GBq median | MS=10.6 mo | Leukopenia, hyperbilirubinemia, transaminitis |
| Sofocleous et al (77) | 2014 | 19 | Y90 | 1.19 GBq median | MS=14.9 mo, 3 mo CT response 53% | Liver failure, hyperbilirubinemia, thrombocytopenia, renal injury |
| Abott et al (78) | 2015 | 68 | Y90 | 135 Gy median | MS=11.6 mo, 2 y OS 34% | Nausea, emesis, abdominal pain, fatigue, hyperbilirubinemia, transaminitis |
| Maleux et al (79) | 2015 | 71 | Y90 | 7.81 GBq median | Median TTP 4 mo. Median DFS 3 mo | Fatigue, abdominal discomfort, nausea, fever, transaminitis, diarrhea, gastric ulcer, portal hypertension |
| Kennedy et al (80) | 2015 | 606 | Y90 | 1.17 GBq median | MS, by line of therapy: 13.0, 9.0, and 8.1 | Fatigue, abdominal pain, nausea |
| Wright et al (81) | 2016 | 6 | Y90+resection | Variable | Median disease-free survival 23 months | Bile leak, sepsis, abscess, failure to thrive |
| Van Hazel et al (82) | 2016 | 530 | FOLFOX+/−Y90 | 1.4 GBq median | Median TTP, 20.5 mo (SIRT) vs. 12.6mo | Treatment emergent AE in 85.4% SIRT vs 73.3% no SIRT |
| Rosenbaum et al (83) | 2016 | 42 | Y90 | 43–45 Gy | MS=9.2 months | Fever, fatigue |
| Jakobs et al (84) | 2017 | 104 | Y90 | 1.6 GBq median | MS=10.2 months | Fatigue, abdominal pain, ulcer, cholecystitis, hyperbilirubinemia, transaminitis |

*Note:* CEA, carcino-embryonic antigen; FOLFOX, folinic acid, fluorouracil, and oxaliplatin; FUDR, fluorodeoxyuridine; HAC, hepatic artery chemotherapy; MS, median survival; OS, overall survival; PD, progressive disease; SD, stable disease; SIRT, selective internal radiation therapy; TPP, time to progression; Y90, yttrium 90.

(WHO) performance status of 0 to 2, and a Child-Pugh class of less than B7, survival rates were 61.8% versus 27% at 12 months, 44.1% versus 13.9% at 24 months, and 25.2% versus 8.7% at 36 months for SIRT and sorafenib alone, respectively. Additionally, in comparing the SIRT and sorafenib groups, there were significantly different median overall survival times of 18.3 months versus 6.5 months ($P < .001$) and mRECIST overall response rates of 77.8% versus 26.7% favoring radioembolization ($P = .003$). The portal vein thrombosis response was also significantly improved, with an overall subjective response rate of 57.6% compared to 10.5% ($P = .001$) for radioembolization versus sorafenib, respectively (43).

## FUTURE DIRECTIONS

As the efficacy of SIRT has become better demonstrated and subsequently incorporated into treatment guidelines, several ongoing trials have been initiated to potentially expand the indications for radioembolization as well as to understand its place in an expanding armamentarium of treatments for liver cancer. FOXFIRE is an open-label, randomized phase III trial of 4-fluorouracil, oxaliplatin, and folinic acid with or without SIRT as a first-line therapy for patients with liver-dominant or unresectable liver-only metastatic colorectal cancer (44). EPOCH is a large-scale, multinational phase III randomized controlled trial seeking to compare PFS in patients with liver metastases from colorectal carcinoma who received second-line chemotherapy with or without SIRT after the failure of oxaliplatin or irinotecan. SARAH is a prospective, multicenter, open-label randomized controlled phase III trial comparing sorafenib with or without SIRT in patients with advanced HCC (BCLC class C or recurrent HCC after surgical or thermoablative treatment only) with end points for efficacy, safety, quality of life, and cost-effectiveness. SIRveNIB (AHCC06) is a multicenter Australasian open-label phase III randomized controlled trial comparing SIRT and sorafenib treatment, with end points for overall survival, in BCLC class B or C patients with good performance status (ECOG 0–1), locally advanced HCC, and no evidence of extrahepatic disease (45).

## References


1. Muller JH, Rossier PH. *Experientia.* Publisher unknown. 1947;3:75.
2. Salem R, Thurston KG. Radioembolization with 90yttrium microspheres: a state-of-the-art brachytherapy treatment for primary and secondary liver malignancies. *J Vasc Interv Radiol.* 2006;17:1251–1278.
3. Lewandowski RJ, Sato KT, Atassi B, et al. Radioembolization with 90y microspheres: angiographic and technical considerations. *Cardiovasc Intervent Radiol.* 2007;30:571–592.

4. Dezarn WA, Cessna JT, DeWerd LA, et al. Recommendations of the American Association of Physicists in medicine on dosimetry, imaging, and quality assurance procedures for 90y microsphere brachytherapy in the treatment of hepatic malignancies. *Med Phys.* 2011;38:4824–4845.

5. Seidensticker R, Seidensticker M, Damm R, et al. Hepatic toxicity after radioembolization of the liver using 90y-microspheres: sequential lobar versus whole liver approach. *Cardiovasc Intervent Radiol.* 2012;35:1109–1118.

6. Elschot M, Vermolen BJ, Lam MGEH, et al. Quantitative comparison of pet and bremsstrahlung spect for imaging the in vivo yttrium-90 microsphere distribution after liver radioembolization. *PLOS One.* 2013;8:e55742.

7. Salem R, Lewandowski RJ, Sato KT, et al. Technical aspects of radioembolization with 90y microspheres. *Tech Vasc Interv Radiol.* 2007;10:12–29.

8. Gray BN, Burton MA, Kelleher D, et al. Tolerance of the liver to the effects of yttrium-90 radiation. *Int J Radiat Oncol Biol Phys.* 1990;18:619–623.

9. Kennedy AS, McNeillie P, Dezarn WA, et al. Treatment parameters and outcome in 680 treatments of internal radiation with resin 90y-microspheres for unresectable hepatic tumors. *Int J Radiat Oncol Biol Phys.* 2009;74:1494–1500.

10. Kennedy AS, Nutting C, Coldwell D, et al. Pathologic response and microdosimetry of (90)y microspheres in man: review of four explanted whole livers. *Int J Radiat Oncol Biol Phys.* 2004;60:1552–1563.

11. Jiao LR, Szyszko T, Al-Nahhas A, et al. Clinical and imaging experience with yttrium-90 microspheres in the management of unresectable liver tumours. *Eur J Surg Oncol.* 2007;33:597–602.

12. Goin JE, Salem R, Carr BI, et al. Treatment of unresectable hepatocellular carcinoma with intrahepatic yttrium 90 microspheres: factors associated with liver toxicities. *J Vasc Interv Radiol.* 2005;16:205–213.

13. Naymagon S, Warner RRP, Patel K, et al. Gastroduodenal ulceration associated with radioembolization for the treatment of hepatic tumors: an institutional experience and review of the literature. *Digest Dis Sci.* 2010;55:2450–2458.

14. Crowder CD, Grabowski C, Inampudi S, et al. Selective internal radiation therapy-induced extrahepatic injury: An emerging cause of iatrogenic organ damage. *Am J Surg Pathol.* 2009;33:963–975.

15. Lawrence TS, Robertson JM, Anscher MS, et al. Hepatic toxicity resulting from cancer treatment. *Int J Radiat Oncol Biol Phys.* 1995;31:1237–1248.

16. Dawson LA, Ten Haken RK. Partial volume tolerance of the liver to radiation. *Semin Radiat Oncol.* 2005;15:279–283.

17. McMillan DC, McArdle CS. Epidemiology of colorectal liver metastases. *Surg Oncol.* 2007;16:3–5.

18. Van Hazel G, Blackwell A, Anderson J, et al. Randomised phase 2 trial of sir-spheres plus fluorouracil/leucovorin chemotherapy versus fluorouracil/leucovorin chemotherapy alone in advanced colorectal cancer. *J Surg Oncol.* 2004;88:78–85.

19. van Hazel GA, Pavlakis N, Goldstein D, et al. Treatment of fluorouracil-refractory patients with liver metastases from colorectal cancer by using yttrium-90 resin microspheres plus concomitant systemic irinotecan chemotherapy. *J Clin Oncol.* 2009;27:4089–4095.

20. Gray B, Van Hazel G, Hope M, et al. Randomised trial of sir-spheres plus chemotherapy vs. Chemotherapy alone for treating patients with liver metastases from primary large bowel cancer. *Ann Oncol.* 2001;12:1711–1720.

21. van Hazel GA, Heinemann V, Sharma NK, et al. Sirflox: Randomized phase iii trial comparing first-line mfolfox6 (plus or minus bevacizumab) versus mfolfox6 (plus or minus

bevacizumab) plus selective internal radiation therapy in patients with metastatic colorectal cancer. *J Clin Oncol.* 2016;34:1723–1731.

22. Sofocleous CT, Garcia AR, Pandit-Taskar N, et al. Phase i trial of selective internal radiation therapy for chemorefractory colorectal cancer liver metastases progressing after hepatic arterial pump and systemic chemotherapy. *Clin Colorectal Cancer.* 2014;13:27–36.

23. Hong K, McBride JD, Georgiades CS, et al. Salvage therapy for liver-dominant colorectal metastatic adenocarcinoma: Comparison between transcatheter arterial chemoembolization versus yttrium-90 radioembolization. *J Vasc Interv Radiol.* 2009;20:360–367.

24. Abdel-Rahman OM, Elsayed Z. Yttrium-90 microsphere radioembolisation for unresectable hepatocellular carcinoma. *Cochrane Database Syst Rev.* 2016;2:CD011313.

25. Forner A, Reig ME, de Lope CR, et al. Current strategy for staging and treatment: The bclc update and future prospects. *Semin Liver Dis.* 2010;30:61–74.

26. Poon RT-P, Fan ST, Lo CM, et al. Long-term survival and pattern of recurrence after resection of small hepatocellular carcinoma in patients with preserved liver function: Implications for a strategy of salvage transplantation. *Ann Surg.* 2002;235:373–382.

27. Lo CM, Ngan H, Tso WK, et al. Randomized controlled trial of transarterial lipiodol chemoembolization for unresectable hepatocellular carcinoma. *Hepatology.* 2002;35:1164–1171.

28. Llovet JM, Bruix J. Systematic review of randomized trials for unresectable hepatocellular carcinoma: Chemoembolization improves survival. *Hepatology.* 2003;37:429–442.

29. Salem R, Lewandowski RJ, Mulcahy MF, et al. Radioembolization for hepatocellular carcinoma using yttrium-90 microspheres: A comprehensive report of long-term outcomes. *Gastroenterology.* 2010;138:52–64.

30. Llovet JM, Ricci S, Mazzaferro V, et al. Sorafenib in advanced hepatocellular carcinoma. *N Engl J Med.* 2008;359:378–390.

31. Gramenzi A, Golfieri R, Mosconi C, et al. Yttrium-90 radioembolization vs sorafenib for intermediate-locally advanced hepatocellular carcinoma: A cohort study with propensity score analysis. *Liver Int.* 2015;35:1036–1047.

32. Salem R, Lewandowski RJ, Kulik L, et al. Radioembolization results in longer time-to-progression and reduced toxicity compared with chemoembolization in patients with hepatocellular carcinoma. *Gastroenterology.* 2011;140:497–507, e492.

33. Kolligs FT, Bilbao JI, Jakobs T, et al. Pilot randomized trial of selective internal radiation therapy vs. Chemoembolization in unresectable hepatocellular carcinoma. *Liver Int.* 2015;35:1715–1721.

34. Fujiki M, Aucejo F, Choi M, et al. Neo-adjuvant therapy for hepatocellular carcinoma before liver transplantation: Where do we stand? *World J Gastroenterol.* 2014;20:5308–5319.

35. Lewandowski RJ, Kulik LM, Riaz A, et al. A comparative analysis of transarterial downstaging for hepatocellular carcinoma: Chemoembolization versus radioembolization. *Am J Transplant.* 2009;9:1920–1928.

36. Ettorre GM, Vennarecci G, Santoro R, et al. Bridging and downstaging to transplantation in hcc. *EJC Suppl.* 2012;10:41–43.

37. Kennedy AS, Dezarn WA, McNeillie P, et al. Radioembolization for unresectable neuroendocrine hepatic metastases using resin 90y-microspheres: Early results in 148 patients. *Am J Clin Oncol.* 2008;31:271–279.

38. Yao JC, Shah MH, Ito T, et al. Everolimus for advanced pancreatic neuroendocrine tumors. *N Engl J Med.* 2011;364:514–523.

39. Strosberg J, El-Haddad G, Wolin E, et al. Phase 3 trial of 177lu-dotatate for midgut neuroendocrine tumors. *N Engl J Med.* 2017;376:125–135.

40. Memon K, Lewandowski RJ, Mulcahy MF, et al. Radioembolization for neuroendocrine liver metastases: Safety, imaging, and long-term outcomes. *Int J Radiat Oncol Biol Phys.* 2012;83:887–894.

41. Saxena A, Chua TC, Bester L, et al. Factors predicting response and survival after yttrium-90 radioembolization of unresectable neuroendocrine tumor liver metastases: A critical appraisal of 48 cases. *Ann Surg.* 2010;251:910–916.

42. Kokabi N, Camacho JC, Xing M, et al. Open-label prospective study of the safety and efficacy of glass-based yttrium 90 radioembolization for infiltrative hepatocellular carcinoma with portal vein thrombosis. *Cancer.* 2015;121:2164–2174.

43. Edeline J, Crouzet L, Campillo-Gimenez B, et al. Selective internal radiation therapy compared with sorafenib for hepatocellular carcinoma with portal vein thrombosis. *Eur J Nucl Med Mol Imaging.* 2016;43:635–643.

44. Dutton SJ, Kenealy N, Love SB, et al. Foxfire protocol: An open-label, randomised, phase iii trial of 5-fluorouracil, oxaliplatin and folinic acid (oxmdg) with or without interventional selective internal radiation therapy (sirt) as first-line treatment for patients with unresectable liver-only or liver-dominant metastatic colorectal cancer. *BMC Cancer.* 2014;14:497.

45. Gandhi M, Choo SP, Thng CH, et al. Single administration of selective internal radiation therapy versus continuous treatment with sorafenib in locally advanced hepatocellular carcinoma (sirvenib): Study protocol for a phase iii randomized controlled trial. *BMC Cancer.* 2016;16:856.

46. Gray BN, Anderson JE, Burton MA, et al. Regression of liver metastases following treatment with yttrium-90 microspheres. *Aust N Z J Surg.* 1992;62:105–110.

47. Anderson JH, Goldberg JA, Bessent RG, et al. Glass yttrium-90 microspheres for patients with colorectal liver metastases. *Radiother Oncol.* 1992;25:137–139.

48. Andrews JC, Walker SC, Ackermann RJ, et al. Hepatic radioembolization with yttrium-90 containing glass microspheres: Preliminary results and clinical follow-up. *J Nucl Med.* 1994;35:1637–1644.

49. Stubbs RS, Cannan RJ, Mitchell AW. Selective internal radiation therapy with 90yttrium microspheres for extensive colorectal liver metastases. *J Gastrointest Surg.* 2001;5:294–302.

50. Gray B, Van Hazel G, Hope M, et al. Randomised trial of sir-spheres plus chemotherapy vs. Chemotherapy alone for treating patients with liver metastases from primary large bowel cancer. *Ann Oncol.* 2001;12:1711–1720.

51. Wong CY, Salem R, Raman S, et al. Evaluating 90y-glass microsphere treatment response of unresectable colorectal liver metastases by [18f]fdg pet: A comparison with CT or MRI. *Eur J Nucl Med Mol Imag.* 2002;29:815–820.

52. Herba MJ, Thirlwell MP. Radioembolization for hepatic metastases. *Semin Oncol.* 2002;29:152–159.

53. Van Hazel G, Blackwell A, Anderson J, et al. Randomised phase 2 trial of sir-spheres plus fluorouracil/leucovorin chemotherapy versus fluorouracil/leucovorin chemotherapy alone in advanced colorectal cancer. *J Surg Oncol.* 2004;88:78–85.

54. Goin JE, Salem R, Carr BI, et al. Treatment of unresectable hepatocellular carcinoma with intrahepatic yttrium 90 microspheres: Factors associated with liver toxicities. *J Vasc and Interven Radiol.* 2005;16:205–213.

55. Lim L, Gibbs P, Yip D, et al. A prospective evaluation of treatment with selective internal radiation therapy (sir-spheres) in patients with unresectable liver metastases from colorectal cancer previously treated with 5-fu based chemotherapy. *BMC Cancer* 2005;5:132.

56. Lewandowski RJ, Thurston KG, Goin JE, et al. 90y microsphere (therasphere) treatment for unresectable colorectal cancer metastases of the liver: Response to treatment at targeted doses of 135–150 gy as measured by [18f]fluorodeoxyglucose positron emission tomography and computed tomographic imaging. *J Vasc Interv Radiol.* 2005;16: 1641–1651.

57. Murthy R, Xiong H, Nunez R, et al. Yttrium 90 resin microspheres for the treatment of unresectable colorectal hepatic metastases after failure of multiple chemotherapy regimens: Preliminary results. *J Vasc Interv Radiol.* 2005;16:937–945.

58. Popperl G, Helmberger T, Munzing W, et al. Selective internal radiation therapy with sir-spheres in patients with nonresectable liver tumors. *Cancer Biother Radiopharm.* 2005;20:200–208.

59. Kennedy AS, Coldwell D, Nutting C, et al. Resin 90y-microsphere brachytherapy for unresectable colorectal liver metastases: Modern USA experience. *Int J Radiat Oncol Biol Phys.* 2006;65:412–425.

60. Mancini R, Carpanese L, Sciuto R, et al. A multicentric phase ii clinical trial on intra-arterial hepatic radiotherapy with 90yttrium sir-spheres in unresectable, colorectal liver metastases refractory to i.V. Chemotherapy: Preliminary results on toxicity and response rates. *In Vivo* 2006;20:711–714.

61. Stubbs RS, O'Brien I, Correia MM. Selective internal radiation therapy with 90y microspheres for colorectal liver metastases: Single-centre experience with 100 patients. *ANZ J Surg.* 2006;76:696–703.

62. Sharma RA, Van Hazel GA, Morgan B, et al. Radioembolization of liver metastases from colorectal cancer using yttrium-90 microspheres with concomitant systemic oxaliplatin, fluorouracil, and leucovorin chemotherapy. *J Clin Oncol.* 2007;25:1099–1106.

63. Jakobs TF, Hoffmann RT, Poepperl G, et al. Mid-term results in otherwise treatment refractory primary or secondary liver confined tumours treated with selective internal radiation therapy (sirt) using (90)yttrium resin-microspheres. *Eur Radiol.* 2007;17:1320–1330. response. *EJNMMI Res.* 2016;6:92.

64. Sato KT, Lewandowski RJ, Mulcahy MF, et al. Unresectable chemorefractory liver metastases: Radioembolization with 90y microspheres—safety, efficacy, and survival. *Radiology* 2008;247:507–515.

65. Cianni R, Urigo C, Notarianni E, et al. Selective internal radiation therapy with sir-spheres for the treatment of unresectable colorectal hepatic metastases. *Cardiovasc Intervent Radiol* 2009;32:1179–1186.

66. Mulcahy MF, Lewandowski RJ, Ibrahim SM, et al. Radioembolization of colorectal hepatic metastases using yttrium-90 microspheres. *Cancer* 2009;115:1849–1858.

67. van Hazel GA, Pavlakis N, Goldstein D, et al. Treatment of fluorouracil-refractory patients with liver metastases from colorectal cancer by using yttrium-90 resin microspheres plus concomitant systemic irinotecan chemotherapy. *J Clin Oncol* 2009;27: 4089–4095.

68. Cosimelli M, Golfieri R, Cagol PP, et al.Italian Society of Locoregional Therapies in O. Multi-centre phase ii clinical trial of yttrium-90 resin microspheres alone in unresectable, chemotherapy refractory colorectal liver metastases. *Br J Cancer* 2010;103:324–331.

69. Evans KA, Richardson MG, Pavlakis N, et al. Survival outcomes of a salvage patient population after radioembolization of hepatic metastases with yttrium-90 microspheres. *J Vasc Interv Radiol* 2010;21:1521–1526.

70. Hendlisz A, Van den Eynde M, Peeters M, et al.Phase iii trial comparing protracted intravenous fluorouracil infusion alone or with yttrium-90 resin microspheres radioembolization for liver-limited metastatic colorectal cancer refractory to standard chemotherapy. *J Clin Oncol* 2010;28:3687–3694.

71. Kosmider S, Tan TH, Yip D, et al. Radioembolization in combination with systemic chemotherapy as first-line therapy for liver metastases from colorectal cancer. *J Vasc Interv Radiol* 2011;22:780–786.

72. Nace GW, Steel JL, Amesur N, et al. Yttrium-90 radioembolization for colorectal cancer liver metastases: A single institution experience. *Int J Surg Oncol* 2011;2011:571261.

73. Bester L, Meteling B, Pocock N, Saxena A, Chua TC, Morris DL. Radioembolisation with yttrium-90 microspheres: An effective treatment modality for unresectable liver metastases. *J Med Imaging Radiat Oncol* 2013;57:72–80.

74. Martin LK, Cucci A, Wei L, et al.Yttrium-90 radioembolization as salvage therapy for colorectal cancer with liver metastases. *Clin Colorectal Cancer* 2012;11:195–199.

75. Turkmen C, Ucar A, Poyanli A, et al. Initial outcome after selective intraarterial radionuclide therapy with yttrium-90 microspheres as salvage therapy for unresectable metastatic liver disease. *Cancer Biother Radiopharm* 2013;28:534–540.

76. Lewandowski RJ, Memon K, Mulcahy MF, et al. Twelve-year experience of radioembolization for colorectal hepatic metastases in 214 patients: Survival by era and chemotherapy. *Eur J Nucl Med Mol Imaging* 2014;41:1861–1869.

77. Sofocleous CT, Garcia AR, Pandit-Taskar N, et al. Phase i trial of selective internal radiation therapy for chemorefractory colorectal cancer liver metastases progressing after hepatic arterial pump and systemic chemotherapy. *Clin Colorectal Cancer* 2014;13:27–36.

78. Abbott AM, Kim R, Hoffe SE, et al. Outcomes of therasphere radioembolization for colorectal metastases. *Clin Colorectal Cancer* 2015;14:146–153.

79. Maleux G, Deroose C, Laenen A, et al. Yttrium-90 radioembolization for the treatment of chemorefractory colorectal liver metastases: Technical results, clinical outcome and factors potentially influencing survival. *Acta Oncol* 2016;55:486–495.

80. Kennedy AS, Ball D, Cohen SJ, et al. Multicenter evaluation of the safety and efficacy of radioembolization in patients with unresectable colorectal liver metastases selected as candidates for (90)y resin microspheres. *J Gastrointest Oncol* 2015;6:134–142.

81. Wright GP, Marsh JW, Varma MK, et al. Liver resection after selective internal radiation therapy with yttrium-90 is safe and feasible: A bi-institutional analysis. *Ann Surg Oncol* 2017;24:906–913.

82. van Hazel GA, Heinemann V, Sharma NK, et al. Sirflox: Randomized phase iii trial comparing first-line mfolfox6 (plus or minus bevacizumab) versus mfolfox6 (plus or minus bevacizumab) plus selective internal radiation therapy in patients with metastatic colorectal cancer. *J Clin Oncol* 2016;34:1723–1731.

83. Rosenbaum CE, van den Hoven AF, Braat MN, et al. Yttrium-90 radioembolization for colorectal cancer liver metastases: A prospective cohort study on circulating angiogenic factors and treatment response. *EJNMMI Res* 2016;6:92.

84. Jakobs TF, Paprottka KJ, Raessler F, et al. Robust evidence for long-term survival with 90y radioembolization in chemorefractory liver-predominant metastatic colorectal cancer. *Eur Radiol* 2017;27:113–119.

# Radiogenomics 11



*Barry S. Rosenstein*

## THE RECOGNITION AND SEARCH FOR GENOMIC FACTORS ASSOCIATED WITH RADIATION RESPONSE

*Radiogenomics* is the study of the link between germline genotypic variations and the large clinical variability observed in response to cancer radiotherapy (1). Although the genomic factors influencing tumor radiosensitivity are assuredly of great importance (2–8), research efforts in radiogenomics have primarily focused on the genetic alterations that influence the susceptibility to developing adverse effects from radiotherapy (9–11). This emphasis has been placed on normal tissue effects because adverse effects following radiation treatment are relatively common, with roughly 2% to 5% of patients developing some form of severe complication and approximately 10% to 20% exhibiting a moderate form of toxicity (12). These complications can have a significant adverse effect upon the quality of life, particularly for those cancer patients who have a favorable prognosis and may live for several decades following treatment. For example, the 10-year relative survival rate, which adjusts for the expected mortality from other causes of death, exceeds 90% for people treated for either early-stage localized prostate or breast cancer (13,14). Even though substantial technological improvements have enabled a more precise localization of the treatment dose to the tumor, some normal tissue is inevitably exposed to radiation, which may lead to injuries to those tissues or surrounding organs. In addition, the financial costs associated with managing the chronic complications resulting from cancer treatment are substantial and place a significant burden on both individuals and the healthcare system (15).

For much of the history involving the use of radiation for cancer treatment, it was generally thought that the large variability in response among patients who developed normal tissue toxicities was essentially a random process. Nevertheless, radiation oncologists were often perplexed as to why certain patients displayed severe complications even though they received a treatment that was nearly identical to other patients showing little or minimal toxicity. However, in the past 20 years, it has come to be recognized that 80% to 90% of the basis for the development of adverse effects is related to patient characteristics, including genetic or genomic factors (16–18). Additionally, cellular studies suggest that upward of 80% of the variance in response to radiation can be attributed to genetic variations (19,20). Furthermore, with the launch of the human genome project in the 1990s came a recognition that genomic factors play a significant role in the development of many phenotypic traits and thus may include susceptibility to experiencing adverse effects from exposure to the large doses of radiation used in cancer treatment (21).

## SINGLE NUCLEOTIDE POLYMORPHISMS

Most of the research in radiogenomics has focused on the genomic alterations called *single nucleotide polymorphisms* (SNPs). These variants represent a major source of the genetic variation between individuals, as roughly one in every 1,000 nucleotides or more than 5% of people have an alternate base pair at a particular nucleotide location, although the incidence of particular SNPs varies with ethnic, racial, and geographic location. Consequently, approximately 10 million common SNPs are present in the human population (22). For those SNPs that influence the incidence of certain phenotypes, the impact is typically modest, with effect sizes usually less than 1.5. This is in contrast to the relatively rare mutations that when possessed, often in the homozygous configuration, have high penetrance and greatly increase the risk for developing a variety of "Mendelian" diseases (23). However, it is unusual for a common SNP to dramatically alter the risk for a particular phenotype (Figure 11.1). It must also be noted that in addition to common SNPs, many rare variants exist that could represent a substantial portion of the inherited susceptibility for the development of a specific trait (24). Since the cost for whole exome and whole genome sequencing using next-generation techniques has substantially reduced the cost of genotyping (25), these rare variants will increasingly be identified (26). Because they are rare, however, new statistical techniques will be required to identify those genetic alterations associated with specific outcomes. This relates to the debate regarding whether common variants with relatively low phenotypic

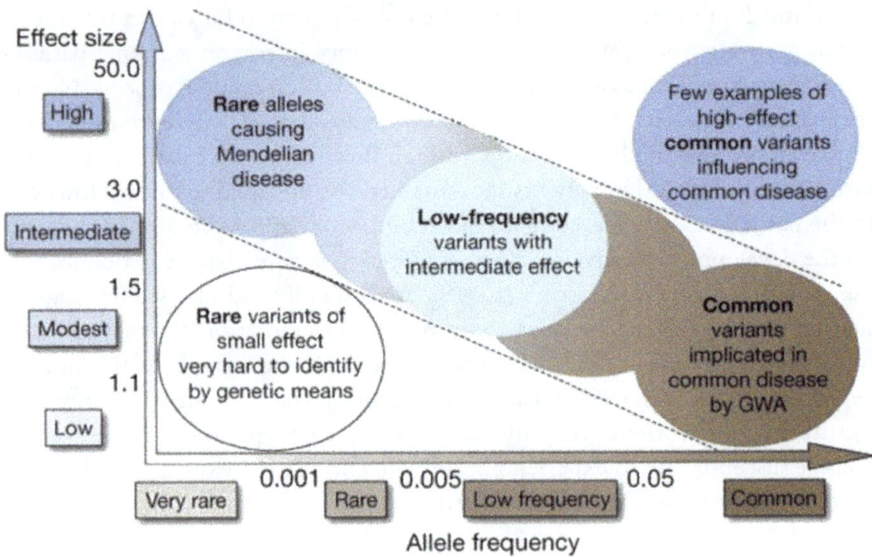


**FIGURE 11.1**  Effect sizes of common and rare variants

penetrance or rare genetic alterations with high penetrance are responsible for most inherited disease susceptibility. Although the "missing heritability" that common variants have not yet explained leaves room for the importance of rare variants, both the common disease–common variant and common disease–rare variant models are generally considered to be valid and likely to contribute to the inherited basis of most phenotypes (27).

## RADIATION RESPONSE REPRESENTS A COMPLEX POLYGENIC TRAIT

The hypothesis formulated from initial radiogenomics research consisted of several basic concepts (28,29). The first is that normal tissue radiosensitivity is a complex trait contingent upon the collective impact of sequence variants in many genes. Thus, normal tissue radiosensitivity lies along a spectrum, which is typical of polygenic inheritance since the response of normal tissues to radiation is complex and involves multiple genes that encode for products that play roles in a variety of molecular pathways. Hence, it is likely that numerous genetic loci could potentially be affected, which would result in a manifestation of clinical radiosensitivity. The second point is that SNPs make up at least a proportion of the inherited basis of radiosensitivity, although many other factors could also influence radiosensitivity. A third concept is that the genetic alterations of importance are expressed selectively in certain organs and tissues, although some may have a global effect. Even though the mutations observed in radiosensitivity syndromes appear to affect most tissues in the body, the results of genome-wide association studies (GWAS) seem to indicate that the genetic variants associated with complications arising from radiotherapy may be specific to the tissue or organ for which the association was discovered. This is in fact consistent with observations from clinical studies that have examined normal tissue radiosensitivity. They indicate that the risk for developing different types of adverse reactions is not strongly correlated (18).

## THE GOALS OF RADIOGENOMICS

The goals of radiogenomics are essentially twofold. The main goal, which has been the initial focus of research in this field, is to identify SNPs that could form the basis of an assay capable of predicting, with a high degree of sensitivity and specificity, the risk for developing specific complications from radiotherapy on an individual patient basis. In this regard it should be recognized that SNPs clearly do not represent the only genomic factor that can influence radiosensitivity. It is likely that epigenetic factors, both inherited and acquired, as well as many other factors, are also important (30). Thus, it is envisioned that any predictive assay will not be static but will be continuously modified and improved to include not only new SNPs as yet undiscovered but also epigenetic, proteomic, and metabolomic factors and the whole range of "panomic" factors. It is anticipated that identifying increasing numbers of the SNPs and the genes associated with adverse effects from radiotherapy will result in a greater understanding of the molecular pathways underlying the development of these adverse effects, leading to the creation of pharmacologic agents to prevent or mitigate these toxicities.

Figure 11.2 (11) outlines the goals of radiogenomics. Typically, patients receiving radiotherapy are treated to a tolerance dose, whose determination is a reflection of the incidence and severity of the complications caused by this dose, balanced against the aggressiveness of the cancer being treated. Unfortunately, the risk for severe toxicity in a minority of patients may limit potentially curative doses that could be prescribed to the majority. A predictive instrument would permit patients to be separated into groups at either high or low genetic risk for developing these toxicities. Thus, the results of this assay would be actionable since alternate measures could be employed to treat the radiosensitive patients, including a nonradiation treatment if it presents an effective option for controlling the cancer undergoing treatment. Alternatively, modified radiation dose parameters may be employed, or there may be justification for using a more conformal form of radiotherapy, such as protons or carbon

# Goals of Radiogenomics

**Research Focus:** Genome-wide approach to identify single nucleotide polymorphisms (SNPs) associated with the development of adverse effects resulting from radiation therapy.

**Two overall goals:**

1) Develop an assay capable of predicting which cancer patients are most likely to develop radiation injuries resulting from treatment with a standard RT protocol

2) Obtain information to assist with the elucidation of the molecular pathways responsible for radiation-induced normal tissue toxicities

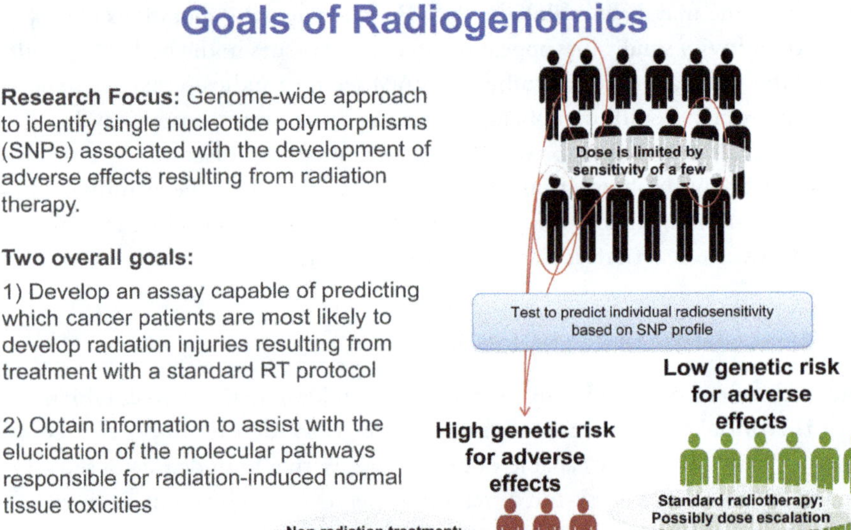


**FIGURE 11.2** Goals of radiogenomics

ions. Men diagnosed with prostate cancer but displaying borderline prostate-specific antigen (PSA) and Gleason scores may give additional consideration to active surveillance (31) if the assay predicts an elevated risk for complications following treatment with radiation. Those women diagnosed with breast cancer who are expected to have a high probability of experiencing adverse effects may decide to receive a mastectomy followed by breast reconstruction rather than a lumpectomy with radiotherapy. In contrast, the majority of individuals predicted to be at low genetic risk for adverse effects can be more confident about receiving radiotherapy, possibly even with dose escalation. Data based upon skin toxicity have shown that it may be possible to dose escalate the most resistant 40% of patients by as much as 20% (12). Thus, the use of a predictive assay could improve the therapeutic index.

Another way to view the usefulness of an assay to predict radiosensitivity is shown in Figure 11.3, which displays a theoretical normal tissue complication probability (NTCP) curve. If it is assumed that a dose of 50 Gy is necessary to achieve an acceptable level of tumor control, then this dose would result in approximately a 20% rate of complications in the overall patient population. However, with a putative predictive test, the patients could be stratified to either a low- or high-risk SNP profile. The rate of complications for patients in the

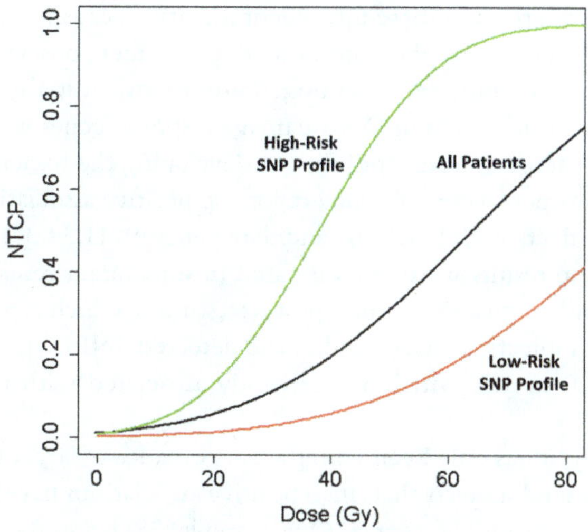



**FIGURE 11.3** Normal tissue complication probability curves for individuals with either a low–risk or a high-risk SNP profile

*Note:* SNP, single nucleotide polymorphism.

low-risk group may be at an acceptable 10% level, and they may safely proceed with this form of treatment. In contrast, patients with a high-risk SNP profile would be predicted to have toxicity rates in the range of 80%. Depending upon the type and severity of complications, this information would likely provide useful guidance to patients and their physicians and influence them to consider an alternative treatment to radiotherapy.

## CANDIDATE GENE STUDIES

Research in radiogenomics and the search for genetic markers associated with the development of adverse effects following radiotherapy began nearly 20 years ago (10,11,32). Initially, the research focused on genes whose products play a role in radiation response, such as proteins associated with DNA damage response pathways. It should be noted that when these studies began in the mid-1990s, the cost of genotyping was several orders of magnitude greater than it is today. Thus, from a technical and financial feasibility viewpoint, work was initially restricted to genotyping only a relatively small number of SNPs in just a few candidate genes. Another rationale for this approach was to identify syndromes characterized by radiation hypersensitivity in which there is an alteration in a gene that encodes a product involved in DNA damage response, such as ataxia–telangiectasia, Nijmegen breakage syndrome, and ataxia–telangiectasia–like disorder (33). Even though these infrequent mutations causing rare syndromes clearly cannot account for the common adverse effects observed in patients treated with radiotherapy, early radiogenomics work initially hypothesized that possessing certain SNPs in DNA damage response genes would result in a relatively large increase in susceptibility to developing the toxicity being studied. Numerous papers were published reporting positive associations for a variety of adverse effects with SNPs in candidate genes (9–11,34,35), but with few exceptions, these results were not validated in subsequent research. In retrospect, it was unlikely that these underpowered studies, which typically involved a few hundred subjects at most, could have detected SNPs with effect sizes in the range of 1.0 to 1.5, which are generally associated with most common SNPs (29,36,37).

Consequently, it has only been with the performance of larger studies involving several thousand subjects that small positive associations have been reported for SNPs in certain candidate genes. One example (38) is a study in which SNPs in genes related to transforming growth factor beta (TGFβ) signaling were screened in more than 2,000 patients. In a combined analysis, homozygosity for the rare allele increased the overall toxicity ($P=.001$) and the chance of being in the upper quartile of risk with an odds ratio (OR) of 2.46 (95% CI [1.52–3.98]). The most strongly associated SNPs genotyped were in the tumor necrosis factor-alpha (*TNFα*) gene rs1800629 and rs2857595, which are in the same linkage disequilibrium (LD) block and in the major histocompatibility complex (MHC) class III region. In another example, SNPs in a series of genes related to oxidative stress and DNA repair were assessed (39). This study identified rs2682585, an SNP in the *XRCC1* gene whose product plays a role in DNA repair. Carriers of the minor allele had a reduced risk of late skin toxicity (multivariate OR 0.77, 95% CI [0.61–0.96], $P=.02$) and overall toxicity (regression coefficient −0.08, 95% CI [−0.15 to −0.02], $P=.02$). In another large candidate gene study, samples from more than 5,000 people treated with radiotherapy for either breast or prostate cancer were genotyped for the *ATM* rs1801516 SNP (29,40). It was reported that possession of the minor allele was associated with an increased risk for toxicity, with an OR of 1.5 for acute toxicity and 1.2 for late toxicity.

## GENOME-WIDE ASSOCIATION STUDIES AND THE CREATION OF THE RADIOGENOMICS CONSORTIUM

With the development of microarrays capable of providing genotyping information for large numbers of SNPs at a reasonable cost, the focus of radiogenomics research shifted toward GWAS. Many areas of medicine have demonstrated that

GWAS represent a powerful method to identify the genetic factors associated with many diseases and other phenotypic traits (41,42). It is now possible to genotype on the order of 1 million SNPs for less than $100, and the amount of data can be routinely increased at least 10-fold through genotype imputation, which determines missing genotypes based on haplotype structure in reference populations, such as the 1000 Genomes Project (43). This also provides a robust method to permit the harmonization of genetic data sets obtained using different genotyping platforms. One large advantage to using a genome-wide approach is that no a priori assumptions need be made as to the genes involved in the occurrence of specific normal tissue toxicities. This is important since relatively little is definitively known about the molecular pathways involved in the development of most adverse effects resulting from radiotherapy.

It should be noted that important characteristics of radiogenomics research facilitate work in this field, among which are that: (a) complications are relatively common in that roughly 2% to 5% of patients treated with radiotherapy for a particular type of cancer develop some form of grade 3 toxicity, while approximately 10% to 20% exhibit a grade 2 adverse effect that nevertheless may still have an impact upon their quality of life (12); (b) the outcome of interest occurs in response to a specific agent, radiation, which is in contrast to most other traits, including disease susceptibility, for which many different environmental, behavioral, or dietary factors may produce the effect; and (c) the findings of genetic studies may be actionable in that a predictive instrument can guide treatment and help to elucidate the biological understanding of the molecular pathways leading to the adverse effect. This increased knowledge of the molecular biology of normal tissue toxicities could lead to the discovery of agents to prevent or mitigate these effects.

Nevertheless, significant challenges are associated with conducting radiogenomic studies, including (a) the requirement for detailed diametric information associated with the radiotherapy since the doses received by particular volumes of normal tissues and organs are important in terms of risk for certain adverse effects; (b) the necessity of enrolling patients in radiogenomic studies prior to the start of radiotherapy since baseline symptom scores are essential; (c) the fact that long-term follow-up, generally of at least 2 years, is crucial since many late or chronic effects may take at least this long to appear; (d) the difficulty of data harmonization for studies involving multiple subject enrollment centers since different instruments are often used to assess toxicity; (e) the multiple toxicities that may result from radiotherapy for a particular type of cancer and the generally limited understanding of the etiology associated with their development; (f) the variety of factors that can affect toxicity besides the dose and the volume irradiated, including comorbid conditions, body habitus, use of chemotherapy or surgery, time, etc; and (g) the requirement of biospecimens and detailed clinical data for large numbers of patients from multiple cohorts. In addition, a general challenge for all GWAS is the problem of false positives. Typically, roughly 1 million SNPs are examined in such a study for association with a specific outcome. Thus, the use of a $P$ value of .05 would result in approximately 50,000 SNPs being incorrectly identified as positively associated with the outcome. To reduce the rate of false positives, various statistical techniques are used, including a Bonferroni correction in which the desired $P$ value is divided by the number of tests performed (44). Thus, an SNP is usually thought to meet genome-wide significance only if the $P$ value for its association with the outcome is less than $5 \times 10^{-8}$.

Notwithstanding all of the challenges associated with the performance of radiogenomic studies, substantial progress has been made in this field, primarily due to the creation of the Radiogenomics Consortium (RGC) in 2009 (45). Researchers realized that to conduct definitive studies, it would be necessary to both substantially increase the size of cohorts being examined and to include multiple cohorts in any project in order to perform meta-analyses and replication studies. To achieve this aim, the RGC was established and has become a National Cancer Institute/NIH–supported Cancer Epidemiology Consortium through the Epidemiology and Genomics Research Program (46). It currently consists of 202 investigators at 119 institutions in 29 countries. In conjunction, the RGC investigators aim to identify SNPs associated with radiotherapy adverse effects and to develop predictive assays ready for clinical implementation. The goal of the RGC is to bring collaborators together to pool samples and data for increased statistical power in radiogenomic studies. In addition, the RGC has enabled cross-center validation studies to be performed, which is essential for a predictive instrument to achieve widespread clinical implementation (47). It should also be noted that the RGC has issued a set of guidelines for reporting the results of radiogenomic studies, and all investigators performing research in the field are encouraged to follow these guidelines (48).

A major focus of GWAS has been to identify SNPs associated with the adverse effects resulting from prostate cancer radiotherapy. The main reason for this is because the 5-year survival rate is high—greater than 95%—for men with localized disease, and approximately 50% of men diagnosed with prostate cancer receive radiotherapy (13). However, late/chronic effects are common, and the complications that may develop following prostate cancer radiotherapy are classified into three general categories: (a) gastrointestinal, leading to urinary frequency, retention, obstruction, dysuria, hematuria, and cystitis; (b) genito-urinary, resulting in rectal urgency, incontinence, bleeding, and proctitis; and

(c) sexual, manifested as erectile dysfunction, loss of libido, and poor ejaculation. As reported in an analysis of 20 publications reporting toxicity outcomes for 11,835 men treated with radiotherapy for prostate cancer, it was estimated that either moderate or severe late gastrointestinal toxicity was observed in 15% and 2%, respectively, of these men (49). In addition, either moderate or severe genitourinary complications arose in 17% and 3%, respectively, of these patients. Thus, overall, approximately 25% to 30% and 4% to 5% of patients with prostate cancer who received radiotherapy develop either moderate or severe, respectively, gastrointestinal and genitourinary complications. In addition, sexual functioning is affected for a considerable number of prostate cancer patients following radiotherapy, and it has been estimated that roughly half of men with prostate cancer who receive radiation treatment develop erectile dysfunction (50).

The first genome-wide association (GWA) study performed in radiogenomics focused upon identifying SNPs associated with erectile dysfunction following prostate cancer radiotherapy in a cohort of African American patients. Even though this study involved a relatively small cohort, an SNP (rs2268363) was identified that approached ($P = 5.5 \times 10^{-8}$) genome-wide significance and tags a locus in the *FSHR* gene, which encodes the follicle-stimulating hormone receptor (FSHR). The product of this gene is expressed in testis Sertoli cells and is involved in testis development and function (51,52). Disruption of the FSHR signaling pathway can lead to abnormal spermatogenesis, small testis size, and infertility. Thus, it is plausible that the product of this gene is associated with erectile dysfunction following exposure to a high dose of radiation.

The next GWA study focused on prostate cancer radiotherapy patients involved roughly 800 patients from several institutions who were assessed for urinary toxicity, rectal bleeding, and erectile dysfunction (53–55). The data set was split into a discovery set and a replication set. In this study, an eight-SNP haplotype block on chromosome 9p21.2 exhibited an association with a change in the American Urological Association Symptom Score (AUASS). SNP rs17779457 displayed the strongest signal, with a beta coefficient of 2.7 (95% CI [1.2–4.1]) in the discovery cohort and 2.4 (95% CI [1.1–3.6]) in the replication cohort (combined $P = 6.5 \times 10^{-7}$). When patients were stratified by rs17779457, those with the risk genotype experienced a mean AUASS increase of 4.7 points at the 2- to 3-year follow-up period, which is of clinical significance (56). This haplotype block lies within the interferon kappa (*INFK*) gene, which encodes for a type I interferon and modulates cytokine release. This may play a role in urinary symptoms following radiotherapy, which are thought to be a manifestation of an inflammatory response to radiation tissue damage through immune modulation (57). In addition, SNP rs13035033 on chromosome

2q31.1 displayed a strong association with the AUASS question on straining (beta coefficient 0.9; 95% CI [0.6, 1.2]; $P = 5.0 \times 10^{-9}$). This SNP lies within the *MYO3B* gene, which encodes the actin-based motor protein myosin IIIB and is highly expressed in the kidney (58).

Twelve SNPs were identified in the discovery cohort and validated in the replication cohort located within or near genes associated with the development of erectile dysfunction following radiation therapy (Fisher's combined $P$ values $= 2.1 \times 10^{-5} - 6.2 \times 10^{-4}$). For example, SNP rs11648233, associated with erectile dysfunction, lies within the 17-beta-hydroxysteroid dehydrogenase II (*HSD17B2*) gene that catalyzes the oxidative metabolism of androgens and estrogens with an OR of 1.8 and a $P$ value of $9.1 \times 10^{-5}$ (59). This study also identified other SNPs with similar $P$ values involved in cellular growth, cell signaling, and tissue development.

The locus most strongly associated with rectal bleeding contained two SNPs in linkage disequilibrium on chromosome 11q14.3, rs7120482 and rs17630638, with $P$ values of $5.4 \times 10^{-8}$ and $6.9 \times 10^{-7}$, respectively. This locus lies upstream of the solute carrier family 36 member 4 (*SLC36A4*) gene, whose product can modulate the activity of the mTOR complex 1 (mTORC1) signaling cascade that affects angiogenesis, proliferation, cell survival, and cellular radiosensitization (60–63)

In addition, a three-stage GWA study was performed for men treated with radiotherapy for prostate cancer (64). The outcome for this study was overall toxicity measured using the standardized total average toxicity (STAT) score (65). This project involved a discovery cohort of 741 men treated for prostate cancer with radiotherapy and replication cohorts consisting of 633 and 368 prostate cancer patients. One SNP (rs264663) in the identified locus at chromosome 2q24.1, which comprised the tetratricopeptide repeat, ankyrin repeat and coiled-coil containing 1 (*TANC1*) gene, was associated with overall late toxicity with a combined $P$ value of $4.64 \times 10^{-11}$ and an OR of approximately 6. The study also showed that the most strongly associated SNP has a probable expression quantitative trait locus that affects the expression of TANC1. In addition, an interaction was shown between this SNP and the biologically effective dose. TANC1 is vital for the recruitment of fusion-competent myoblasts during myotube formation, an essential process for the regeneration of adult muscle in response to local damage (66). Therefore, it is biologically plausible that TANC1 is involved in regenerating muscle tissue damaged by radiation.

The largest GWA study performed to date involved over 3,000 subjects (67) who received either adjuvant breast radiotherapy or radical prostate radiotherapy. The quantile-quantile (Q-Q) plots from this study demonstrated a larger number of associations at the level when $P$ is less than $5 \times 10^{-7}$ than expected by chance, which provides evidence that common genetic variants are associated with a risk of toxicity. The strongest associations were for individual end points rather than an overall measure of toxicity, which is consistent with previous evidence that specific SNPs are associated with adverse effects in each organ or tissue rather than a common set of SNPs being linked with toxicity regardless of the organ irradiated. One notable SNP, which was strongly associated with late rectal incontinence with a relative risk of 9.91 ($P = 1.05 \times 10^{-12}$), is located in the potassium voltage-gated channel, Shal-related subfamily, member 3 (*KCND3*) gene and is expressed in smooth muscle. It therefore may be involved in sphincter function.

A GWAS meta-analysis of data from multiple cohorts is yet another approach to radiogenomics research (68). Figure 11.4 displays the capacity of this approach, in which a locus of SNPs on chromosome 8 is powerfully identified from meta-analyzing the data. This contrasts with an analysis on an individual cohort basis in which the associations are much weaker and uncertain. In addition, meta-analysis across multiple GWAS data sets can address confounding by the so-called center effect (69) and enable the identification of SNPs that display a consistent association with a particular form of toxicity among cohorts with differing treatment, clinical, and patient-specific factors. In addition, tests of heterogeneity can assist in the determination of methods for combining data sets and examining whether variability across data sets affects the strength of particular SNP associations (70,71).

One example involves the meta-analysis of data from four GWAS focusing on men treated with radiotherapy for prostate cancer. It sought to identify SNPs associated with either increased urinary frequency, decreased urine stream, rectal bleeding, or overall toxicity. Two SNPs were discovered that met genome-wide significance for associations with urinary toxicity [(72) and personal communication]. rs17599026 is located on 5q31.2 and was associated with increased urinary frequency (OR 3.12, 95% CI [2.08–4.69], $P$ value $= 4.16 \times 10^{-8}$) whereas rs7720298 is on 5p15.2 and is associated with a decreased urine stream (OR 2.71, 95% CI [1.90–3.86], $P$ value $= 3.21 \times 10^{-8}$). rs17599026 tags a region of LD that contains part of *KDM3B*, which encodes the lysine-specific demethylase 3B protein, a histone demethylase. Consequently, it may exert its function on chromatin conformation, which could lead to direct effects via sensitivity to DNA damage or indirect effects through modifying gene expression. This gene is highly expressed in bladder tissue, suggesting it might be involved in normal bladder function, and potentially dysfunction, following damage from radiation exposure (73). rs7720298 tags a 39kb region of LD that includes *DNAH5*, which encodes the dynein, axonemal, heavy chain 5 protein that is part of a microtubule-associated motor protein complex and is expressed in both

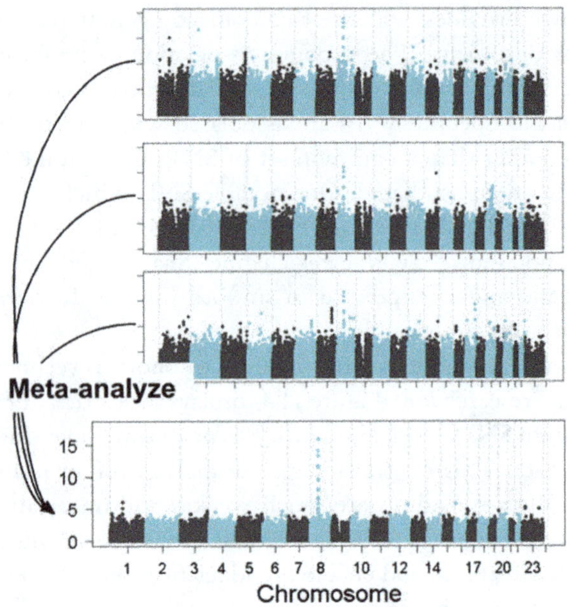



**FIGURE 11.4** Improved power to detect a hypothetical locus on chromosome 8 from meta-analysis of three individual GWAS

*Note:* GWAS, genome-wide association studies.

kidney and bladder tissue, implying a biologic role in the normal function of the urinary tract. Thus, these SNPs reside within genes that are expressed in tissues adversely affected by pelvic radiotherapy, including the bladder, kidney, rectum, and small intestine. This SNP tags a region containing several sites of transcription factor binding and DNase hypersensitivity as measured in ENCODE cell lines (74), signifying that it may be associated with a site affecting transcriptional regulation.

A main finding of the GWAS conducted so far is that genes associated with a particular normal tissue's toxicities produce products that play a role in the function of the tissue or organ affected by the radiation, rather than in a gene encoding a protein involved specifically in response to radiation. It is also interesting to note that most of the SNPs discovered to be associated with adverse effects following radiotherapy reside within noncoding regions of the genome. When research in radiogenomics began, it was assumed that most SNPs of importance would be located in coding sequences, since the majority of traits that follow a Mendelian pattern of inheritance are associated with alterations in coding sequences. However, with increasing numbers of GWAS has come the realization that the preponderance of the sequence variants, primarily SNPs, that affect complex traits are located in noncoding regions (75). The importance of genomic regions that do not encode proteins is being increasingly recognized since these noncoding regions exert critical regulatory functions (76). It is also crucial to remember that the SNPs identified using microarrays used for GWAS are selected on the basis of an ability to tag a large number of SNPs that are in linkage. Thus, the SNP identified in a GWAS is likely not the functional SNP whose alteration produces the impact that renders an individual more likely to develop a complication from radiotherapy. In order to identify the causal variant, it is necessary to perform fine mapping for the region in which the tag SNP is situated to pinpoint the SNP most strongly associated with the toxicity of interest (75). Identification of the causal SNP is of importance both for functional studies and for improving the performance of a predictive model. A variety of computerized annotation and prediction tools are available to rank SNPs and verify the likely functional impact of the variant.

## DEVELOPMENT OF SINGLE NUCLEOTIDE POLYMORPHISM–BASED PREDICTIVE MODELS

As research is progressing to identify SNPs associated with various outcomes following radiotherapy, the development of models that incorporate this information is critical to form the basis of a predictive instrument. One approach utilizes as its basis normal tissue complication (NTCP) models, whose goal is to estimate the risk of complications based on dosimetric parameters (77). However, existing NTCP models are limited and likely to be improved through the addition of patient-specific factors, including genetic information. In this way, a predictive instrument could be formulated that would help guide treatment for patients and their healthcare providers by offering a genetically tailored approach. It is expected that robust multiparametric methods incorporating patient, dosimetric, clinical, and genomic data will be more successful at estimating risk for adverse effects than single-parameter models (69). Validation represents a critical aspect in the identification of genetic markers that warrant inclusion in a predictive assay. Models developed using data from a single cohort may perform well for that patient group but tend to overfit and are often not replicated using an independent patient population. Standard statistical approaches are available to prevent this potential problem (78). Examples of methods that could be used include leave one out cross-validation, bootstrapping analyses that involve sampling data points randomly with replacement, and an independent external validation cohort.

Among models proposed to evaluate radiation-induced toxicities based upon clinical and dosimetric information are Lyman-Kutcher-Berman (79), logit equivalent uniform dose and relative seriality (80), and nearest-neighbor risk prediction (81). The incorporation of SNP information has been shown to improve the predictive ability for radiation pneumonitis using the Lyman-Kutcher-Berman model (79). Another statistical method used for model building is the EMLasso technique (82), and several predictive models using this approach have been developed, including for esophagitis after lung cancer chemoradiotherapy (83), genitourinary complications following prostate cancer radiotherapy (84), and dysphagia associated with head and neck cancer treatment (85). EMLasso is attractive because it selects models with the smallest number of parameters, includes cross-validation, helps to avoid overfitting or underfitting, and is well suited for data sets with missing values, which are common in radiogenomic studies. Decision analytic methods—for example, net benefit and decision curve analysis—can help to quantify clinical usefulness (86,87).

Model building can also help to provide an approximate sense of the number of SNPs required to substantially improve upon the performance of an NTCP model, which can be approached through the use of simulation data (88). For example, simulation analyses (9) could address the issue of how well predictive models would discriminate between those individuals susceptible to the development of a specific radiation-induced toxicity and those who are unlikely to develop that complication. The results of simulation experiments have demonstrated that (a) increasing numbers of SNPs included in the risk model improve discrimination accuracy as measured by the area under the receiver-operating characteristic curve (AUC); (b) the inclusion of SNPs with larger effect sizes and/or higher risk allele frequency improves the accuracy of the model; and (c) relatively high AUC values can be achieved with roughly 50 to 100 common risk SNPs with effect sizes in the range of 1.05 to 1.5 (of course, discovery and validation of common risk SNPs with larger effect sizes would reduce the number of SNPs required to substantially improve the AUC). The results of these simulation experiments are encouraging, since they suggest that a relatively small number of SNPs could form the basis of an assay that would markedly improve the ability to predict a particular patient's risk for developing an adverse effect from radiotherapy. As outlined previously, approximately 10 SNPs associated with the risk for experiencing complications following prostate cancer radiotherapy have already been discovered and validated, and it is likely that a large number of additional SNPs will be identified through ongoing studies. Thus, an assay to predict the risk for complications resulting from prostate cancer radiotherapy is likely to be ready for clinical implementation in the near future.

## BEYOND SINGLE NUCLEOTIDE POLYMORPHISMS

In addition to SNPs, copy number variations (CNVs) and insertions and deletions (INDELS) may be of importance in terms of predicting individual radiosensitivity. It has been reported that CNVs in *XRCC1* were found to be associated with rectal bleeding following prostate cancer radiotherapy (89) and a splice variant of DNA-PKcs linked with radiosensitivity (90). Another significant genomic factor is the role of epigenetic alterations, which can modify transcriptional activity and posttranslational modulation. This generally occurs from the silencing of genes by the methylation of cytosine in the CpG island, and epigenetic modifications have been identified in fibrotic disease and radiation response (91). It has been reported that the decreased DNA methylation of an enhancing region for the diacylglycerol kinase alpha (*DGKA*) gene was found to be associated with a risk of developing fibrosis after adjuvant radiotherapy in patients treated for breast cancer (92). Transcriptional activity also depends upon opening the chromatin structure to permit access to transcription factors, which is achieved through the acetylation of histones in transcriptionally active euchromatin by histone acetyltransferases. Deacetylation by histone deacetylases (HDAC) results in a more condensed chromatin and gene silencing. Thus, HDAC inhibitors can activate gene transcription and alter radiosensitivity (93). MicroRNAs (miRNAs) are another means of gene silencing. They are small (20–22 base) noncoding RNAs that exert a posttranslational regulatory function by mediating mRNA cleavage, destabilization, and translational repression (94). It has been reported that irradiation alters the expression of multiple miRNAs, many of which affect radiosensitivity (95). In addition to genomic parameters, it is likely that proteomic, metabolomic, and other panomic factors could affect radiosensitivity (96–100).

## FUTURE DIRECTIONS

Several important projects currently in progress should substantially advance the translation of research findings in radiogenomics into a predictive instrument ready for routine clinical use. In one project, multiple cohorts obtained through the RGC are being used to expand the number of prostate patients screened to roughly 7,000 subjects. The goals for this project are to (a) validate the SNPs identified in previous GWAS and discover additional SNP associations with adverse effects resulting from radiotherapy for prostate cancer through GWAS meta-analysis using detailed radiotherapy and genotyping data; (b) build clinically useful multi-SNP predictive models for each form of radiation injury that incorporate radiation dosimetric and clinical factors; and (c) create a low-cost, high-performance genetic assay and companion risk assessment tool that physicians in practice and/or genetic testing laboratories could use to predict the risk for developing adverse effects following radiotherapy. Related to this project is support from the Small Business Innovation Research Program of the National Institutes of Health (NIH) to help advance the results of this research into a predictive assay ready for implementation in the clinic (101).

Another important project is termed REQUITE: validating predictive models and biomarkers of radiotherapy toxicity to reduce side effects and improve quality of life in cancer survivors (102). This represents a multicenter study involving member investigators of the RGC. One of the main issues this study addresses is the challenge of data harmonization faced in previous radiogenomic projects, for which patients were often assessed using a variety of toxicity evaluation instruments in addition to the collection of diverse types of clinical, treatment, and dosimetric data. In contrast, REQUITE requires that all centers use identical case report forms so that standardization is maintained for all data collected. The objectives of REQUITE are to (a) perform a multicenter, observational cohort study in which epidemiologic, treatment, longitudinal toxicity, and quality of life data are collected from 5,300 patients treated with radiotherapy for either breast, prostate, or lung cancer; (b) produce a centralized biobank in which DNA is isolated from patients enrolled in the observational study and create a centralized data management system for the secure collection, integration, mining, sharing, and archiving of all project data; (c) validate published SNP biomarkers of radiosensitivity and discover new variants associated with specific forms of adverse effects following radiotherapy; (d) validate clinical and dosimetric predictors of radiotherapy toxicity and incorporate biomarker data; (e) design interventional trials to reduce long-term adverse cancer treatment effects; and (f) deliver interventional trial protocols using validated models incorporating biomarkers to identify patient subpopulations likely to benefit from interventions and serve as an exploitable resource for future studies that will use developing technologies, such as next-generation sequencing, to explore the relationships between adverse effects resulting from radiotherapy and the genetics of radiosensitivity.

It is important to note that radiogenomics represents a prime example of research that makes use of "big data," which in essence are large, complex, and linkable sets of information (103). This is largely feasible due to advances in computer storage, computing power, and statistical methods as well as the ability to associate multiple types of data from a variety of sources. In this regard, although an initial predictive assay will likely focus primarily on the use of SNPs, ultimately, an algorithm will probably be developed

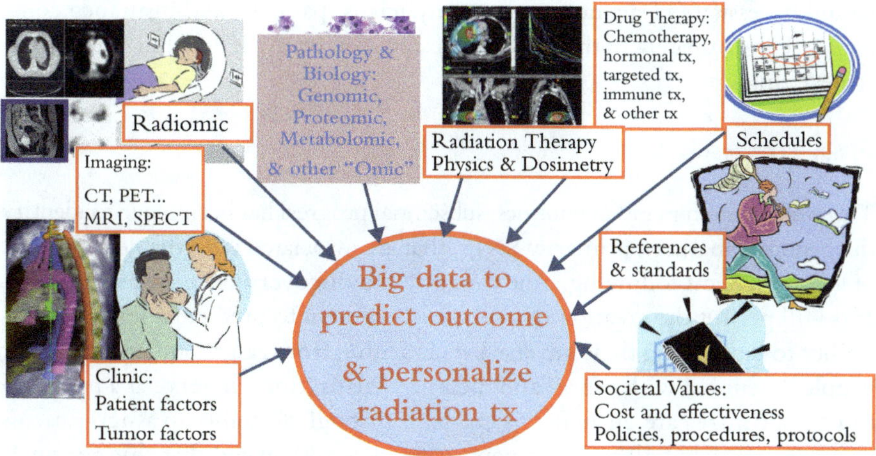



**FIGURE 11.5** Knowledge-guided radiotherapy (KGRT)

that could be incorporated into treatment-planning software that includes a variety of other relevant information and may be termed *knowledge-guided radiotherapy* (KGRT), as outlined in Figure 11.5 (103). This might include other genomic information, such as alterations in the level of expression for certain genes as well as epigenetic information. In addition, proteomic and metabolomic information could well be informative and improve the sensitivity and specificity performance of this test. Beyond that, imaging; dosimetry; drug therapy; references and standards; imaging; clinical information; and the incorporation of societal values, including the cost and effectiveness of treatment, will all be utilized to help formulate the optimal treatment plan for a particular patient.

The development and the application of genetic biomarkers clearly represent critical aspects of patient-centered oncology care and are therefore foundations of precision medicine. However, a better alignment of patient needs and physician-provided information will be essential to advance precision radiation oncology. Thus, shared decision making must occur between patients and their radiation oncologists that weigh the probabilities for the occurrence of adverse effects against tumor progression. This type of information is increasingly desired by patients, providers, and insurers (104). Therefore, a patient decision aid that incorporates a set of validated genomic markers, as well as patient values, would be of great benefit to help personalize radiotherapy (105). It must be recognized, however, that impediments may hinder the routine clinical use of such a predictive instrument since its implementation would necessitate clear interest from physicians, patients, and insurance companies. Unfortunately, at this time the incentive structure is not clearly aligned to achieve this aim.

## CONCLUSIONS

Through research in radiogenomics, substantial progress has been made to identify the genomic markers, primarily SNPs, that are associated with the development of adverse effects following radiotherapy. The discovery of these genetic variants will permit the creation of a robust instrument to predict patients' susceptibility to developing these adverse events arising from cancer radiotherapy. For people diagnosed with cancer and their physicians, this will serve as a powerful tool to optimize care on an individual basis through an ability to assign patients to more precisely tailored treatment plans. It is anticipated that this personalized approach to cancer management will reduce treatment-related toxicities, improve outcomes for individuals diagnosed with cancer, and thereby advance precision radiation oncology.

## References


1. Rosenstein BS, West CM, Bentzen SM, et al. Radiogenomics: radiobiology enters the era of big data and team science. *Int J Radiat Oncol Biol Phys*. 2014;89(4):709–713.
2. Kim JC, Ha YJ, Roh SA, et al. Novel single-nucleotide polymorphism markers predictive of pathologic response to preoperative chemoradiation therapy in rectal cancer patients. *Int J Radiat Oncol Biol Phys*. 2013;86(2):350–357.
3. Yin M, Liao Z, Huang YJ, et al. Polymorphisms of homologous recombination genes and clinical outcomes of non-small cell lung cancer patients treated with definitive radiotherapy. *PLoS One*. 2011;6(5):e20055.
4. Terrazzino S, Agostini M, Pucciarelli S, et al. A haplotype of the methylenetetrahydrofolate reductase gene predicts poor tumor response in rectal cancer patients receiving preoperative chemoradiation. *Pharmacogenet Genomics*. 2006;16(11):817–824.
5. Ahmed KA, Chinnaiyan P, Fulp WJ, et al. The radiosensitivity index predicts for overall survival in glioblastoma. *Oncotarget*. 2015;6(33):34414–34422.
6. Ahmed KA, Fulp WJ, Berglund AE, et al. Differences between colon cancer primaries and metastases using a molecular assay for tumor radiation sensitivity suggest implications for potential oligometastatic SBRT patient selection. *Int J Radiat Oncol Biol Phys*. 2015;92(4):837–842.
7. Strom T, Hoffe SE, Fulp W, et al. Radiosensitivity index predicts for survival with adjuvant radiation in resectable pancreatic cancer. *Radiother Oncol*. 2015;117(1):159–164.
8. Torres-Roca JF, Fulp WJ, Caudell JJ, et al. Integration of a radiosensitivity molecular signature into the assessment of local recurrence risk in breast cancer. *Int J Radiat Oncol Biol Phys*. 2015;93(3):631–638.
9. Kerns SL, Kundu S, Oh JH, et al. The prediction of radiotherapy toxicity using single nucleotide polymorphism-based models: a step toward prevention. *Semin Radiat Oncol*. 2015;25(4):281–291.

10. Kerns SL, West CM, Andreassen CN, et al. Radiogenomics: the search for genetic predictors of radiotherapy response. *Future Oncol.* 2014;10(15):2391–2406.

11. Kerns SL, Ostrer H, Rosenstein BS. Radiogenomics: using genetics to identify cancer patients at risk for development of adverse effects following radiotherapy. *Cancer Discov.* 2014;4(2):155–165.

12. Scaife JE, Barnett GC, Noble DJ, et al. Exploiting biological and physical determinants of radiotherapy toxicity to individualize treatment. *Br J Radiol.* 2015;88(1051):20150172.

13. DeSantis CE, Lin CC, Mariotto AB, et al. Cancer treatment and survivorship statistics, 2014. *CA Cancer J Clin.* 2014;64(4):252–271.

14. Narod SA, Javaid I, Miller AB. Why have breast cancer mortality rates declined? *J Cancer Policy.* 2015;5:8–17.

15. Peppercorn J. The financial burden of cancer care: do patients in the US know what to expect? *Expert Rev Pharmacoecon Outcomes Res.* 2014;14(6):835–842.

16. Safwat A, Bentzen SM, Turesson I, et al. Deterministic rather than stochastic factors explain most of the variation in the expression of skin telangiectasia after radiotherapy. *Int J Radiat Oncol Biol Phys.* 2002;52(1):198–204.

17. Bentzen SM, Overgaard J. Patient-to-patient variability in the expression of radiation-induced normal tissue injury. *Semin Radiat Oncol.* 1994;4(2):68–80.

18. Bentzen SM, Overgaard M, Overgaard J. Clinical correlations between late normal tissue endpoints after radiotherapy: implications for predictive assays of radiosensitivity. *Eur J Cancer.* 1993;29A(10):1373–1376.

19. Finnon P, Robertson N, Dziwura S, et al. Evidence for significant heritability of apoptotic and cell cycle responses to ionising radiation. *Hum Genet.* 2008;123(5):485–493.

20. Roberts SA, Spreadborough AR, Bulman B, et al. Heritability of cellular radiosensitivity: a marker of low-penetrance predisposition genes in breast cancer? *Am J Hum Genet.* 1999;65(3):784–794.

21. Wilson BJ, Nicholls SG. The Human Genome Project, and recent advances in personalized genomics. *Risk Manag Healthc Policy.* 2015;8:9–20.

22. Erichsen HC, Chanock SJ. SNPs in cancer research and treatment. *Br J Cancer.* 2004;90(4):747–751.

23. Manolio TA, Collins FS, Cox NJ, et al. Finding the missing heritability of complex diseases. *Nature.* 2009;461(7265):747–753.

24. Kosmicki JA, Churchhouse CL, Rivas MA, et al. Discovery of rare variants for complex phenotypes. *Hum Genet.* 2016;135(6):625–634.

25. Hayden EC. Technology: The $1,000 genome. Nature. 2014;507(7492):294–295.

26. Goodwin S, McPherson JD, McCombie WR. Coming of age: ten years of next-generation sequencing technologies. *Nat Rev Genet.* 2016;17(6):333–351.

27. Gibson G. Rare and common variants: twenty arguments. *Nat Rev Genet.* 2011;13(2):135–145.

28. Andreassen CN. Can risk of radiotherapy-induced normal tissue complications be predicted from genetic profiles? *Acta Oncol.* 2005;44(8):801–815.

29. Andreassen CN, Schack LM, Laursen LV, et al. Radiogenomics—current status, challenges and future directions. *Cancer Lett.* 2016;382(1):127–136.

30. Herskind C, Talbot CJ, Kerns SL, et al. Radiogenomics: a systems biology approach to understanding genetic risk factors for radiotherapy toxicity? *Cancer Lett.* Mar 2016;382(1):127–136.

31. Tosoian JJ, Carter HB, Lepor A, et al. Active surveillance for prostate cancer: current evidence and contemporary state of practice. *Nat Rev Urol.* 2016;13(4):205–215.

32. Iannuzzi CM, Atencio DP, Green S, et al. ATM mutations in female breast cancer patients predict for an increase in radiation-induced late effects. *Int J Radiat Oncol Biol Phys.* 2002;52(3):606–613.

33. Pollard JM, Gatti RA. Clinical radiation sensitivity with DNA repair disorders: an overview. *Int J Radiat Oncol Biol Phys.* 2009;74(5):1323–1331.

34. Andreassen CN. Searching for genetic determinants of normal tissue radiosensitivity—are we on the right track? *Radiother Oncol.* 2010;97(1):1–8.

35. Andreassen CN, Alsner J. Genetic variants and normal tissue toxicity after radiotherapy: a systematic review. *Radiother Oncol.* 2009;92(3):299–309.

36. Barnett GC, Coles CE, Elliott RM, et al. Independent validation of genes and polymorphisms reported to be associated with radiation toxicity: a prospective analysis study. *Lancet Oncol.* 2012;13(1):65–77.

37. Barnett GC, Elliott RM, Alsner J, et al. Individual patient data meta-analysis shows no association between the SNP rs1800469 in TGFB and late radiotherapy toxicity. *Radiother Oncol.* 2012;105(3):289–295.

38. Talbot CJ, Tanteles GA, Barnett GC, et al. A replicated association between polymorphisms near TNFalpha and risk for adverse reactions to radiotherapy. *Br J Cancer.* 2012;107(4):748–753.

39. Seibold P, Behrens S, Schmezer P, et al. XRCC1 Polymorphism associated with late toxicity after radiation therapy in breast cancer patients. *Int J Radiat Oncol Biol Phys.* 2015;92(5):1084–1092.

40. Andreassen CN, Kerns S, Rosenstein B, et al. Possession of the ATM codon 1853 SNP is associated with an increased risk for radiation-induced toxicity. *Int J Radiat Oncol Biol Phys.* 2014;90:S148-S149.

41. Manolio TA. Bringing genome-wide association findings into clinical use. *Nat Rev Genet.* 2013;14(8):549–558.

42. Manolio TA, Chisholm RL, Ozenberger B, et al. Implementing genomic medicine in the clinic: the future is here. *Genet Med.* 2013;15(4):258–267.

43. Abecasis GR, Auton A, Brooks LD, et al; Genomes Project C. An integrated map of genetic variation from 1,092 human genomes. *Nature.* 2012;491(7422):56–65.

44. Johnson RC, Nelson GW, Troyer JL, et al. Accounting for multiple comparisons in a genome-wide association study (GWAS). *BMC Genomics.* 2010;11:724.

45. West C, Rosenstein BS. Establishment of a radiogenomics consortium. *Radiother Oncol.* 2010;94(1):117–118.

46. http://epi.grants.cancer.gov/Consortia/single/rgc.html.

47. Lambin P, van Stiphout RG, Starmans MH, et al. Predicting outcomes in radiation oncology—multifactorial decision support systems. *Nat Rev Clin Oncol.* 2013;10(1):27–40.

48. Kerns SL, de Ruysscher D, Andreassen CN, et al. STROGAR—strengthening the reporting of genetic association studies in radiogenomics. *Radiother Oncol.* 2014;110(1):182–188.

49. Ohri N, Dicker AP, Showalter TN. Late toxicity rates following definitive radiotherapy for prostate cancer. *Can J Urol.* 2012;19(4):6373–6380.

50. Zelefsky MJ, Chan H, Hunt M, et al. Long-term outcome of high dose intensity modulated radiation therapy for patients with clinically localized prostate cancer. *J Urol.* 2006;176(4, pt 1):1415–1419.

51. Simoni M, Weinbauer GF, Gromoll J, et al. Role of FSH in male gonadal function. *Ann Endocrinol (Paris).* 1999;60(2):102–106.

52. Themmen APN, Huhtaniemi IT. Mutations of gonadotropins and gonadotropin receptors: elucidating the physiology and pathophysiology of pituitary-gonadal function. *Endocr Rev.* 2000;21(5):551–583.

53. Kerns SL, Stock R, Stone N, et al. A 2-stage genome-wide association study to identify single nucleotide polymorphisms associated with development of erectile dysfunction following radiation therapy for prostate cancer. *Int J Radiat Oncol Biol Phys*. 2013;85(1): e21–e28.

54. Kerns SL, Stock RG, Stone NN, et al. Genome-wide association study identifies a region on chromosome 11q14.3 associated with late rectal bleeding following radiation therapy for prostate cancer. *Radiother Oncol*. 2013;107(3):372–376.

55. Kerns SL, Stone NN, Stock RG, et al. A 2-stage genome-wide association study to identify single nucleotide polymorphisms associated with development of urinary symptoms after radiotherapy for prostate cancer. *J Urol*. 2013;190(1):102–108.

56. Cesaretti JA, Stone NN, Stock RG. Urinary symptom flare following I-125 prostate brachytherapy. *Int J Radiat Oncol Biol Phys*. 2003;56(4):1085–1092.

57. Nardelli B, Zaritskaya L, Semenuk M, et al. Regulatory effect of IFN-kappa, a novel type I IFN, on cytokine production by cells of the innate immune system. *J Immunol*. 2002;169(9):4822–4830.

58. Nambiar R, McConnell RE, Tyska MJ. Myosin motor function: the ins and outs of actin-based membrane protrusions. *Cell Mol Life Sci*. 2010;67(8):1239–1254.

59. Wu L, Einstein M, Geissler WM, et al. Expression cloning and characterization of human 17 beta-hydroxysteroid dehydrogenase type 2, a microsomal enzyme possessing 20 alpha-hydroxysteroid dehydrogenase activity. *J Biol Chem*. 1993;268(17):12964–12969.

60. Heublein S, Kazi S, Ogmundsdottir MH, et al. Proton-assisted amino-acid transporters are conserved regulators of proliferation and amino-acid-dependent mTORC1 activation. *Oncogene*. 2010;29(28):4068–4079.

61. Pillai SM, Meredith D. SLC36A4 (hPAT4) is a high affinity amino acid transporter when expressed in Xenopus laevis oocytes. *J Biol Chem*. 2011;286(4):2455–2460.

62. Ausborn NL, Le QT, Bradley JD, et al. Molecular profiling to optimize treatment in non-small cell lung cancer: a review of potential molecular targets for radiation therapy by the translational research program of the radiation therapy oncology group. *Int J Radiat Oncol Biol Phys*. 2012;83(4):e453–e464.

63. Schiewer MJ, Den R, Hoang DT, et al. mTOR is a selective effector of the radiation therapy response in androgen receptor-positive prostate cancer. *Endocr Relat Cancer*. 2012;19(1):1–12.

64. Fachal L, Gomez-Caamano A, Barnett GC, et al. A three-stage genome-wide association study identifies a susceptibility locus for late radiotherapy toxicity at 2q24.1. *Nat Genet*. 2014;46(8):891–894.

65. Barnett GC, West CM, Coles CE, et al. Standardized total average toxicity score: a scale- and grade-independent measure of late radiotherapy toxicity to facilitate pooling of data from different studies. *Int J Radiat Oncol Biol Phys*. 2012;82(3):1065–1074.

66. Avirneni-Vadlamudi U, Galindo KA, Endicott TR, et al. Drosophila and mammalian models uncover a role for the myoblast fusion gene TANC1 in rhabdomyosarcoma. *J Clin Invest*. 2012;122(1):403–407.

67. Barnett GC, Thompson D, Fachal L, et al. A genome wide association study (GWAS) providing evidence of an association between common genetic variants and late radiotherapy toxicity. *Radiother Oncol*. 2014;111(2):178–185.

68. Manolio TA. Genomewide association studies and assessment of the risk of disease. *N Engl J Med*. 2010;363(2):166–176.

69. Andreassen CN, Barnett GC, Langendijk JA, et al. Conducting radiogenomic research— do not forget careful consideration of the clinical data. *Radiother Oncol*. 2012;105(3): 337–340.

70. Higgins J, Thompson S, Deeks J, et al. Statistical heterogeneity in systematic reviews of clinical trials: a critical appraisal of guidelines and practice. *J Health Serv Res Policy.* 2002;7(1):51–61.

71. Petitti DB. Approaches to heterogeneity in meta-analysis. *Stat Med.* 2001;20(23): 3625–3633.

72. Kerns S, Barnett G, Dorling L, et al. Identification of single nucleotide polymorphisms (SNPs) associated with late toxicity following radiation therapy for prostate cancer through a meta-analysis of genome-wide association studies (GWAS). *Int J Radiat Oncol Biol Phys.* 2014;90:S55-S.

73. Uhlen M, Fagerberg L, Hallstrom BM, et al. Proteomics. Tissue-based map of the human proteome. *Science.* 2015;347(6220):1260419.

74. Consortium EP. An integrated encyclopedia of DNA elements in the human genome. *Nature.* 2012;489(7414):57–74.

75. Edwards SL, Beesley J, French JD, et al. Beyond GWASs: illuminating the dark road from association to function. *Am J Hum Genet.* 2013;93(5):779–797.

76. Albert FW, Kruglyak L. The role of regulatory variation in complex traits and disease. *Nat Rev Genet.* 2015;16(4):197–212.

77. Bentzen SM, Constine LS, Deasy JO, et al. Quantitative Analyses of Normal Tissue Effects in the Clinic (QUANTEC): an introduction to the scientific issues. *Int J Radiat Oncol Biol Phys.* 2010;76(suppl 3):S3-S9.

78. Good PI, Hardin JW. *Common Errors in Statistics (and How to Avoid Them).* Hoboken, NJ: Wiley; 2009.

79. Tucker SL, Li M, Xu T, et al. Incorporating single-nucleotide polymorphisms into the Lyman model to improve prediction of radiation pneumonitis. *Int J Radiat Oncol Biol Phys.* 2013;85(1):251–257.

80. Bakhshandeh M, Hashemi B, Mahdavi SR. Normal tissue complication probability modeling of radiation-induced hypothyroidism after head-and-neck radiation therapy. *Int J Radiat Oncol Biol Phys.* 2013;85(2):514–521.

81. Saligan LN, Fernandez-Martinez JL, deAndres-Galiana EJ, et al. Supervised classification by filter methods and recursive feature elimination predicts risk of radiotherapy-related fatigue in patients with prostate cancer. *Cancer Inform.* 2014;13:141–152.

82. Sabbe N, Thas O, Ottoy JP. EMLasso: logistic lasso with missing data. *Stat Med.* 2013;32(18):3143–3157.

83. De Ruyck K, Sabbe N, Oberije C, et al. Development of a multicomponent prediction model for acute esophagitis in lung cancer patients receiving chemoradiotherapy. *Int J Radiat Oncol Biol Phys.* 2011;81(2):537–544.

84. De Langhe S, De Meerleer G, De Ruyck K, et al. Integrated models for the prediction of late genitourinary complaints after high-dose intensity modulated radiotherapy for prostate cancer: making informed decisions. *Radiother Oncol.* 2014;112(1):95–99.

85. De Ruyck K, Duprez F, Werbrouck J, et al. A predictive model for dysphagia following IMRT for head and neck cancer: introduction of the EMLasso technique. *Radiother Oncol.* 2013;107(3):295–299.

86. Van Calster B, Vickers AJ, Pencina MJ, et al. Evaluation of markers and risk prediction models: overview of relationships between NRI and decision-analytic measures. *Med Decis Making.* 2013;33(4):490–501.

87. Steyerberg EW, Vickers AJ, Cook NR, et al. Assessing the performance of prediction models: a framework for traditional and novel measures. *Epidemiology.* 2010;21(1):128–138.

88. Janssens AC, Aulchenko YS, Elefante S, et al. Predictive testing for complex diseases using multiple genes: fact or fiction? *Genet Med.* 2006;8(7):395–400.

89. Coates J, Jeyaseelan AK, Ybarra N, et al. Contrasting analytical and data-driven frameworks for radiogenomic modeling of normal tissue toxicities in prostate cancer. *Radiother Oncol.* 2015;115(1):107–113.

90. Abbaszadeh F, Clingen PH, Arlett CF, et al. A novel splice variant of the DNA-PKcs gene is associated with clinical and cellular radiosensitivity in a patient with xeroderma pigmentosum. *J Med Genet.* 2010;47(3):176–181.

91. Weigel C, Schmezer P, Plass C, et al. Epigenetics in radiation-induced fibrosis. *Oncogene.* 2015;34(17):2145–2155.

92. Weigel C, Veldwijk MR, Oakes CC, et al. Epigenetic regulation of diacylglycerol kinase alpha promotes radiation-induced fibrosis. *Nat Commun.* 2016;7:10893.

93. Groselj B, Sharma NL, Hamdy FC, et al. Histone deacetylase inhibitors as radiosensitisers: effects on DNA damage signalling and repair. *Br J Cancer.* 2013;108(4):748–754.

94. Jonas S, Izaurralde E. Towards a molecular understanding of microRNA-mediated gene silencing. *Nat Rev Genet.* 2015;16(7):421–433.

95. Mao A, Liu Y, Zhang H, et al. microRNA expression and biogenesis in cellular response to ionizing radiation. *DNA Cell Biol.* 2014;33(10):667–679.

96. Coy SL, Cheema AK, Tyburski JB, et al. Radiation metabolomics and its potential in biodosimetry. *Int J Radiat Biol.* 2011;87(8):802–823.

97. Eichner J, Rosenbaum L, Wrzodek C, et al. Integrated enrichment analysis and pathway-centered visualization of metabolomics, proteomics, transcriptomics, and genomics data by using the InCroMAP software. *J Chromatogr B Analyt Technol Biomed Life Sci.* 2014;966:77–82.

98. Guipaud O. Serum and plasma proteomics and its possible use as detector and predictor of radiation diseases. *Adv Exp Med Biol.* 2013;990:61–86.

99. Oh JH, Craft JM, Townsend R, et al. A bioinformatics approach for biomarker identification in radiation-induced lung inflammation from limited proteomics data. *J Proteome Res.* 2011;10(3):1406–1415.

100. Cai XW, Shedden KA, Yuan SH, et al. Baseline plasma proteomic analysis to identify biomarkers that predict radiation-induced lung toxicity in patients receiving radiation for non-small cell lung cancer. *J Thorac Oncol.* 2011;6(6):1073–1078.

101. Prasanna PG, Narayanan D, Hallett K, et al. Radioprotectors and radiomitigators for improving radiation therapy: the Small Business Innovation Research (SBIR) gateway for accelerating clinical translation. *Radiat Res.* 2015;184(3):235–248.

102. West C, Azria D, Chang-Claude J, et al. The REQUITE project: validating predictive models and biomarkers of radiotherapy toxicity to reduce side-effects and improve quality of life in cancer survivors. *Clin Oncol (R Coll Radiol).* 2014;26(12):739–742.

103. Rosenstein BS, Capala J, Efstathiou JA, et al. How will big data improve clinical and basic research in radiation therapy? *Int J Radiat Oncol Biol Phys.* 2016; 95(3):895–904.

104. Feldman-Stewart D, Brundage MD, Tong C. Information that affects patients' treatment choices for early stage prostate cancer: a review. *Can J Urol.* 2011;18(6):5998–6006.

105. Feldman-Stewart D, Tong C, Siemens R, et al. The impact of explicit values clarification exercises in a patient decision aid emerges after the decision is actually made: evidence from a randomized controlled trial. *Med Decis Making.* 2012;32(4):616–626.

# Combined Effects of Immunotherapy and Radiation Therapy

*Sachin Jhawar and Ann W. Silk*

## INTRODUCTION

Although radiation is generally thought of as a cytocidal local therapy working through DNA damage and mitotic catastrophe, there is increasing evidence that at least part of its antitumor effect is through immune modulation. Radiation therapy triggers multiple cellular and chemical signaling pathways, resulting in both immune-activating and immune-suppressive effects. Many open questions remain regarding the factors that may enhance the immune response, including the appropriate dose, fractionation, timing, and modality of radiation, as well as how to best combine radiation therapy with systemic immunotherapies to maximize these effects.

The human immune system plays a central role in the prevention of clinical cancer. Specifically, the adaptive immune system is able to recognize and attack cells that have undergone a malignant transformation (1,2). Indirect clinical evidence for this comes from the increased incidence of cancers observed in immunosuppressed patients (3–6). It is even argued that clinically measurable malignancy only emerges when immune surveillance has been subverted (7). The notion of cancer *immunosurveillance* was first posited by Burnet and Thomas (8,9) and later modified by Dunn et al. This later group described immunosurveillance as one of the three steps involved in the more general process of cancer "immunoediting." The first step (the elimination or immunosurveillance phase), they wrote, occurs when transformed cells are recognized and killed by CD8+ cytotoxic T cells. The second step (the equilibrium phase) occurs when the elimination of the transformed cells is incomplete, so the most highly resistant strains of transformed cells survive. In step three (the escape phase), these surviving cancer cells evade the cytotoxic response and undergo further and faster mutations that allow for tumor growth, invasion, and metastasis (9).

The major goal of immune therapy for cancer is the creation of antitumor cytotoxic T lymphocytes (CTL). These cells can recognize and attack cancer cells and are thought to be primarily responsible for cancer elimination and equilibrium, although the innate immune response, made up of components such as natural killer (NK) cells, may also be important. The generation of a cytotoxic immune response requires several important steps. The previously mentioned ideas have led to the advent of a multitude of immunotherapies that work by either trying to enhance the immune response through stimulatory factors, such as cytokines, or to dampen the effects of inhibitory molecules, such as checkpoint blockade.

## IMMUNE AVOIDANCE AND THE TUMOR MICROENVIRONMENT: MELANOMA AS A MODEL SYSTEM

Although melanoma represents only 4% of all skin cancers, it is the leading cause of death related to skin cancer. Approximately 75,000 new cases of melanoma and 10,000 deaths attributed to melanoma occur in the United States annually. Radiation therapy (RT) has traditionally been used for the palliation of painful or bleeding melanoma metastases. More recently, however, RT has also been used for oligometastatic disease in an attempt to cure this patient population, and interest is now growing in better elucidating the immune response that RT induces in those with melanoma (10).

It has long been recognized that the immune system plays a role in the pathogenesis of melanoma. Halpern and Schuchter created multivariate logistic regression models to predict survival in patients with primary melanoma. They found that tumor infiltration by lymphocytes was an independent predictor of survival in patients with vertical growth phase melanomas (11). Tumor mechanisms for immune evasion include the downregulation of major histocompatibility complex (MHC) class I, which makes them poor targets for CTLs (12,13). Specifically, in melanoma more advanced disease tends to be associated with the reduced expression or variable amounts of MHC class I expression (14–16). The loss of MHC class I and II expression in a subset of cells in an individual or the loss of other tumor-specific antigens (gp-100 or melanoma antigen reacting to T cell [MART-1]) may be associated with mixed responses in some patients, driven by tumor progression in lesions with downregulated antigens recognized by CTLs (17–21). Al-Batran et al performed immunohistochemistry on samples from 124 stage IV melanoma patients and determined that T cell infiltration is associated with prolonged survival. They found that intratumoral CD4+ and CD8+ T cell infiltration is related to the expression of MHC class I molecules ($P < .0001$) but not any other antigen tested, including cancer-associated antigens or MHC class II molecules (22).

In the tumor microenvironment, the dendritic cells tend to be immature and suppressive and are called *regulatory dendritic cells* (regDC). Therefore, the presentation of tumor antigens occurs without the costimulation and priming of T cells, which can result in cross-tolerance to certain antigenic epitopes (23,24). There is a blockade of CTL effector function by the immunosuppressive microenvironment, characterized by an increase in regulatory T cells (Tregs), tumor-associated macrophages (TAMs), and myeloid-derived suppressor cells (MDSCs). The TAMs and the MDSCs make and secrete anti-inflammatory transforming growth factor-beta (TGF-β) and interleukin-10 (IL-10) and can express programmed death-ligand (PD)-L1 and PD-L2, which can lead to the decreased proliferation of T cells (25,26). Finally, the vasculature of tumors has anti-immunogenic properties that tend to favor the recruitment of immunosuppressive cells, including MDSCs, regDCs, and Tregs (27).

As an end result of this immunosuppressive environment, tumors escape immune surveillance and elimination. Because RT triggers many proinflammatory signals, it has been hypothesized as a way to reverse this immunosuppressive power and force the unmasking of the tumor cells.

## THE IMMUNOMODULATORY EFFECTS OF RADIATION

Although the mechanism of radiation treatment has traditionally been thought to be via local control by direct cytotoxicity through DNA damage and apoptosis, a plethora of evidence suggests that radiation can lead to an immunogenic form of cell death. In fact, the effect of radiation on the tumor microenvironment and vasculature can directly counteract many of the previously mentioned escape mechanisms. Even the local effects of radiation seem to be, at least in part, mediated by the immune system, as CD8+ T cells are required for tumor regression after radiation (28). Lee et al showed that using an ablative 20-Gy dose to treat B16 melanoma in mice led to tumor regression associated with an influx of T cells into the tumor microenvironment. The effect was abrogated when mice undergoing the same treatment had their CD8+ T cells depleted.

Multiple mechanisms lead to immunogenic tumor cell death after radiation. Radiation damage unmasks previously unseen tumor antigens that initiate an immune response, and direct DNA damage causes new mutations to occur, leading to the creation of neoantigens. The radiation-induced translocation of calreticulin to the cell membrane serves as a phagocytosis signal to dendritic cells. The subsequent cell death also causes the release of certain danger- associated molecular patterns (DAMP), such as adenosine triphosphate (ATP) and high-mobility group box 1 (HMGB1), along with uric acid and heat shock protein release. These molecules can act as adjuvants that signal through toll-like receptors (TLRs), which lead to dendritic cell maturation and the priming of antitumor CTLs, counteracting the anergic effect usually seen in the tumor microenvironment described earlier. Furthermore, RT promotes tumor antigen uptake and cross-presentation on MHC class I molecules by dendritic cells. It causes MHC-I expression to increase in both tumors and normal tissue, which allows for better potentiation of and recognition by CTLs. RT leads to the increased expression of multiple cell signaling molecules, including intercellular adhesion molecules (ICAMs), chemokines, and cytokines, that can mediate naïve dendritic cells to subvert immune tolerance in tumors (27) (Figure 12.1). Radiation induces the production of CXCL16, which mediates the recruitment of effector T cells to tumors (29). The effects of radiation on the vascular endothelium induce cell adhesion and promote the recruitment of antitumor T cells as well (30). There can be a dose-dependent augmentation of cell surface molecules (eg, ICAM-1, mucin-1, MHC class I, MHC class II, and tumor-associated antigens) and a lag between when radiation is given and when these cells eventually die (31–33). This time lag between cell death, with an increased expression of immune-stimulatory molecules, could provide a chance for the immune system to recognize these cells and provide a window of opportunity for immunotherapeutic agents to exploit this increased immune recognition.

All these described effects of radiation activate the immune response, supporting the role that the immune system is thought to play in the abscopal effect (*ab* = away, *scopus* = from the target), in which a primary tumor is irradiated, and distant sites outside the path of the radiation show a clinical response. As discussed in the excellent review article by Vatner and colleagues, there are multiple preclinical examples and case reports of the abscopal effect. Unfortunately, however, it seems that the immunostimulatory effects of radiation alone do not seem to be enough in most cases to overcome the immunosuppressive effects of the cancer (27). In addition to cancer-specific factors, some radiation-associated factors may prevent the abscopal effect from occurring. Multiple local immunosuppressive effects of radiation exist, including the activation of anti-inflammatory TGF-β, increased Tregs, and the preferential differentiation of macrophages into the anti-inflammatory M2 subtype (34). The radiation can have a direct cytocidal effect on many of the CTLs and NKs in the area (27). In addition to these effects in the tumor microenvironment, evidence shows that radiation can cause systemic lymphopenia, as lymphocytes are exquisitely

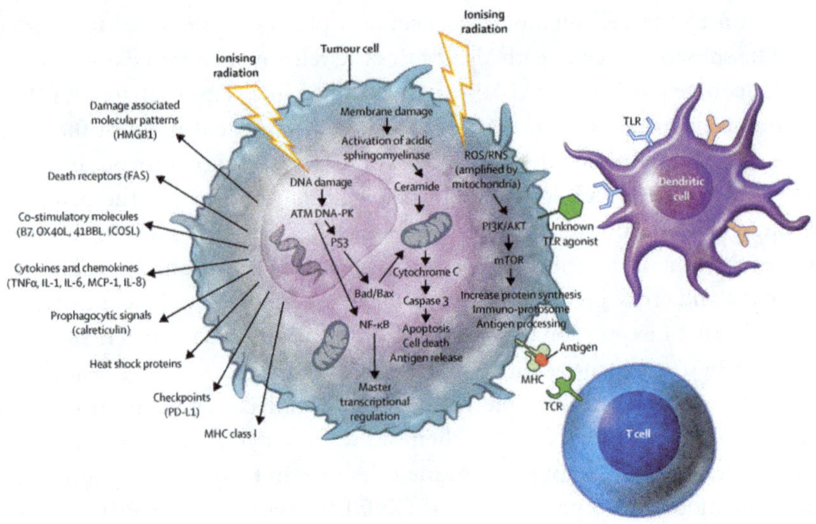



**FIGURE 12.1**  Immunomodulatory effects of radiation therapy

Radiation leads to immunogenic tumor cell death and immune activation through a variety of well-described mechanisms. Radiation damage unmasks previously unseen tumor antigens and causes new mutations, leading to the creation of neoantigens. The translocation of calreticulin to the cell membrane serves as a phagocytosis signal to dendritic cells. The release of certain DAMPs, such as ATP and HMGB1, along with uric acid and heat shock protein leads to signaling through TLRs, causing dendritic cell maturation and the priming of antitumor CTLs. This counteracts the immunosuppressive tumor microenvironment. The upregulation of costimulatory molecules and proinflammatory cytokines and chemokines also occurs. The increased MHC class I expression allows for the increased presentation of tumor antigens and easier recognition by immune effector cells. Conversely, radiation can also lead to the release of anti-inflammatory cytokines (eg, TGF-β, not pictured) and inhibitory cell surface molecules (eg, PD-L1), complicating the overall effects on immune modulation.

*Note:* ATP, adenosine triphosphate; CTL, cytotoxic T lymphocytes; DAMP, danger-associated molecular patterns; HMGB1, high-mobility group box 1; MHC, major histocompatibility complex; PD, programmed death-ligand; TGF-β, transforming growth factor-beta; TLR, toll-like receptors.

*Source:* Reprinted from Sharabi AB, Lim M, DeWeese TL, et al. Radiation and checkpoint blockade immunotherapy: radiosensitisation and potential mechanisms of synergy. *Lancet Oncol.* 2015;16(13):e498–e509, with permission from Elsevier.

radiosensitive and require doses of as little as 0.5 Gy to die. Because of the large volume often irradiated in the traditional treatment of locally advanced tumors and the fact that radiation is repeated every day, a large percentage of the circulating lymphocytes get exposed to radiation. Macrophages, on the other hand, are relatively radioresistant and can survive higher doses.

Lastly, any T cell activation in response to neoantigens takes 1 or more weeks after initial exposure to RT, and any T cell activation that may occur could lead to an influx of new T cells into the tumor microenvironment. Because these new T cells tend to come in the normal regimen of long-course radiation, they may be killed (35–37).

These opposing downstream effects of radiation may explain the rarity of the abscopal effect but also point to different targetable mechanisms for synergy between radiation and immunotherapy.

## RADIATION-SPECIFIC FACTORS

Many studies investigating the combination of radiation and immunotherapies have examined the order of radiation and immunotherapy as well as the dose and fractionation of radiation that acts as the best immune adjuvant.

### Timing

In regard to the question of order, a review of the open protocols in melanoma specifically reveals the differences in opinion about whether immunotherapy should be given before, after, or during radiation therapy (27). Mechanistically speaking, it is not surprising that the best timing for certain treatments may differ. One example of this is the tumor necrosis factor receptor superfamily member 4 ligand (OX40) costimulatory molecule, which is a short-lived molecule that is only upregulated for approximately 24 hours after a naïve T cell becomes activated. Crittenden's group studied an OX40 agonist in combination with hypofractionated radiotherapy. As hypothesized, the optimal administration time of immunotherapy targeting this pathway in a mouse model was 1 day following radiation therapy. In the same study, they looked at the optimal timing of targeting cytotoxic T lymphocyte antigen 4 (CTLA-4), an inhibitory molecule that tends to be upregulated on activated T cells approximately 2 to 4 days after antigen presentation. Surprisingly, the best treatment results occurred when anti-CTLA-4 therapy was given prior to radiation (38). They proposed that this could be because CTLA-4 also results in Treg depletion. A retrospective review of patients receiving the anti-CTLA-4 antibody ipilimumab confirmed this finding and showed that patients who received RT after the first cycle of ipilimumab had longer survival than those who received a concurrent administration with the first cycle of ipilimumab (39). This difficulty in predicting the effects based on the suspected mechanism of action highlights the need for in-depth preclinical studies to inform the design of clinical trials.

### Dose Fractionation

The appropriate dose fractionation is another important variable in the optimal combination of multimodality therapy. A great deal of preclinical data can be found on this subject. Klein et al took tumor samples and exposed them to radiation doses from 0 Gy to 2,000 cGy in 200 cGy per fraction increments.

Dose–related augmentation of human leukocyte antigen (HLA) class I expression was seen in glioblastomas and meningiomas. The optimal dose for inducing HLA expression in this study was at 1200 cGy (32). A study by Garnett et al assessed the effects of sublethal doses of irradiation on human tumor cells and found a more frequent upregulation of the surface molecules involved in T cell–mediated attacks, including Fas (CD95), ICAM-1, mucin-1, carcino-embryonic antigen (CEA), and MCH class-1, as well as increased HLA-A2 restricted CD8+CTL- mediated cell kill in certain cell lines (31). Santin et al assessed four different ovarian cancer cell lines for the expression of cell surface antigens. They found that exposure to high doses of radiation (5–10 Gy) increased the expression of all cell surface antigens, including MHC class I and tumor-specific antigens, that were present prior to irradiation and further showed that this upregulation persisted until cell death (33). In a mouse model of high-grade glioma, single-fraction stereotactic radiosurgery (SRS) proved to be optimal for combined treatment with a PD-1 blockade (40). Therefore, the in vitro data have examined multiple intermediate outcomes, and no clear prescription has arisen out of this work, making dose an open question in animal and early clinical studies of combination therapy.

Although curative RT must be performed within clinical guidelines, there is room to explore different schedules in palliative radiation, and the standard of care is wide in this space. Different groups have addressed this problem using various strategies. When assessing combination radiation and anti-PD1 therapy in a mouse model, Srivastava et al were able to show that multiple small doses of RT (2 Gy×10 fractions) resulted in better antitumor immune responses, tumor shrinkage, PD-L1 expression, and tumor antigen-specific T cells compared to a large single 12-Gy fraction (41). Similar results were seen with combination radiation and anti-CTLA-4 therapy in mice with breast cancer. Dewan et al devised a study in which mice injected with two tumors received one of three different radiation fractionation schemes (20 Gy×1, 8 Gy×3, or 6 Gy×5) to only one of the tumors in combination with a CTLA-4 antagonist. They showed that fractionated therapy led to a better response in the radiated field and could lead to an increase in CD8+T cells and a clinical abscopal effect in the untreated tumor (42). Other investigators have chosen to focus on stereotactic doses, however, which have also shown positive results. A phase I clinical trial by Seung et al showed that high-dose interleukin-2 (IL-2) combined with stereotactic body radiation therapy (SBRT) of 20 Gy per fraction in patients with melanoma or renal cell carcinoma can result in the increased proliferation of activated CD4+T cells and improved clinical response rates in nonirradiated lesions. There was a 66.6% response rate in patients, which was significantly higher than historical controls (43). These data make it difficult to assess the correct course of action when trying to determine the best fractionation schemes for clinical trials. Both preclinical and early clinical results seem to point to different optimal regimens for various immunotherapeutic agents and a variety of malignancies. Many more studies will be required to assess the best treatment regimens.

The effect on lymphocyte count is more straightforward. Clinical data suggest that fractionated radiation worsens lymphopenia in the circulation. A model developed by Yovino et al showed that in patients given the standard fractionated treatment for glioma, over 99% of the circulating lymphocytes were likely to receive more than 0.5 Gy of radiation (37). A study that assessed chemoradiotherapy (CRT) versus SBRT in a retrospective cohort treated for pancreatic cancer found that SBRT led to less severe lymphopenia (~14%), whereas standard CRT led to much worse (~72%), which lasted for at least 2 months (44). Another prospective study in pancreatic cancer showed that hypofractionated radiotherapy avoided the lymphopenia seen with chemoradiation in borderline resectable patients (35). A study in lung cancer showed that a twice-daily fractionation of radiation led to lower circulating lymphocyte nadirs (36).

### Field Size and Treatment Techniques

Field size also affects circulating immune cells. A study by Yovino et al that modeled radiation doses to circulating lymphocytes in glioma patients found that changes in the size of the planning target volume (PTV) affected the dose to circulating cells. However, it found no significant difference when using intensity-modulated radiation therapy (IMRT) or three-dimensional conformal techniques or with changing the dose rate of delivery (37). Another study in lung cancer compared the radiation treatment plan parameters to circulating immune cell levels. It found that larger gross tumor volumes (GTVs) and stage III disease were associated with lower lymphocyte nadirs independent of concurrent chemotherapy administration. Interestingly, no association was seen with total leukocyte, neutrophil, or monocyte nadirs with RT (36).

So far there are scarce data on the effects of linear energy transfer (LET) and the dose rate on the immunogenicity of tumors. Preclinical data presented in abstract form only report that while immune biomarkers increase in a dose-dependent manner, no evidence indicates that the alteration of LET or the dose rate affects tumor immunogenicity (45). Early preclinical data on the dose rate suggests that lower dose rates lead to increases in the amount of lymphocytes in the blood pool receiving potentially lethal doses, but these data have not yet been correlated to clinical outcomes (37).

### Treatment Site

At this time it is unclear whether there is any benefit to treating tumors in specific organs to spur the optimal immune-stimulatory response. There would be a theoretical benefit to giving some radiation to every lesion, as each lesion may represent different clones and therefore be able to release a host of different neoantigens that could then be used for T cell priming. It could be that certain areas are more immune privileged or have their own local immune milieu (eg, the liver and the lungs) and therefore respond differently to immunotherapy. The attempt to answer some these questions is just beginning with ongoing clinical trials (46).

## Concurrent Chemoradiation

Research on the concurrent administration of chemoradiation in combination with immunotherapy is still in its infancy. Adding chemotherapy to combination radiation and immunotherapy has both theoretical risks and benefits. For example, certain chemotherapeutic agents may selectively deplete inhibitory or regulatory immune cell populations. A preclinical model of breast cancer showed that low-dose cyclophosphamide prior to imiquimod, a toll-like receptor TLR7 agonist, and radiation led to better tumor inhibition and less tumor recurrence. The authors of this study suggest that this could be secondary to Treg reduction or increased proimmugenic cell death (47). Some clinical data have shown that immunotherapy can be added to chemotherapy to improve outcomes. A phase II study of ipilimumab in combination with paclitaxel and carboplatin in advanced non–small cell lung cancer (NSCLC) showed that phased but not concurrent ipilimumab improved immune-related progression-free survival (irPFS) and progression-free survival (48). A similar study in extensive-stage small cell lung cancer showed that phased ipilimumab led to improved irPFS (49).

In contrast, there is the risk that adding chemotherapy to radiation can lead to decreased global immunity. It is well known that chemotherapy can lead to cytopenias in multiple immune cell lines. A study by Tang et al showed that concurrent chemotherapy with radiation in lung cancer leads to worse lymphopenia with lower nadirs (36).

More research on this topic will be necessary to understand the interaction of concurrent CRT and immunotherapy. This is a significant complicating factor to many clinical trials, as the standard of care often includes combined chemoradiation.

## IMMUNOTHERAPY IN COMBINATION WITH RADIATION

The goal of immunotherapy is to harness the patient's own immune system to fight the ever-evolving cancer cells, which may be the most important factor to consider when looking at combinations with radiation. Formenti et al have reviewed the literature on radiation as an immune adjuvant, along with combinations of immunotherapy and radiation in the preclinical and early clinical setting (27,34,50). Many of these combinations with radiation therapy have been shown to have additive or even synergistic benefits.

## Checkpoint Inhibitors

Checkpoint inhibitors have been an extremely active area of research and excitement in recent years. Immune checkpoints, such as CTLA-4 and PD-1, normally serve to counteract excessive immune responses from T cells fighting infection, thereby acting as a safeguard against autoimmunity. With malignancy, however, the tumor cells often prevent the costimulation of activated T cells to suppress T cell proliferation and function. PD-1 and PD-L1 inhibitors have been approved by the Food and Drug Administration (FDA) for advanced melanoma, renal cell carcinoma, NSCLC, Hodgkin lymphoma, squamous cell carcinoma of the head and neck, urothelial carcinoma, and Merkel cell carcinoma. During treatment, palliative RT is often needed for symptomatic tumors at the primary site or for bone or brain metastases.

Many completed studies have looked at the combinations of radiation with anti–CTLA-4 (42,51,52) and anti–PD-1 therapy (41). On clinicaltrials.gov there are currently over 50 clinical trials with anti–PD1 or PD-L1 plus RT that are ongoing or planned. In fact, there is now evidence of using RT with dual checkpoint blockade with combined anti–CTLA-4 and anti–PD-L1 therapy (53). These authors have shown that single-agent checkpoint blockade may allow escape through another immune checkpoint, and combined therapy may allow for the abrogation of the second escape pathway. This is particularly important given that a multitude of T cell modulators, including checkpoints and agonists, are currently being investigated as targets for therapy and could be potential avenues for future combination therapies to increase objective response rates and decrease tolerance and escape.

## Cytokines

Cytokines have been used to bolster the effect of tumor-specific T cells that have been induced by radiation, including interferons (54), TNF-$\alpha$ (55), and interleukins. An excellent response rate of 67% was achieved in a small phase I study of SBRT followed by high-dose interleukin-2 in 12 subjects with melanoma or renal cell carcinoma (43). This response rate exceeded the expected response rates of around 20%. An increased number of CD4+ effector memory T cells were observed in the blood of the responding subjects. Thus, the trial data illustrate an important principle—that exposure to high-dose RT followed by cytokine therapy may increase the chances of response. Furthermore, studies looking at the enhancement of T cell costimulation with radiation have assessed molecules that affect the B7/CD28 immunoglobulin family and the TNF/TNFR family (27). The overlap between these discrete subgroups further displays the complexity of these mechanisms of immunotherapy that continue to be elucidated.

## Oncolytic Viruses

The oncolytic viruses are a particularly interesting treatment paradigm because of their dual mechanism of action in which they directly lyse cancer cells, activating an immune response against the malignant cells (56). These viruses preferentially replicate in tumor cells, causing an immunogenic cell death with the release of tumor neoantigens and the attraction of immune cells. The only FDA-approved virus to date, talimogene laherparepvec (T-VEC) has been shown in preclinical models to increase circulating MART-1-specific T cells and intralesional tumor-infiltrating lymphocytes (TILs) while decreasing the number of intralesional Tregs, suppressor T cells (Ts), and MDSCs. There may be a reciprocal benefit in combining radiation and oncolytic virus therapy, as early preclinical work has shown that radiation may enhance oncolytic virus replication, and viral infection may have radiosensitizing effects (57,58). An early-phase dose-finding trial in locally advanced head and neck cancer with combination T-VEC and chemoradiation has been completed. In this trial, patients were treated with intratumoral viral injection concurrently with chemoradiation on the days of cisplatin administration. Of these, 93% were found to have a pathologic complete response at the time of neck dissection, and the disease specific survival was 82.4% at a median follow-up of 29 months (59). Combination therapy is also being studied in melanoma, Merkel cell carcinoma, and other solid tumors (NCT02819843), as well as soft tissue sarcoma (NCT02453191, NCT02923778).

## EMERGING ADDITIONAL TARGETS OF IMMUNOTHERAPY

### Dendritic Cells

The cross-priming of CTLs is an important step in the activation of the immune system. CTLs require antigen presentation by professional antigen-presenting cells; that is, dendritic cells. The mechanisms of cross-priming in combination with RT include cancer tumor–specific vaccine therapy (60,61), the injection of growth factors to recruit dendritic cells (62,63), the injection of autologous dendritic cells (64,65), and dendritic cell activation using toll-like receptor agonists (47,66,67).

### Tumor-Associated Macrophages

Although most of the studies to date have focused on harnessing the adaptive immune response and the creation of tumor-specific T cells, targeting the innate immune response and myeloid cells may also be beneficial. Macrophages can generally be split into a proinflammatory M1 subtype and an anti-inflammatory M2 subtype. They respond to apoptotic cells and can drive an anti-inflammatory response by differentiating to an M2 macrophage phenotype. This can lead to suppression of the adaptive immune response and tissue repair. An animal study of pancreatic tumors in mice showed that radiation induced a macrophage phenotype that suppressed T cell responses (68). When used in combination with agents that modulate macrophage phenotype or decrease macrophages, however, outcomes can be improved. Combining this regimen with T cell–activating therapies, in turn, provides an even greater advantage (69–71).

## IMPLICATIONS FOR RESPONSE ASSESSMENT

Response assessment can be challenging, as occasionally tumors can appear to grow in size on initial posttreatment imaging due to the infiltration of immune-effector cells, commonly referred to as *pseudoprogression* (72). The inflammation may be more pronounced when RT is given to the lesion at the same time as immunotherapy, potentially further complicating response assessment. Up to 15% of patients receiving immunotherapy who are believed to have progression may actually respond (73). A study assessing a group of pooled patients who continued to receive anti–PD1 therapy despite progression showed that 8% experienced subsequent shrinkage, with a more than 30% decrease in tumor burden (74). This has led to the description of immune-related response criteria (irRC) (72) and more recently, Response Evaluation Criteria in Solid Tumors (iRECIST) (75). Interestingly, patients who improve according to both traditional RECIST criteria and irRC may have better survival (73). A clinical evaluation, including performance status, can be helpful to distinguish pseudo-progression from true tumor progression, and some centers perform biopsies to evaluate for TILs. In the absence of clinical deterioration, patients often remain on the treatment until the next restaging scan is performed.

## CONCLUSIONS

The ability of radiation therapy to potentiate the effectiveness of immunotherapies has become widely recognized, as evidenced by numerous opening and ongoing clinical trials (46,76). Although a number of promising clinical trials have shown improvements in both local and distant control, many unanswered questions remain, especially regarding the optimal radiation dose, fractionation, site, and timing relative to immunotherapy, as well as the changing role of traditional chemotherapeutic agents in this context. It is possible that studies of each malignancy type will suggest their own optimal mix of techniques, which may not only be tumor site–specific but target the molecular and immunologic phenotype of each individual patient. A continued investment in clinical and translational research will be necessary to ascertain the best treatments for our individual patients. It is clear that RT will not be outmoded in the era of immuno-oncology but will instead be a crucial partner.

## References


1. Arstila TP, Casrouge A, Baron V, et al. A direct estimate of the human alphabeta T cell receptor diversity. *Science.* 1999;286(5441):958–961.
2. Gabrilovich D. Mechanisms and functional significance of tumour-induced dendritic-cell defects. *Nat Rev Immunol.* 2004;4(12):941–952.
3. Curtis RE, Rowlings PA, Deeg HJ, et al. Solid cancers after bone marrow transplantation. *N Engl J Med.* 1997;336(13):897–904.
4. Haverkos HW, Drotman DP. Prevalence of Kaposi's sarcoma among patients with AIDS. *N Engl J Med.* 1985;312(23):1518.
5. Kasiske BL, Snyder JJ, Gilbertson DT, et al. Cancer after kidney transplantation in the United States. *Am J Transplant.* 2004;4(6):905–913.
6. Pape JW, Liautaud B, Thomas F, et al. Characteristics of the acquired immunodeficiency syndrome (AIDS) in Haiti. *N Engl J Med.* 1983;309(16):945–950.
7. Hanahan D, Weinberg RA. Hallmarks of cancer: the next generation. *Cell.* 2011;144(5):646–674.
8. Burnet FM. The concept of immunological surveillance. *Prog Exp Tumor Res.* 1970;13: 1–27.
9. Dunn GP, Bruce AT, Ikeda H, et al. Cancer immunoediting: from immunosurveillance to tumor escape. *Nat Immunol.* 2002;3(11):991–998.
10. Yoshimoto Y, Kono K, Suzuki Y. Anti-tumor immune responses induced by radiotherapy: a review. *Fukushima J Med Sci.* 2015;61(1):13–22.
11. Halpern AC, Schuchter LM. Prognostic models in melanoma. *Semin Oncol.* 1997;24(suppl 4):S2-S7.
12. Campoli M, Chang CC, Ferrone S. HLA class I antigen loss, tumor immune escape and immune selection. *Vaccine.* 2002;20(suppl 4):A40-A45.
13. Seliger B. Molecular mechanisms of MHC class I abnormalities and APM components in human tumors. *Cancer Immunol Immunother.* 2008;57(11):1719–1726.
14. Munzarova M, Zemanova D, Rejthar A, et al. HLA-DR antigen expression on melanoma metastases and the course of the disease. *Cancer Immunol Immunother.* 1989;30(3): 185–189.
15. Taramelli D, Fossati G, Mazzocchi A, et al. Classes I and II HLA and melanoma-associated antigen expression and modulation on melanoma cells isolated from primary and metastatic lesions. *Cancer Res.* 1986;46(1):433–439.
16. Geertsen RC, Hofbauer GF, Yue FY, et al. Higher frequency of selective losses of HLA-A and -B allospecificities in metastasis than in primary melanoma lesions. *J Invest Dermatol.* 1998;111(3):497–502.
17. Jager E, Ringhoffer M, Altmannsberger M, et al. Immunoselection in vivo: independent loss of MHC class I and melanocyte differentiation antigen expression in metastatic melanoma. *Int J Cancer.* 1997;71(2):142–147.

18. Khong HT, Wang QJ, Rosenberg SA. Identification of multiple antigens recognized by tumor-infiltrating lymphocytes from a single patient: tumor escape by antigen loss and loss of MHC expression. *J Immunother.* 2004;27(3):184–190.

19. Maeurer MJ, Gollin SM, Storkus WJ, et al. Tumor escape from immune recognition: loss of HLA-A2 melanoma cell surface expression is associated with a complex rearrangement of the short arm of chromosome 6. *Clin Cancer Res.* 1996;2(4):641–652.

20. Garrido C, Paco L, Romero I, et al. MHC class I molecules act as tumor suppressor genes regulating the cell cycle gene expression, invasion and intrinsic tumorigenicity of melanoma cells. *Carcinogenesis.* 2012;33(3):687–693.

21. Ahmad M, Rees RC, Ali SA. Escape from immunotherapy: possible mechanisms that influence tumor regression/progression. *Cancer Immunol Immunother.* 2004;53(10):844–854.

22. Al-Batran SE, Rafiyan MR, Atmaca A, et al. Intratumoral T-cell infiltrates and MHC class I expression in patients with stage IV melanoma. *Cancer Res.* 2005;65(9):3937–3941.

23. Cuenca A, Cheng F, Wang H, et al. Extra-lymphatic solid tumor growth is not immunologically ignored and results in early induction of antigen-specific T-cell anergy: dominant role of cross-tolerance to tumor antigens. *Cancer Res.* 2003;63(24):9007–9015.

24. Shurin GV, Ma Y, Shurin MR. Immunosuppressive mechanisms of regulatory dendritic cells in cancer. *Cancer Microenviron.* 2013;6(2):159–167.

25. Gajewski TF, Schreiber H, Fu YX. Innate and adaptive immune cells in the tumor microenvironment. *Nat Immunol.* 2013;14(10):1014–1022.

26. Ostrand-Rosenberg S, Sinha P, Beury DW, et al. Cross-talk between myeloid-derived suppressor cells (MDSC), macrophages, and dendritic cells enhances tumor-induced immune suppression. *Semin Cancer Biol.* 2012;22(4):275–281.

27. Vatner RE, Cooper BT, Vanpouille-Box C, et al. Combinations of immunotherapy and radiation in cancer therapy. *Front Oncol.* 2014;4:325.

28. Lee Y, Auh SL, Wang Y, et al. Therapeutic effects of ablative radiation on local tumor require CD8+ T cells: changing strategies for cancer treatment. *Blood.* 2009;114(3): 589–595.

29. Matsumura S, Wang B, Kawashima N, et al. Radiation-induced CXCL16 release by breast cancer cells attracts effector T cells. *J Immunol.* 2008;181(5):3099–3107.

30. Mole RH. Whole body irradiation; radiobiology or medicine? *Br J Radiol.* 1953;26(305): 234–241.

31. Garnett CT, Palena C, Chakraborty M, et al. Sublethal irradiation of human tumor cells modulates phenotype resulting in enhanced killing by cytotoxic T lymphocytes. *Cancer Res.* 2004;64(21):7985–7994.

32. Klein B, Loven D, Lurie H, et al. The effect of irradiation on expression of HLA class I antigens in human brain tumors in culture. *J Neurosurg.* 1994;80(6):1074–1077.

33. Santin AD, Hiserodt JC, Fruehauf J, et al. Effects of irradiation on the expression of surface antigens in human ovarian cancer. *Gynecol Oncol.* 1996;60(3):468–474.

34. Formenti SC, Demaria S. Combining radiotherapy and cancer immunotherapy: a paradigm shift. *J Natl Cancer Inst.* 2013;105(4):256–265.

35. Crocenzi T, Cottam B, Newell P, et al. A hypofractionated radiation regimen avoids the lymphopenia associated with neoadjuvant chemoradiation therapy of borderline resectable and locally advanced pancreatic adenocarcinoma. *J Immunother Cancer.* 2016;4:45.

36. Tang C, Liao Z, Gomez D, et al. Lymphopenia association with gross tumor volume and lung V5 and its effects on non-small cell lung cancer patient outcomes. *Int J Radiat Oncol Biol Phys.* 2014;89(5):1084–1091.

37. Yovino S, Kleinberg L, Grossman SA, et al. The etiology of treatment-related lymphopenia in patients with malignant gliomas: modeling radiation dose to circulating

lymphocytes explains clinical observations and suggests methods of modifying the impact of radiation on immune cells. *Cancer Invest.* 2013;31(2):140–144.

38. Young KH, Baird JR, Savage T, et al. Optimizing timing of immunotherapy improves control of tumors by hypofractionated radiation therapy. *PLoS One.* 2016;11(6):e0157164.

39. Barker CA, Postow MA, Khan SA, et al. Concurrent radiotherapy and ipilimumab immunotherapy for patients with melanoma. *Cancer Immunol Res.* 2013;1(2):92–98.

40. Zeng J, See AP, Phallen J, et al. Anti-PD-1 blockade and stereotactic radiation produce long-term survival in mice with intracranial gliomas. *Int J Radiat Oncol Biol Phys.* 2013;86(2):343–349.

41. Srivastava R, Clump D, Ferris R. Anti-PD-1 mAb pre-radiotherapy (RT) loading dose and fractionated RT induce better tumor-specific immunity and tumor shrinkage than sequential administration in an HPV+ head and neck cancer model. *J ImmunoTher Cancer.* 2015;3(suppl 2):P314.

42. Dewan MZ, Galloway AE, Kawashima N, et al. Fractionated but not single-dose radiotherapy induces an immune-mediated abscopal effect when combined with anti-CTLA-4 antibody. *Clin Cancer Res.* 2009;15(17):5379–5388.

43. Seung SK, Curti BD, Crittenden M, et al. Phase 1 study of stereotactic body radiotherapy and interleukin-2—tumor and immunological responses. *Sci Transl Med.* 2012;4(137): 137ra74.

44. Wild AT, Herman JM, Dholakia AS, et al. Lymphocyte-sparing effect of stereotactic body radiation therapy in patients with unresectable pancreatic cancer. *Int J Radiat Oncol Biol Phys.* 2016;94(3):571–579.

45. Ng J, Golden E, Stuff D, et al. LET effects on in vitro markers of immunogenic cell death. *Int J Radiat Oncol Biol Phys.* 2016;96(2):e576-e577.

46. Kang J, Demaria S, Formenti S. Current clinical trials testing the combination of immunotherapy with radiotherapy. *J Immunol Cancer.* 2016;4(1):51.

47. Dewan MZ, Vanpouille-Box C, Kawashima N, et al. Synergy of topical toll-like receptor 7 agonist with radiation and low-dose cyclophosphamide in a mouse model of cutaneous breast cancer. *Clin Cancer Res.* 2012;18(24):6668–6678.

48. Lynch TJ, Bondarenko I, Luft A, et al. Ipilimumab in combination with paclitaxel and carboplatin as first-line treatment in stage IIIB/IV non-small-cell lung cancer: results from a randomized, double-blind, multicenter phase II study. *J Clin Oncol.* 2012;30(17): 2046–2054.

49. Reck M, Bondarenko I, Luft A, et al. Ipilimumab in combination with paclitaxel and carboplatin as first-line therapy in extensive-disease-small-cell lung cancer: results from a randomized, double-blind, multicenter phase 2 trial. *Ann Oncol.* 2013;24(1):75–83.

50. Demaria S, Pilones KA, Vanpouille-Box C, et al. The optimal partnership of radiation and immunotherapy: from preclinical studies to clinical translation. *Radiat Res.* 2014;182(2): 170–181.

51. Kwon ED, Drake CG, Scher HI, et al. Ipilimumab versus placebo after radiotherapy in patients with metastatic castration-resistant prostate cancer that had progressed after docetaxel chemotherapy (CA184–043): a multicentre, randomised, double-blind, phase 3 trial. *Lancet Oncol.* 2014;15(7):700–712.

52. Hodi FS, O'Day SJ, McDermott DF, et al. Improved survival with ipilimumab in patients with metastatic melanoma. *N Engl J Med.* 2010;363(8):711–723.

53. Twyman-Saint Victor C, Rech AJ, Maity A, et al. Radiation and dual checkpoint blockade activate non-redundant immune mechanisms in cancer. *Nature.* 2015;520(7547):373–377.

54. Schmidt J, Abel U, Debus J, et al. Open-label, multicenter, randomized phase III trial of adjuvant chemoradiation plus interferon Alfa-2b versus fluorouracil and folinic acid for patients with resected pancreatic adenocarcinoma. *J Clin Oncol.* 2012;30(33):4077–4083.

55. Herman JM, Wild AT, Wang H, et al. Randomized phase III multi-institutional study of TNFerade biologic with fluorouracil and radiotherapy for locally advanced pancreatic cancer: final results. *J Clin Oncol.* 2013;31(7):886–894.

56. Sathyanarayanan V, Neelapu SS. Cancer immunotherapy: Strategies for personalization and combinatorial approaches. *Mol Oncol.* 2015;9(10):2043–2053.

57. Harrington KJ, Melcher A, Vassaux G, et al. Exploiting synergies between radiation and oncolytic viruses: current opinion in molecular therapeutics. *Curr Opin Mol Ther.* 2008;10(4):362–370.

58. McEntee G, Kyula JN, Mansfield D, et al. Enhanced cytotoxicity of reovirus and radiotherapy in melanoma cells is mediated through increased viral replication and mitochondrial apoptotic signalling. *Oncotarget.* 2016;7(30):48517–48532.

59. Harrington KJ, Hingorani M, Tanay MA, et al. Phase I/II study of oncolytic HSV GM-CSF in combination with radiotherapy and cisplatin in untreated stage III/IV squamous cell cancer of the head and neck. *Clin Cancer Res.* 2010;16(15):4005–4015.

60. Tan AC, Goubier A, Kohrt HE. A quantitative analysis of therapeutic cancer vaccines in phase 2 or phase 3 trial. *J Immunother Cancer.* 2015;3:48.

61. Dranoff G, Jaffee E, Lazenby A, et al. Vaccination with irradiated tumor cells engineered to secrete murine granulocyte-macrophage colony-stimulating factor stimulates potent, specific, and long-lasting anti-tumor immunity. *Proc Natl Acad Sci U S A.* 1993;90(8): 3539–3543.

62. Golden EB, Chhabra A, Chachoua A, et al. Local radiotherapy and granulocyte-macrophage colony-stimulating factor to generate abscopal responses in patients with metastatic solid tumours: a proof-of-principle trial. *Lancet Oncol.* 2015;16(7):795–803.

63. Formenti SC, Demaria S. Systemic effects of local radiotherapy. *Lancet Oncol.* 2009;10(7):718–726.

64. Finkelstein SE, Rodriguez F, Dunn M, et al. Serial assessment of lymphocytes and apoptosis in the prostate during coordinated intraprostatic dendritic cell injection and radiotherapy. *Immunotherapy.* 2012;4(4):373–382.

65. Finkelstein SE, Iclozan C, Bui MM, et al. Combination of external beam radiotherapy (EBRT) with intratumoral injection of dendritic cells as neo-adjuvant treatment of high-risk soft tissue sarcoma patients. *Int J Radiat Oncol Biol Phys.* 2012;82(2):924–932.

66. Kim YH, Gratzinger D, Harrison C, et al. In situ vaccination against mycosis fungoides by intratumoral injection of a TLR9 agonist combined with radiation: a phase 1/2 study. *Blood.* 2012;119(2):355–363.

67. Milas L, Mason KA, Ariga H, et al. CpG oligodeoxynucleotide enhances tumor response to radiation. *Cancer Res.* 2004;64(15):5074–5077.

68. Seifert L, Werba G, Tiwari S, et al. Radiation therapy induces macrophages to suppress t-cell responses against pancreatic tumors in mice. *Gastroenterology.* 2016;150(7):1659–1572.e5.

69. Zhu Y, Knolhoff BL, Meyer MA, et al. CSF1/CSF1R blockade reprograms tumor-infiltrating macrophages and improves response to T-cell checkpoint immunotherapy in pancreatic cancer models. *Cancer Res.* 2014;74(18):5057–5069.

70. Shiao SL, Ruffell B, DeNardo DG, et al. TH2-polarized CD4(+) T Cells and macrophages limit efficacy of radiotherapy. *Cancer Immunol Res.* 2015;3(5):518–525.

71. Xu J, Escamilla J, Mok S, et al. CSF1R signaling blockade stanches tumor-infiltrating myeloid cells and improves the efficacy of radiotherapy in prostate cancer. *Cancer Res.* 2013;73(9):2782–2794.

72. Wolchok JD, Hoos A, O'Day S, et al. Guidelines for the evaluation of immune therapy activity in solid tumors: immune-related response criteria. *Clin Cancer Res.* 2009;15(23): 7412–7420.

73. Hodi FS, Hwu WJ, Kefford R, et al. Evaluation of immune-related response criteria and RECIST v1.1 in patients with advanced melanoma treated with pembrolizumab. *J Clin Oncol.* 2016;34(13):1510–1517.

74. Kazandjian DG, Blumenthal GM, Khozin S, et al. Characterization of patients treated with a programmed cell death protein 1 inhibitor (anti-PD-1) past RECIST progression from a metastatic non-small cell lung cancer (mNSCLC) trial. Paper presented at: 2016 ASCO Annual Meeting; 2016.

75. Seymour L, Bogaerts J, Perrone A, et al. iRECIST: guidelines for response criteria for use in trials testing immunotherapeutics. *Lancet Oncol.* 2017;18(3):e143–e52.

76. Johnson CB, Jagsi R. The promise of the abscopal effect and the future of trials combining immunotherapy and radiation therapy. *Int J Radiat Oncol Biol Phys.* 2016;95(4):1254–1256.

77. Sharabi AB, Lim M, DeWeese TL, et al. Radiation and checkpoint blockade immunotherapy: radiosensitisation and potential mechanisms of synergy. *Lancet Oncol.* 2015;16(13):e498–e509.

# Radiomics 13

*Ke Nie and Min-Ying Lydia Su*

## INTRODUCTION

The concept of "precision medicine" differs from conventional medicine, a one-size-fits-all approach that leads to the possibility of under- or overtreating patients. The core of precision medicine is to tailor the treatment based on the individual patient and disease profile. Current discussions have focused on molecular characterization using genomic and proteomic technologies. However, it is known that multiple subclonal populations coexist within tumors. This heterogeneous nature might create a barrier for the biopsy-based or current genome-based techniques, as the obtained mutation does not represent the entire population of cancer cells. In contrast, this situation seems ideally suitable to imaging analytics, as imaging is able to capture a comprehensive view of the tissue noninvasively.

With the recent advances in imaging acquisition and analysis, imaging can now provide much more insightful information than one might suspect from daily practice. For example, Kuo et al reported that following a complete manual extraction of more than 100 imaging features, a subset of 14 features predicted nearly 80% of the gene expression pattern in hepatocellular carcinoma using CT images (1). Diehn et al reported a similar finding, showing that a combination of only 28 imaging features was sufficient to reconstruct the variation of 116 gene expression modules in glioblastoma multiforme (GBM) using MRI (2). These studies have prompted a rapidly expanding research field—*radiomics*.

In this chapter, we will review the current state of the art in the radiomics research field, along with its challenges and its potentials in the era of precision medicine.

## What Is Radiomics

The current practice of imaging interpretation in clinical oncology remains subjective—for example, "a peripherally enhanced spiculated mass in the lower left lobe." And even when quantitative analysis is performed, the sole measurement is only one-dimensional, such as maximum tumor diameter (Response Evaluation Criteria in Solid Tumors [RECIST]), or two-dimensional, such as long-axis measurement (World Health Organization [WHO]). These measures neither reflect the complexity of tumor morphology or behavior nor, in many cases, predict therapeutic benefits. In contrast, radiomics considers medical imaging to be data instead of pictures. It refers to the extraction and analysis of large amounts of advanced imaging features with high-throughput computing. The obtained information is then mined into descriptive and predictive models relating to gene-protein signatures or therapy outcomes. Further, these data are designed to be extracted from standard-of-care medical images as CT, MRI, PET, et cetera. The creation of databases that combine vast quantities of radiomics data from millions of patients is foreseeable.

## The Rebirth of Radiomics

The quantitative analysis of medical image features is not new; it has been in development for decades. The majority of the previous work focused on the detection of small nodules (3–9) or the differentiation between malignant and benign lesions (10–16), with the help of computer-aided detection or diagnosis (CAD). Early success has been the greatest in breast cancer imaging. For example, the Food and Drug Administration (FDA) approved the R2 CAD system for cancer detection on mammography. It is used as a "second pair of eyes" to detect mammographic findings that radiologists might otherwise overlook, thus increasing cancer detection. The FDA also approved several systems for breast MRI interpretation, such as CADstream (Merge Healthcare Inc., Chicago, IL) and DynaCAD (Invivo, Gainesville, FL). These image-processing systems are designed to display critical information from hundreds of acquired MR images to assist radiologists in the visualization, analysis, and reporting of breast MRI studies. MRI CAD systems for other organs are also widely used in the clinic to assist radiologists' interpretations and improve their specificity while maintaining a high sensitivity. Radiomics is a natural extension of CAD systems, yet the methodologies and applications are distinct. It is explicitly a process designed to extract the maximum amount of information from images and subsequently mine the data for hypothesis testing to determine a correlation with genomics information or with therapy response, treatment outcome, et cetera.

The modern rebirth of radiomics was articulated in two papers by Kuo and colleagues. In an analysis of patients with hepatocellular carcinoma, the investigators compared radiologist-defined features extracted from contrast-enhanced CT images to gene expression patterns using a neural network–based machine-learning approach. They found that a combined small subset of imaging traits was able to reconstruct 78% of the global gene expression profiles, which were in turn related to cell proliferation, liver synthetic function, and patient prognosis (1). In a subsequent study, they compared image features from MRI with global gene expression patterns in patients with GBM (2). They found that the tumor mass effect predicted the proliferation gene expression pattern, while the internal contrast enhancement was related to the activation of specific hypoxia. Further, they found that patients with an "infiltrative" imaging phenotype had a greater tendency to have multiple tumor foci and significantly shorter survival rates. Their findings demonstrated the capacity to use imaging to provide an in vivo portrait of global gene expression, which in turn makes a new research area—radiomics—possible.

## Insight Into Tumor Heterogeneity

The rationale of precision medicine is that significant genomic heterogeneity exists among and even within tumors, and those differences are the key causes of a heterogeneous treatment response (17–20). In addition, human tumors have been shown to have clones that evolve over time; for example, clonal mutations occur early in tumorigenesis, and subclonal mutations occur later (21–22). Phenomena such as the presence of drug-resistant cells could be explained by the emergence of subclones of malignant cells later. Successful personalized medicine requires a clear understanding of each tumor's heterogeneity and each individual patient's situation. However, taking multiple biopsies to truly understand the spatial heterogeneity is not a simple or practical solution. Further, given the evidence for the evolution of subclones over time, the sampling bias involved in the current biopsy-based or genome-based approaches limits our capability to accurately identify biomarkers for clinical use. Yet this situation might be suitable for imaging analytics. Radiomics is a noninvasive approach that can be repeatedly used to monitor disease progression and capture a comprehensive view of the tissue at a macroscopic level. Thus, imaging radiomics, alongside demographics, blood biomarkers, genomics, and combinations thereof, is expected to improve individualized treatment selection.

## THE PROCESS AND CHALLENGE OF RADIOMICS

The goal of radiomics is to convert images into minable data with high-throughput computing. Generally, it involves following the steps, each with its own challenges: (a) image acquisition, (b) volume of interest (VOI) identification and segmentation, (c) quantitative image feature extraction, and (d) data mining and informatics analysis.

## Image Acquisition

Radiomics data are generally captured from daily, routinely used imaging, such as CT, MRI, and PET. These devices are designed so that clinicians can interpret the images to identify the presence of lesions, which is usually qualitative. Technical innovation has largely focused on improving image quality, shortening the scanning time, or enhancing the user interface as matters of convenience. How these improvements affect the quantification of imaging features is not the first priority. Moreover, the standardization of imaging acquisition protocols is typically lacking. Wide variations in reconstruction or acquisition parameters have made imaging biomarker translation problematic. For example, Goh et al have investigated variations in quantifying perfusion parameters from dynamic contrast–enhanced CT of colorectal cancer using commercialized software. These variances are due to differences in vendors or kinetic tracer models (23), software versions (24), image acquisition intervals (25), image acquisition length (26), and contrast agent volume (27). Identical data can have order-of-magnitude differences, and the results are not interchangeable. Galavis et al have assessed the variability of radiomics features extracted from PET due to differing acquisition modes, reconstruction algorithms, postfiltering widths, and iteration numbers. Out of 50 features, 40 were shown to have substantial variability of up to 30% (28). Results from MRI could vary even more due to the gradient strength of the scanner, pulse sequence used, method of contrast agent administration, k-space trajectory, and beyond. In recent years multiple efforts have been made to standardize the acquisition protocols. The major efforts come from the Quantitative Imaging Network (QIN) and the Quantitative Imaging Biomarker Alliance (QIBA). Other professional societies, such as the Radiological Society of North America (RSNA), the American Association of Physicists in Medicine (AAPM), the International Society of Magnetic Resonance in Medicine (ISMRM), and the Society of Nuclear Medicine and Molecular Imaging (SNMMI), are increasingly including aspects of the bedrock of quantitative imaging in their guidelines. Nevertheless, the stability of radiomics features must be evaluated across various imaging acquisitions, and standardization is needed to build reliable imaging biomarkers for clinical use.

## Volume of Interest Identification and Segmentation

All the subsequent radiomics analyses, such as morphological or contrast heterogeneity features, rely on the accurate identification and segmentation of the volume of interest (VOI). Manual outlining by experienced radiologists or oncologists is often treated as the gold standard. Yet it is labor-intensive and suffers from high interoperator or even intraoperator variations. Many automatic and semiautomatic segmentation methods have been developed across various anatomical sites, such as thresholding, region growing, clustering, and knowledge-based machine-learning approaches. The segmentation of normal structures such as the brain, lung, or skeleton can practically be achieved by automation. But any diseased structures, especially when due to tumors, require operator input because of their usually indistinct and irregular boundaries.

## Quantitative Image Feature Extraction

The core of radiomics is the extraction of high-dimensional feature sets to quantify volumes of interest. These features can be divided into several categories as morphology-based, intensity-based, and model-based.

*Morphology-based features* are used to capture three-dimensional morphological characteristics, such as volume, surface area, circularity, compactness, et cetera (15,29). For example, *compactness* is defined as the ratio of surface area to the volume. A lower compactness ratio indicates a more smooth and spherical tumor. A higher ratio means a more irregular tumor with a spiculated margin. *Circularity* is defined as the ratio of the actual tumor inside a sphere of its equivalent volume. The higher the circularity index, the more spherical is the shape of the tumor. Other disease-specific features can also be extracted. For example, *rim enhancement*, a typical sign of a malignant breast tumor, can be quantified by the enhancement rate between the peripheral regions to the internal core. Integrating tumor volume and density can also measure *tumor mass*, a parameter for the early detection of lung cancer.

*Intensity-based features* are used to quantify the gray-level distribution inside the VOI. The first-order intensity-based features are histogram-based. They reduce the three-dimensional volume data into a single histogram without concern for their spatial relationships. Multiple first-order statistics—mean, median, standard deviation, percentile, kurtosis, skewness, and more—can be acquired. Second-order intensity-based features are able to take the spatial relationships among voxels into account. They are also referred to as *texture* features, which include the gray-level co-occurrence matrix (GLCM), the run-length matrix, and Law's energy texture features. Higher-order statistical methods, such as fractal analyses or wavelet transformations, assess repetitive patterns after applying different filter grids onto the image.

*Model-based features* refer to fitting the data using mathematical models. For example, different kinetic models can be used to describe the image signal changes on dynamic contrast–enhanced (DCE) CT or DCE-MRI images. These include the conventional compartmental models; the adiabatic tissue homogeneity model; the distributed parameter model; and a generalized kinetic model, such as a standard or modified Toft's model, to derive model-dependent parameters, regional blood flow (RBF), regional blood volume (rBV), mean transit time (MTT), extraction fraction, permeability surface area product, and most frequently volume transfer constant (Ktrans) and extravascular extracellular volume (ve).

Although tumor characteristics can be potentially quantified using numerous radiomics features, their reliability needs to be studied. However, relevant research is still limited. For instance, the computation of radiomics features may be implemented differently. Typically, the volume data are acquired on a cross-sectional slice and then reconstructed into an entire volume. The radiomics features can be captured from either on a two-dimensional slice basis or from reconstructed three-dimensional volume (15,30). Another example, GLCM texture analysis, usually prerequires normalizing the image intensity into a limited range with reduced discrete levels. It can then be calculated by averaging either the values of the matrices computed for 13 distinct directions or a single matrix that accounts for tumor co-occurrence information in all 13 directions (31,32). The impact of different feature implementation/computation methods on the predictive values of radiomics features needs to be carefully studied. Further, many features are often found to be unstable between imaging scans acquired within weeks—or even minutes—of each other. Leijennar et al assessed the reproducibility of 219 radiomics features extracted from two separate lung CT scans taken on the same patient 15 minutes apart (33,34). Only one quarter were found to have good correlation. Although tumor heterogeneity can be potentially quantified using numerous radiomics features extracted from medical imaging, in order to identify reliable radiomics features, their reproducibility between scans must be further evaluated.

## Data Mining and Informatics Analysis

As hundreds or thousands of imaging features are extracted, important principles of data science must be applied to interpret those data. First, radiomics data are usually highly correlated with each other. Feature selection is needed to remove redundant information for better classification performance. Numerous methods can be applied to reduce the dimension of the radiomics features (35). Clusters of highly correlated features can be generated and then collapsed into one representative feature. Or, a generic algorithm (GA) can be used as a search engine to score a feature subset according to its predictive power. Another way to reduce their dimension is to rank features within separate categories representing different classes, such as morphological-, texture-, or kinetic-based algorithms (36,37). To avoid overfitting, a reasonable rule of thumb is that 10 samples (patients) are needed for each feature selected for binary classification.

For example, radiomics analysis can be performed for 100 patients, resulting in no more than 10 features being selected for the final prediction of different groups (eg, benign vs. malignant or responder vs. nonresponder) (35,38). Second, computational methods must be applied to build accurate classifiers. These include supervised and unsupervised machine-learning approaches. The distinction is that unsupervised analysis provides summary information of the data, not outcome variables. The most frequently used graphical display is a heat map, which simultaneously reveals cluster structures in a data matrix. This cluster heat map is a synthesis of various graphic displays developed by statisticians over more than a century (39). Supervised analysis, in contrast, creates models that attempt to separate the data with respect to phenotype or outcome, such as malignant versus benign or pathological complete response (pCR) versus non-pCR. The supervised machine-learning algorithms include artificial neural networks (ANN), support vector machines (SVM), and Bayesian networks, et cetera. Indeed, prognostic biomarkers developed using these machine-learning methods have increased performance when compared with conventional statistical methods, such as logistic regression or multivariate analysis, in lung (40,41), breast (42), and head and neck cancer (43). In one study, Parmar et al (43) investigated the prognostic values of 440 radiomic features using 14 feature selection methods and 12 feature classification models in over 460 lung cancer patients. They found that the choice of feature selection only led to variations of 6% in predictive power but choosing different feature classification algorithms could result in variations up to 30%.

In the current iteration of radiomics, image features must be extracted with high throughput, putting a premium on novel machine-learning algorithm development. However, methods that generate understandable decisions need to accommodate clinical patient information besides imaging, with covariates of genomic profiles, histology, biomarkers, patient histories, and more. In addition, not all information is expected to be available for all patients; hence, models should also be designed to accommodate sparse data.

## CURRENT STATUS OF RADIOMICS

With the advancement of new techniques, imaging has extended its role to the whole spectrum of cancer management, from screening and diagnosis to treatment monitoring and further surveillance. The clinical application of radiomics is expected to play important roles in every aspect.

### Cancer Screening and Tumor Diagnosis

Radiomic features have been very successful in discriminating malignant from benign tumors in many disease types. Nie et al showed that combining morphological and texture features from DCE-MRI while using ANN could differentiate malignant breast cancer from benign diseases. They observed that malignant tumors had relatively more spiculated boundaries, a more irregular shape, and higher enhancement compared to benign lesions (15). Wibmer et al demonstrated that texture features can discriminate between prostate cancer versus a benign lesion in the peripheral zone with 93% accuracy using T2 weighted and diffusion-weighted MRI (44,45). Besides MRI, radiomics from CT images have a long history of use for classifying a pulmonary nodule as benign or malignant (46–49). Commercialized products are also available for lung nodule detection and classification, including Lung VCAR (GE Health-care), ImageChecker CT (Hologic), syngo.via (Siemens Healthineers), et cetera. The recent International Early Lung Cancer Action Program (I-ELCAP) trial showed that these clinically used commercial tools discovered most of the lung cancers that radiologists initially missed (50). The radiomics information extracted from PET-CT was also found to be useful. Xu et al reported that the $^{18}$F-FDG uptake of malignant lesions in 103 patients was more heterogeneous than for benign bone and soft-tissue lesions (51). The classification results of their texture-based diagnosis method performed much better diagnostically compared to the histological method in terms of sensitivity (86% vs. 64%), specificity (77% vs. 61%), and accuracy (83% vs. 63%). In addition to cancer diagnosis, imaging features can assist in determining various histological or molecular types of tumors. Li et al suggested that mammographic images contain computer-extractable information, which may help to distinguish between breast cancer antigen (BRCA) 1 and 2 mutation carriers and noncarriers (52). Grimm et al extracted 56 imaging features (kinetic, morphologic, and texture analytics) on preoperative DCE-MRIs from 275 breast cancer patients (53). They found the imaging features to be strongly associated with luminal A and luminal B hormonal receptor positive molecular subtypes but saw no association with the imaging features for either human epidermal growth factor receptor family 2 (HER2 [HER2+]) or basal (ER [estrogen receptor]/PR [progester-one receptor]/HER2−) molecular subtypes. Overall, the early identification of tumor types can help physicians to better stratify patients and subsequently select the best treatment for each.

### Treatment Outcome Prediction

Recently, a significant amount of interest in utilizing radiomics for the early prediction of various treatment outcomes has emerged. The results are spread over many disease types. For neoadjuvant chemotherapy treatment in breast cancer, Su et al first showed that morphological and texture radiomics features from DCE-MRI could be used to discriminate breast cancer types as mass,

mass with rim enhancement, and nodular and septal patterns, which in turn might show a heterogeneous response to treatment regimens (54–55). Later, they reported strong associations between the baseline or early response patterns of the radiomics features as morphology/texture features from anatomical MRI (56–57), kinetic features derived from DCE-MRI (58), and MR spectroscopy (59–60) with the pathological complete response (61). ANN analysis was performed separately using (a) morphology/texture features, (b) enhancement kinetic features, and (c) a combination of all. They showed that the kinetic features only achieved an area under the receiver operating characteristic (ROC) curve (AUC) of 0.51, a morphology/texture along the AUC of 0.76, and an improvement in overall performance to 0.85 if combined into different categorical features (57). Pickles et al also determined that an association existed between pretreatment DCE-MRI–based metrics (shape, texture, and kinetic features) and survival intervals for 112 subjects (62). Promising results were reported for other cancer types. Nie et al evaluated multiparametric MRI features in predicting pCR after preoperative chemoradiation therapy (CRT) for locally advanced rectal cancer (37). A total of 103 imaging features (from anatomical, perfusion, and diffusion MRI), analyzed using both volume-averaged and voxelized methods, were extracted for each patient. The conventional volume-averaged analysis could provide an area under the ROC curve ranging from 0.54 to 0.73 in predicting pCR. If a voxelized heterogeneity analysis replaced the models, the prediction accuracy measured by the AUC could be improved to 0.71 up to 0.79. In addition, each subcategory image could generate moderate power in predicting the response, and all this information combined could improve the AUC to 0.84. This study suggested that an improved prognosis value could be achieved using a voxelized radiomics analysis approach over conventional imaging metrics. In patients with lung cancer, Aerts et al assessed the prognostic values of 440 radiomics features on a training data set with 420 patients from two institutes (36). The results were further validated on independent data sets, including another cohort of 225 lung cancer patients and a cohort of 231 head and neck cancer patients. Their results demonstrated the potential use of radiomics features in therapeutic benefit prediction in different disease types. Very recently, Kickingereder et al extracted a total of 4,842 quantitative MRI features of 172 recurrent glioblastoma (GBM) patients on bevacizumab treatment (63). The predictor stratified patients in the training set into a low- or high-risk group and was successfully validated in the validation set. Regarding CT images, Coroller et al identified 35 CT radiomics features to be significant predictors of distant metastasis and 6 features to be predictors of survival in 182 lung cancer patients (64). They concluded that the radiomics features identified may be useful for the early identification of cancer patients who have a high risk of developing distant metastasis, thus allowing physicians to better adapt treatment plans for individual patients. Vasculature measured from DCE–CT or perfusion CT has also demonstrated a strong association with angiogenesis treatment. Tixier et al observed that tumor blood flow measured on DCE–CT was significantly correlated with the metabolically active tumor volume (65). Hayano et al found that the hepatocellular carcinoma patients with longer survival often had lower fractal dimension on the arterial phase DCE–CT image (66).

All these results are very encouraging, suggesting the radiomics-based signature may emerge as a putative imaging biomarker for therapeutic benefit prediction, advance the knowledge in the noninvasive characterization of different diseases, and stress the role of radiomics as a novel tool for improving decision support in cancer treatment at low cost.

## Risk Assessment

Beyond the diagnosis and prognosis, radiomics has been extended to risk assessment. It is well known in the oncology community that mammographic density is an independent risk factor for breast cancer (67–70). A risk model based on breast density alone and adjusted for age and ethnicity was found to be as accurate as the Gail model (71). However, imaging radiomics can provide much more information than breast density alone. Li et al examined breast parenchymal patterns on mammograms from patients with a high risk versus a low risk of breast cancer (72). A total of 456 cases comprised of 53 BRCA 1 and 2 gene carriers, 75 patients with unilateral cancer, and 328 women at low risk were included. The study showed that women at high risk tend to have dense breasts with coarse and low-contrast texture patterns. Sun et al investigated the potential of using the multiscale texture features from mammograms to predict near-term breast cancer risk (73). From a total of 765 features, an optimal feature set of 12 was selected. Applying this feature set, a support vector machine (SVM) classifier yielded an AUC of 0.73. These results showed a moderately high positive association between risk prediction scores generated by the multiscale mammographic texture features. Nielsen et al further demonstrated that mammographic texture resemblance is independent of breast density and more predictive in a case control study with 495 women, of which 245 were diagnosed with breast cancer (74). Haberle et al conducted a case–control study that included 864 cases and 418 controls (75). A total of 470 radiomic features were explored as possible risk factors for breast cancer. These included statistical features, moment-based features, spectral-energy features, and form-based features. An elaborate variable selection process using logistic regression analyses identified those features associated with case–control status. Of the 470 image features explored, 46 remained in the final logistic regression model, while adding mammographic density did not improve the final model.

If a reliable imaging biomarker can be identified, it might be useful to monitor a treatment over time, since imaging can be provided noninvasively and repeatedly. It is reported that a 2% increase in relative breast cancer risk is associated with every 1% increase in mammographic density (76). Cuzick et al analyzed density results from the International Breast Cancer Intervention Study (IBIS-1) trial (77). This trial randomized 7,154 high-risk women to receive tamoxifen or a placebo for 5 years. Women who had a reduction in mammographic density of at least 10% over the first 12 to 18 months of tamoxifen prophylaxis had a 63% reduction in breast cancer risk ($P = .002$), whereas women who had a reduction in mammographic density of less than 10% received no benefit from tamoxifen treatment ($P = .89$). Therefore, a reliable method that could measure small changes of density in individual women would be very helpful for risk management. Because the two-dimensional mammography-based measurement is subject to tissue overlapping and thus cannot provide volumetric information, there is an urgent need to develop reliable, quantitative measurements of breast density three-dimensionally. Nie et al (78) have developed and Lin et al (79) have further refined an automatic segmentation method for reliable breast density measurement on three-dimensional MRI. The same group then observed a decreased fibroglandular tissue volume (FV) after tamoxifen treatment (80). They also showed that the change in FV was correlated with the baseline value and the duration of treatment. Women with a higher baseline FV or a longer treatment duration demonstrated a greater change. An article by Eng-Wong et al found that women receiving raloxifene experienced no change in mammographic density, but the FV measured by MRI showed a significant reduction (81). Overall, these studies suggest that when a woman's baseline density is known and serves as her own control, a reliable method, such as three-dimensional MRI, may be used to measure changes over time. In addition, breast density and parenchymal patterns analyzed from radiomics are sensitive enough to detect small changes; thus, they may provide promising surrogate biomarkers for adjuvant hormonal therapy and should be investigated further in breast cancer prevention trials (82).

## Radiogenomics

Another provocative research area in radiomics research is *radiogenomics*, which links the radiomics phenotype with the genomic profile. The rationale of this science in imaging might provide insight into the tumor phenotypes driven by the heterogeneity of the gene revolution. Radiogenomics is a very young scientific field, and the overlap between image-based phenotype features and genomic characteristics is not currently well established (83). This might be due to a lack of data, consisting of both imaging and genomic measurements, on the same set of tumors. Nevertheless, a few recent studies have pioneered advances in the field. The most active studies concern brain tumors (84–88), lung cancer (89–91), and breast cancer (52–53).

MR-based imaging features are often observed to be associated with somatic mutations and the genetic expression of brain tumors (86–88,92–93). For example, Ellingson et al observed that GBM tumors exhibiting hypermethylation of the O6-methylguanine-DNA-methyltransferase (MGMT) gene usually had smaller volumes on T1 contrast MRI and T2 fluid attenuated inversion recovery (FLAIR) hyperintensity than methylated GBM (92). Zinn et al identified an association between high T2 FLAIR volumes, the upregulation of periostin (POSTN), and the downregulation of miR-219 using data from The Cancer Genome Atlas (TCGA). They noted the high levels of POSTN associated with mesenchymal tumors and shorter survival and concluded that this approach may prove valuable for identifying new targets for molecular inhibition or future therapies (84). In a recent study by Colen et al, invasive imaging phenotypes such as enhancement across the midline, deep white matter tract involvement, and abnormal MR intensity in the internal capsule or brainstem were associated with the upregulation of the MYC oncogene, which is considered a significant regulator of metabolism (93).

Significant genomic heterogeneity that affects the likelihood of metastasis or treatment outcome has also been reported in lung cancer. Gevaert et al demonstrated 243 statistically significant pairwise correlations between CT and PET radiomics features and metagenes in non–small cell lung cancer (NSCLC) (94–95). Of over 180 extracted imaging features, 114 were predictive in terms of metagenes, with an accuracy of 65% to 86%. Aerts et al found that the heterogeneous phenotype described by wavelet texture features was significantly associated with the cell cycle pathway, suggesting that highly proliferative tumors demonstrate complex imaging patterns (36). Nair et al reported strong associations between histogram-based radiomics features from PET images with various gene expressions that related to patient survival in a cohort of over 300 NSCLC patients (96). In general, researchers have shown promising results from the use of lung radiomics to identify radiographic tumor phenotypes that favor specific genetic expressions (36,96–98).

Currently, several commercialized gene-sequencing tests for breast cancer are available at an affordable price that may, if the data can be obtained, provide valuable prognostic information to guide clinical decisions. These include the Oncotype DX® (Genomic Health, Redwood City, CA), which provides both a prognosis score and a prediction of the adjuvant chemotherapy benefit based on the expression of 21 breast genes; the MammaPrint® (Agendia, Amsterdam, The Netherlands), which gives an individual patient's recurrence risk based on a 70-gene assay; and the Prediction Analysis of Microarray 50 ([PAM50], nanoString Technologies, Inc., Seattle, WA), which was developed with the expression of 50 genes. Li et al investigated the relationships between MRI imaging phenotypes and the multigene assays of Oncotype Dx, MammaPrint, and PAM50 in a database of 84 patients with MRI images from The Cancer Imaging Archive (TCIA), along with clinical, histopathologic, and genomic data from TCGA (52). Multiple linear regression analyses demonstrated significant associations between radiomics signatures and multigene assay recurrence scores. The use of radiomics to distinguish between a good and a poor prognosis yielded area under the ROC curve values of 0.88, 0.76, 0.68, and 0.55 for the MammaPrint, Oncotype DX, and PAM50 risk of relapse based on subtype and the PAM50 risk of relapse based on subtype and proliferation, respectively. Other studies by Suttan et al (99) and Ashraf et al (100) used computationally derived radiomics phenotypes to predict the recurrence likelihood score defined by Oncotype DX. All reported that good associations did exist.

Because numerous radiomics features can be extracted from medical images, these studies play an important role in identifying the subset of features that might be most relevant to the underlying tumor biology and genetics. However, the ways in which tumor pathophysiological processes give rise to imaging phenotypes that can be quantified by radiomics features remain unclear. Future studies would need to investigate these associations to further elucidate on the biological meaning of the radiomics features. Another important thing to point out is that these studies are based on genomic data generated by a single tissue sample. Tumors contain spatially heterogeneous cell populations. A single biopsy sample of a tumor usually contains multiple cell subpopulations but typically cannot encompass all the subclones. Therefore, the genomic profile of a single tumor sample may be incomplete and only partially reflect the overall genomic landscape of the entire tumor. All these issues can affect the results obtained through radiogenomic analysis. A comprehensive study would require multiple biopsy samples from the same tumor, which is often costly and labor-intensive in practice. In return, such a study would be more informative and accurate. Nevertheless, radiogenomics, the study of the associations between radiographic and genomic features, represents a new horizon in cancer research that focuses on the intersection of two diagnostic disciplines. A combination of these two, radiogenomics holds great promise regarding the eventual inexpensive, noninvasive phenotyping of tumors for use in individualized patient therapies or treatment strategies by inferring genomic or pathological characteristics from radiographic information.

## CONCLUSIONS

Radiomics is a young discipline that holds great potential for precision medicine. However, it might be suffering from the same slow pace as genomic studies from about 10 years ago. As was noted in a 2009 report, many genomics-based studies published prior to that date contained significant analytical errors, and the results were too incomplete to be reusable (101). Further, scientists reported that they failed to replicate 47 out of 53 landmark studies in the basic science of cancer (102). These issues raise serious concern in the scientific society regarding the accountability of the statistical analysis, the transparency of the raw data access, and the validation of the study results. This will become more critical in the era of big data when navigating complex "-omics" issues. Because the ultimate goal for radiomics study is to build reliable imaging biomarkers to assist in clinical decision making, a prospective investigation must be trained, tested, and validated against a completely independent data set with a systematic study design with uniform treatment options, complete reporting of results, solid statistical analysis, and more.

Nevertheless, our vision of radiomics is still optimistic. Medical imaging is redefining its role as a data source for precision medicine in the guise of image-based phenotyping, which represents the convergence of medical imaging analysis and radiomics. Further, medical imaging can provide information about tumor internal heterogeneity at a macroscopic level—a critical limitation of biopsy-based or current genome-based approaches—which could potentially provide important complementary information for precision medicine. Successfully introducing these methods into clinical care will require much additional research to determine how underlying driving biologic patterns are related to the tumor imaging phenotypes. In the foreseeable future, we expect that the data gleaned from radiology and oncology examinations will be converted into quantitative data, which will then be merged with knowledge bases to improve diagnostic and predictive power in support of clinical decision making.

## References


1. Segal E, Sirlin CB, Ooi C, et al. Decoding global gene expression programs in liver cancer by non-invasive imaging. *Nat Biotechnol*. 2007;25(6);675–680.
2. Diehn M, Nardini C, Wang DS, et al. Identification of noninvasive imaging surrogates for brain tumor gene-expression modules. *Proc Natl Acad Sci U S A*. 2008;105(13):5213–5218. doi:10.1073/pnas.0801279105

3. Javaid M, Javid M, Rehman MZ, et al. A novel approach to CAD system for the detection of lung nodules in CT images. *Comput Methods Programs Biomed.* 2016;135:125–139. doi:10.1016/j.cmpb.2016.07.031

4. Zeng JY, Ye HH, Yang SX, et al. Clinical application of a novel computer-aided detection system based on three-dimensional CT images on pulmonary nodule. *Int J Clin Exp Med.* 2015;8(9):16077–16082.

5. Jacobs C, van Rikxoort EM, Murphy K, et al. Computer-aided detection of pulmonary nodules: a comparative study using the public LIDC/IDRI database. *Eur Radiol.* 2016;26(7):2139–2147. doi:10.1007/s00330-015-4030-7

6. Schalekamp S, van Ginneken B, Koedam E, et al. Computer-aided detection improves detection of pulmonary nodules in chest radiographs beyond the support by bone-suppressed images. *Radiology.* 2014;272(1):252–261. doi:10.1148/radiol.14131315

7. Schalekamp S, van Ginneken B, Heggelman B, et al. New methods for using computer-aided detection information for the detection of lung nodules on chest radiographs. *Br J Radiol.* 2014;87(1036):20140015. doi:10.1259/bjr.20140015

8. Nishio M, Nagashima C. Computer-aided diagnosis for lung cancer: usefulness of nodule heterogeneity. *Acad Radiol.* 2017; 24(3):328–335. pii:S1076–6332(16)30381–30386. doi:10.1016/j.acra.2016.11.007

9. Choi YJ, Baek JH, Park HS, et al. A computer-aided diagnosis system using artificial intelligence for the diagnosis and characterization of thyroid nodules on ultrasound: initial clinical assessment. *Thyroid.* 2017;27(4):5460552. doi:10.1089/thy.2016.0372

10. Moon WK, Chen IL, Chang JM, et al. The adaptive computer-aided diagnosis system based on tumor sizes for the classification of breast tumors detected at screening ultrasound. *Ultrasonics.* 2016;76:70–77. doi:10.1016/j.ultras.2016.12.017

11. Chang RF, Chen HH, Chang YC, et al. Quantification of breast tumor heterogeneity for ER status, HER2 status, and TN molecular subtype evaluation on DCE-MRI. *Magn Reson Imaging.* 2016;34(6):809–819. doi:10.1016/j.mri.2016.03.001

12. Li H, Giger ML, Lan L, et al. Computerized analysis of mammographic parenchymal patterns on a large clinical dataset of full-field digital mammograms: robustness study with two high-risk datasets. *J Digit Imaging.* 2012;25(5):591–598.

13. Yuan Y, Giger ML, Li H, et al. Multimodality computer-aided breast cancer diagnosis with FFDM and DCE-MRI. *Acad Radiol.* 2010;17(9):1158–1167. doi:10.1016/j.acra.2010.04.015

14. Newell D, Nie K, Chen JH, et al. Selection of diagnostic features on breast MRI to differentiate between malignant and benign lesions using computer-aided diagnosis: differences in lesions presenting as mass and non-mass-like enhancement. *Eur Radiol.* 2010;20(4):771–781. doi:10.1007/s00330-009-1616-y

15. Nie K, Chen JH, Yu HJ, et al. Quantitative analysis of lesion morphology and texture features for diagnostic prediction in breast MRI. *Acad Radiol.* 2008;15(12)1513–1525. doi:10.1016/j.acra.2008.06.005

16. Horsch K, Giger ML, Vyborny CJ, et al. Classification of breast lesions with multimodality computer-aided diagnosis: observer study results on an independent clinical data set. *Radiology.* 2006;240(2):357–368.

17. Lawrence MS, Stojanov P, Mermel CH, et al. Discovery and saturation analysis of cancer genes across 21 tumour types. *Nature.* 2014;505:495–501.

18. Kandoth C, McLellan MD, Vandin F, et al. Mutational landscape and significance across 12 major cancer types. *Nature.* 2014;502:333–339.

19. Alexandrov LB, Nik-Zainal S, Wedge DC, et al; Australian Pancreatic Cancer Genome Initiative; ICGC Breast Cancer Consortium; ICGC MMML-Seq Consortium; ICGC

PedBrain, Zucman-Rossi J, Futreal PA, McDermott U, et al. Signatures of mutational processes in human cancer. *Nature*. 2013;500:415–421.

20. Swanton C. Cancer evolution: the final frontier of precision medicine? *Ann Oncol*. 2014; 25(3):549–551.

21. Landau DA, Carter SL, Stojanov P, et al. Evolution and impact of subclonal mutations in chronic lymphocytic leukemia. *Cell*. 2013;152(4):714–726.

22. Marusyk A, Tabassum DP, Altrock PM, et al. Non-cell-autonomous driving of tumour growth supports sub-clonal heterogeneity. *Nature*. 2014:514(7520):54–58.

23. Koh TS, Ng QS, Thng CH, et al. Primary colorectal cancer: use of kinetic modeling of dynamic contrast enhanced CT data to predict clinical outcome. *Radiology*. 2013:267(1): 145–154. doi:10.1148/radiol.12120186

24. Goh V, Shastry M, Engledow A, et al. Commercial software upgrades may significantly alter Perfusion CT parameter values in colorectal cancer. *Eur Radiol*. 2011;21(4):744–749. doi:10.1007/s00330-010-1967-4

25. Goh V, Liaw J, Bartram CI, et al. Effect of temporal interval between scan acquisitions on quantitative vascular parameters in colorectal cancer: implications for helical volumetric perfusion CT techniques. *Am J Roentgenol*. 2008;191(6):W288-W292. doi:10.2214/AJR.07.3985

26. Goh V, Halligan S, Hugill JA, et al. Quantitative colorectal cancer perfusion measurement using dynamic contrast-enhanced multidetector-row computed tomography: effect of acquisition time and implications for protocols. *J Comput Assist Tomogr*. 2005;29(1): 59–63.

27. Goh V, Bartram C, Halligan S. Effect of intravenous contrast agent volume on colorectal cancer vascular parameters as measured by perfusion computed tomography. *Clin Radiol*. 2009;64(4):368–372. doi:10.1016/j.crad.2008.08.018

28. Galavis PE, Hollensen C, Jallow N, et al. Variability of textural features in FDG PET images due to different acquisition modes and reconstruction parameters. *Acta Oncol*. 2010;49(7):1012–1016. doi:10.3109/0284186X.2010.498437

29. Chen W, Giger ML, Bick U, et al. Automatic identification and classification of characteristic kinetic curves of breast lesions on DCE-MRI. *Med Phys*. 2006;33(8): 2878–2887.

30. Chen W, Giger ML, Li H, et al. Volumetric texture analysis of breast lesions on contrast-enhanced magnetic resonance images. *Magn Reson Med*. 2007;58(3):562–571.

31. Fave X, Cook M, Frederick A, et al. Preliminary investigation into sources of uncertainty in quantitative imaging features. *Comput Med Imaging Graph*. 2015;44:54–61.

32. Hatt M, Majdoub M, Vallières M, et al. 18F-FDG PET uptake characterization through texture analysis: investigating the complementary nature of heterogeneity and functional tumor volume in a multi-cancer site patient cohort. *J Nucl Med*. 2015;56(1):38–44.

33. Leijenaar RT, Nalbantov G, Carvalho S, et al. The effect of SUV discretization in quantitative FDG-PET radiomics: the need for standardized methodology in tumor texture analysis. *Sci Rep*. 2015;5:11075.

34. Leijenaar RT, Carvalho S, Velazquez ER, et al. Stability of FDG-PET Radiomics features: an integrated analysis of test-retest and inter-observer variability. *Acta Oncol*. 2013;52(7):1391–1397.

35. Guyon I, André E. An introduction to variable and feature selection. *J Mach Learn Res*. 2003;3:1157–1182.

36. Aerts HJ, Velazquez ER, Leijenaar RT, et al. Decoding tumour phenotype by noninvasive imaging using a quantitative radiomics approach. *Nat Commun*. 2014;5(3):4006. doi:10.1038/ncomms5006

37. Nie K, Shi L, Chen Q, et al. Rectal cancer: assessment of neoadjuvant chemoradiation outcome based on radiomics of multiparametric MRI. *Clin Cancer Res*. 2016;22(21): 5256–5264.

38. Chalkidou A, O'Doherty MJ, et al. False discovery rates in PET and CT studies with texture features: a systematic review. *PLoS One*. 2015;10(5):e0124165. doi:10.1371/journal.pone.0124165

39. Wilkinson L, Friendly M. The history of the cluster heat map. *Am Stat*. 2009;63(2): 179–184

40. Parmar C, Leijenaar RT, Grossmann P, et al. Radiomic feature clusters and prognostic signatures specific for lung and head & neck cancer. *Sci Rep*. 2015;5:11044. doi:10.1038/srep11044

41. Wu W, Parmar C, Grossmann P, et al. Exploratory study to identify radiomics classifiers for lung cancer histology. *Front Oncol*. 2016;6:71. doi:10.3389/fonc.2016.00071

42. McLaren CE, Chen WP, Nie K, et al. Prediction of malignant breast lesions from MRI features: a comparison of artificial neural network and logistic regression techniques. *Acad Radiol*. 2009;16(7):842–851. doi:10.1016/j.acra.2009.01.029

43. Parmar C, Grossmann P, Rietveld D, et al. Radiomic machine-learning classifiers for prognostic biomarkers of head and neck cancer. *Front Oncol*. 2015;5:272. doi:10.3389/fonc.2015.00272

44. Wibmer A, Hricak H, Gondo T, et al. Haralick texture analysis of prostate MRI: utility for differentiating non-cancerous prostate from prostate cancer and differentiating prostate cancers with different Gleason scores. *Eur Radiol*. 2015;25(10):2840–2850. doi:10.1007/s00330-015-3701-8.

45. Nie K, Chen JH, Yu HJ, et al. Quantitative analysis of lesion morphology and texture features for diagnostic prediction in breast MRI. *Acad Radiol*. 2008;15(12)1513–1525. doi: 0.1016/j.acra.2008.06.005

46. McNitt-Gray MF, Hart EM, Wyckoff N, et al. A pattern classification approach to characterizing solitary pulmonary nodules imaged on high resolution CT: preliminary results. *Med Phys*. 1999;26(6):880–888.

47. Kido S, Kuriyama K, Higashiyama M, et al. Fractal analysis of small peripheral pulmonary nodules in thin-section CT: evaluation of the lung-nodule interfaces. *J Comput Assist Tomogr*. 2002;26(4):573–578.

48. Petkovska I, Shah SK, McNitt-Gray MF, et al. Pulmonary nodule characterization: a comparison of conventional with quantitative and visual semi-quantitative analyses using contrast enhancement maps. *Eur J Radiol*. 2006;59(2):244–252.

49. Way TW, Hadjiiski LM, Sahiner B, et al. Computer-aided diagnosis of pulmonary nodules on CT scans: segmentation and classification using 3D active contours. *Med Phys*. 2006;33(7):2323–2337.

50. Liang M, Tang W, Xu DM, et al. Low-dose CT screening for lung cancer: computer-aided detection of missed lung cancers. *Radiology*. 2016;281(1):279–288. doi:10.1148/radiol.2016150063

51. Xu R, Kido S, Suga K, et al. Texture analysis on 18F-FDG PET/CT images to differentiate malignant and benign bone and soft-tissue lesions. *Ann Nucl Med*. 2014;28(9): 926–935.

52. Li H, Zhu Y, Burnside ES, et al. MR imaging radiomics signatures for predicting the risk of breast cancer recurrence as given by research versions of MammaPrint, Oncotype DX, and PAM50 gene assays. *Radiology*. 2016;281(2):382–391.

53. Grimm LJ, Zhang J, Mazurowski MA. Computational approach to radiogenomics of breast cancer: luminal A and luminal B molecular subtypes are associated with imaging

features on routine breast MRI extracted using computer vision algorithms. *J Magn Reson Imaging.* 2015;42(4):902–907. doi:10.1002/jmri.24879

54. Su MY, Yu H, Chiou JY, et al. Measurement of volumetric and vascular changes with dynamic contrast enhanced MRI for cancer therapy monitoring. *Technol Cancer Res Treat.* 2002;1(6):479–488.

55. Su MY, Yu HJ, Chen JH, et al. MRI monitoring of neoadjuvant chemotherapy response in breast cancer of different phenotypes to doxorubicin-cyclophosphamide followed by Taxane + Carboplatin ± Trastuzumab Regimen. In: Proceedings of the 14th ISMRM Annual Meeting, Seattle, WA; 2006; #2889.

56. Chu Y, Nie K, Yu HJ, et al. Artificial neuronal network analysis of neoadjuvant chemotherapy response using quantitative morphological, texture and enhancement kinetic parameters. In: Proceedings of the 14th ISMRM Annual Meeting, Seattle, WA; 2006; #2889.

57. Nie K, Chen JH, Yu HJ, et al. Quantitative analysis of MRI tumor characteristics for neoadjuvant chemotherapy response prediction in breast cancer to the first-line doxorobixin-cyclophosphamide regimen and the AC followed by Taxane regimen. In: Proceedings of the 15th ISMRM Annual Meeting, Berlin; 2007; #558.

58. Yu HJ, Chen JH, Mehta RS, et al. MRI measurements of tumor size and pharmacokinetic parameters as early predictors of response in breast cancer patients undergoing neoadjuvant anthracycline chemotherapy. *J Magn Reson Imaging.* 2007;26(3):615–623.

59. Baek HM, Chen JH, Nalcioglu O, et al. Proton MR spectroscopy for monitoring early treatment response of breast cancer to neo-adjuvant chemotherapy. *Ann Oncol.* 2008;19(5):1022–1024. doi:10.1093/annonc/mdn121

60. Baek HM, Chen JH, Nie K, et al. Predicting pathologic response to neoadjuvant chemotherapy in breast cancer by using MR imaging and quantitative 1H MR spectroscopy. *Radiology.* 2009;251(3):653–662. doi:10.1148/radiol.2512080553

61. Chen JH, Feig B, Agrawal G, et al. MRI evaluation of pathologically complete response and residual tumors in breast cancer after neoadjuvant chemotherapy. *Cancer.* 2008; 112(1):17–26.

62. Pickles MD, Lowry M, Gibbs P. Pretreatment prognostic value of dynamic contrast-enhanced magnetic resonance imaging vascular, texture, shape, and size parameters compared with traditional survival indicators obtained from locally advanced breast cancer patients. *Invest Radiol.* 2016;51(3):177–185.

63. Kickingereder P, Götz M, Muschelli J, et al. Large-scale radiomic profiling of recurrent glioblastoma identifies an imaging predictor for stratifying anti-angiogenic treatment response. *Clin Cancer Res.* 2016;22(23):5765–5771.

64. Coroller TP, Grossmann P, Hou Y, et al. CT-based radiomic signature predicts distant metastasis in lung adenocarcinoma. *Radiother Oncol.* 2015;114(3):345–350. doi:10.1016/j.radonc.2015.02.015

65. Tixier F, Groves AM, Goh V, et al. Correlation of intra-tumor 18F-FDG uptake heterogeneity indices with perfusion CT derived parameters in colorectal cancer. *PLoS One.* 2014;9(6):e99567.

66. Hayano K, Lee SH, Yoshida H, et al. Fractal analysis of CT perfusion images for evaluation of antiangiogenic treatment and survival in hepatocellular carcinoma. *Acad Radiol.* 2014;21(5):654–660. doi:10.1016/j.acra.2014.01.020

67. Boyd NF, Guo H, Martin LJ, et al. Mammographic density and the risk and detection of breast cancer. *N Engl J Med.* 2007;356(3):227–236.

68. Vachon CM, Brandt KR, Ghosh K, et al. Mammographic breast density as a general marker of breast cancer risk. *Cancer Epidemiol Biomarkers Prev.* 2007;16(1):43–49.

69. Titus-Ernstoff L, Tosteson AN, Kasales C, et al. Breast cancer risk factors in relation to breast density (United States). *Cancer Causes Control.* 2006;17(10):1281–1290.

70. Boyd NF, Martin LJ, Sun L, et al. Body size, mammographic density, and breast cancer risk. *Cancer Epidemiol Biomarkers Prev.* 2006;15(11):2086–2092.

71. Tice JA, Cummings SR, Ziv E, et al. Mammographic breast density and the Gail model for breast cancer risk prediction in a screening population. *Breast Cancer Res Treat.* 2005:94(2):115–122.

72. Li H, Giger ML, Lan L, et al. Comparative analysis of image-based phenotypes of mammographic density and parenchymal patterns in distinguishing between BRCA1/2 cases, unilateral cancer cases, and controls. *J Med Imaging (Bellingham).* 2014;1(3):031009. doi:10.1117/1.JMI.1.3.031009

73. Sun W, Tseng TL, Qian W, et al. Using multiscale texture and density features for near-term breast cancer risk analysis. *Med Phys.* 2015;42(6):2853–2862. doi:10.1118/1.4919772

74. Nielsen M, Vachon CM, Scott CG, et al. Mammographic texture resemblance generalizes as an independent risk factor for breast cancer. *Breast Cancer Res.* 2014;16(2):R37.

75. Häberle L, Wagner F, Fasching PA, et al. Characterizing mammographic images by using generic texture features. *Breast Cancer Res.* 2012;14(2):R59.

76. Boyd NF, Lockwood GA, Byng JW, et al. Mammographic densities and breast cancer risk. *Cancer Epidemiol Biomarkers Prev.* 1998;7(12):1133–1144.

77. Cuzick J, Sestak I, Cawthorn S, et al; IBIS-I Investigators. Tamoxifen for prevention of breast cancer: extended long-term follow-up of the IBIS-I breast cancer prevention trial. *Lancet Oncol.* 2015;16(1):67–75. doi:10.1016/S1470-2045(14)71171-4

78. Nie K, Chen JH, Chan S, et al. Development of a quantitative method for analysis of breast density based on 3-dimensional breast MRI. *Med Phys.* 2008;35(12):5253–5262.

79. Lin M, Chan S, Chen JH, et al. A new bias field correction method combining N3 and FCM for improved segmentation of breast density on MRI. *Med Phys.* 2011;38(1):5–14.

80. Chen JH, Chang YC, Chang D, et al. Reduction of breast density following tamoxifen treatment evaluated by 3-D MRI: preliminary study. *Magn Reson Imaging.* 2011;29(1):91–98. doi:10.1016/j.mri.2010.07.009

81. Eng-Wong J, Orzano-Birgani J, Chow CK, et al. Effect of raloxifene on mammographic density and breast magnetic resonance imaging in premenopausal women at increased risk for breast cancer. *Cancer Epidemiol Biomarkers Prev.* 2008;17(7):1696–1701. doi:10.1158/1055-9965

82. Chen JH, Gulsen G, Su MY. Imaging breast density: established and emerging modalities. *Transl Oncol.* 2015;8(6):435–445. doi:10.1016/j.tranon.2015.10.002

83. Gillies RJ, Kinahan PE, Hricak H. Radiomics: images are more than pictures, they are data. *Radiology.* 2016;278(2):563–577.

84. Zinn PO, Mahajan B, Sathyan P, et al. Radiogenomic mapping of edema/cellular invasion MRI-phenotypes in glioblastoma multiforme. *PLoS One.* 2011;6(10):e25451.

85. Gutman DA, Cooper LA, Hwang SN, et al. MR imaging predictors of molecular profile and survival: multi-institutional study of the TCGA glioblastoma data set. *Radiology.* 2013;267(2):560–569.

86. Naeini KM, Pope WB, Cloughesy TF, et al. Identifying themesenchymal molecular subtype of glioblastoma using quantitative volumetric analysis of anatomicmagnetic resonance images. *Neuro Oncol.* 2013;15(5):626–634.

87. Pope WB, Chen JH, Dong J, et al. Relationship between gene expression and enhancement in glioblastoma multiforme: exploratory DNA microarray analysis. *Radiology.* 2008;249(1):268–277.

88. Gutman DA, Dunn WD Jr, Grossmann P, et al. Somatic mutations associated with MRI-derived volumetric features in glioblastoma. *Neuroradiology.* 2015;57(12):1227–1237.

89. Hong SJ, Kim TJ, Choi YW, et al. Radiogenomic correlation in lung adenocarcinoma with epidermal growth factor receptor mutations: Imaging features and histological subtypes. *Eur Radiol.* 2016;26(10):3660–3668. doi:10.1007/s00330-015-4196-z

90. Hsu JS, Huang MS, Chen CY, et al. Correlation between EGFR mutation status and computed tomography features in patients with advanced pulmonary adenocarcinoma. *J Thorac Imaging.* 2014;29(6):357–363.

91. Liu Y, Kim J, Balagurunathan Y, et al. Radiomic features are associated with EGFR mutation status in lung adenocarcinomas. *Clin Lung Cancer.* 2016;17(5):441–448. doi:10.1016/j.cllc.2016.02.001

92. Ellingson BM, Lai A, Harris RJ, et al. Probabilistic radiographic atlas of glioblastoma phenotypes. *Am J Neuroradiol.* 2013;34(3):533–540. doi:10.3174/ajnr.A3253

93. Colen RR, Vangel M, Wang J, et al. Imaging genomic mapping of an invasive MRI phenotype predicts patient outcome and metabolic dysfunction: a TCGA glioma phenotype research group project. *BMC Med Genomics.* 2014;7:30. doi:10.1186/1755-8794-7-30

94. Gevaert O, Echegaray S, Khuong A, et al. Predictive radiogenomics modeling of EGFR mutation status in lung cancer. *Sci Rep.* 2017;7:41674. doi:10.1038/srep41674

95. Gevaert O, Xu J, Hoang CD, et al. Non-small cell lung cancer: identifying prognostic imaging biomarkers by leveraging public gene expression microarray data—methods and preliminary results. *Radiology.* 2012;264(2):387–396. doi:10.1148/radiol.12111607

96. Nair VS, Gevaert O, Davidzon G, et al. Notice of duplicate publication [duplicate publication of Nair VS, Gevaert O, Davidzon G, et al. Prognostic PET 18F-FDG uptake imaging features are associated with major oncogenomic alterations in patients with resected non-small cell lung cancer. *Cancer Res.* 2012;72(15):3725–3734. doi: 10.1158/0008-5472.CAN-11-3943. Erratum in: *Cancer Res.* 2012;72(18):4870–4871.

97. Yoon HJ, Sohn I, Cho JH, et al. Decoding tumor phenotypes for ALK, ROS1, and RET fusions in lung adenocarcinoma using a radiomics approach. *Medicine (Baltimore).* 2015;94(41):e1753. doi:10.1097/MD.0000000000001753

98. Jeong CJ, Lee HY, Han J, et al. Role of imaging biomarkers in predicting anaplastic lymphoma kinase-positive lung adenocarcinoma. *Clin Nucl Med.* 2015;40(1):e34–39. doi:10.1097/RLU.0000000000000581

99. Sutton EJ, Oh JH, Dashevsky BZ, et al. Breast cancer subtype intertumor heterogeneity: MRI-based features predict results of a genomic assay. *J Magn Reson Imaging.* 2015;42(5):1398–1406. doi:10.1002/jmri.24890

100. Ashraf AB, Daye D, Gavenonis S, et al. Identification of intrinsic imaging phenotypes for breast cancer tumors: preliminary associations with gene expression profiles. *Radiology.* 2014;272(2):374–384. doi:10.1148/radiol.14131375

101. Chalmers I, Glasziou P. Avoidable waste in production and reporting of research evidence. *Lancet.* 2009;374(9683):86–89. doi:10.1016/S0140-6736(09)60329-9.

102. Begley CG, Ellis LM. Drug development: raise standards for preclinical cancer research. *Nature.* 2012;483(7391):531–533. doi:10.1038/483531a

# Big Data and Radiation Oncology 14

*Sanjay Aneja and James B. Yu*

## BIG DATA WITHIN RADIATION ONCOLOGY

### Defining "Big Data": Comparative Effectiveness, Data Mining, and Machine Learning

Any discussion of the data science first requires a broad definition of what are considered "big data." A generally accepted definition is "any useful information too large for human study and thus necessitating computer analysis" (1). This definition is vague by design and meant to reinforce the broad applicability of big data to advance all aspects of the field of radiation oncology. However, the definition does address one important delineation between useful data and unusable data. Big data require information that can be translated into some numerical form and effectively interpreted by computer software. A large portion of data in radiation oncology is already numerical and avoids this problem entirely. Data that are already numerical are considered *structured* data and are the most easily analyzed. *Unstructured* nonnumerical data, however, are quite powerful and can still be studied using big data techniques if abstracted accurately (2). Examples of unstructured data include relevant information found in patient charts and nonnumeric clinical and demographic information, the presence of side effects, or other subjective physical findings. With the advent of electronic medical records (EMRs), unstructured data have become less of an obstacle in big data research. Nevertheless, unstructured data do still require the labor-intensive process of abstracting natural language information into numerical form. Later in this chapter, we will describe some techniques currently being piloted within radiation oncology to overcome this obstacle more efficiently.

In addition to defining the type of data used, big data analysis is often further classified based on the methods and purpose for which data are analyzed. Big data methodology has often been divided into three broad categories: a) comparative effectiveness research, b) data mining, and c) machine learning (3–5). Understanding the nuanced relationship between these methodologies is helpful in comprehending how to effectively interpret big data analysis. Although separately emerging fields, all three disciplines possess more similarities than differences. All are founded upon the principles of statistics and employ similar mathematical techniques to interpret information from large data sets. The defining characteristic of each field is the lens through which it studies data. Comparative effectiveness research, which is most familiar to clinical researchers, is hypothesis driven and relies on the principles of statistical inference to answer a specific question. In contrast, data mining is frequently not founded upon a singular hypothesis-driven research question. Data mining is focused upon using large data sets to extract any possible valuable information. Last, machine learning, which is the least frequently used in clinical research, involves building software systems that use data sets to predict future information (6). Some would argue that each discipline has originated from the differences of the individuals who have aligned with each method. Statisticians/epidemiologists often conduct comparative effectiveness research, computer scientists often conduct data mining, and software/computer engineers conduct machine learning (7).

Although the methodologic nuances regarding the diverse types of analysis extend beyond the scope of this chapter, to better illustrate the differences between the three we will present an example of how the various types of big data analysis would utilize health-related data. Suppose one were given data that detailed survival and clinical information for a group of patients treated with two different interventions labeled *A* and *B*. Comparative effectiveness research would ask, "Is intervention A superior to intervention B with respect to survival?" Those who employ data mining would ask more broadly, "What are the factors associated with improved survival?" Data mining may find one of the interventions among a variety of variables associated with prolonged survival but is not only focused on the interventions. Machine learning would help to answer a related but distinctly different question; specifically, "Can we build a prediction tool to inform which intervention prolongs survival for individual patients based on their characteristics?" Machine learning in some ways is tailored for greater complexity because it does not assume either intervention is superior for all patients. Although all three disciplines are founded upon the same statistical principles, over time researchers employing the different techniques have used various software tools to better suit their needs. Com-

**TABLE 14.1**  Comparing comparative effectiveness research, data mining, and machine learning

| | Comparative effectiveness research | Data mining | Machine learning |
|---|---|---|---|
| Research questions | Hypothesis-driven research questions with a specific focus | Broad nonhypothesis-driven questions focused on gathering information | Questions focused around building predictive systems to help gain information |
| Typical investigators | Clinical researchers, epidemiologists, policy makers | Epidemiologists, biostatisticians | Computer scientists, computer engineers |
| Computer software | SPSS, STATA, SAS | SAS, R | Matlab, Python, JAVA |

parative effectiveness research and data mining are often conducted using statistical software packages, such as STATA, SAS, and SPSS (8–10). In contrast, because machine learning may require the construction of software, it often utilizes computer languages such as R, Python, and Java (11–13). Table 14.1 summarizes some important differences between comparative effectiveness research, data mining, and machine learning.

## UTILITY OF BIG DATA WITHIN RADIATION ONCOLOGY

Big data analytics has the potential to revolutionize multiple fields in the coming years. With applications in healthcare, engineering, and public policy, advances in computer technology will only increase the use of data to expand our knowledge in a variety of fields. Radiation oncology is well positioned to capitalize on advances in data analytics. A greater understanding of the data within radiation oncology will serve to transform radiobiology, clinical decision making, and radiation physics.

### Big Data Within Radiobiology

Within radiobiology, big data analytics has been critical to harnessing the power of genetic sequencing. The emergence of *radiogenomics* is founded upon our ability to efficiently study large amounts of sequencing information using advanced computing techniques. The analysis of genetic data within radiation oncology can improve our ability to stratify patients receiving radiation therapy according to risk (14). A marriage between the fields of radiobiology and data science allows for the identification of genetically important targets that could provide insight into potential mechanisms regulating radiation sensitivity and normal tissue toxicity. More importantly, radiogenomics serves as an example of the ability of big data analysis to help accelerate research within radiobiology that is difficult to ascertain from smaller scale studies (15). The identification of genetic sequences and/or genetic biomarkers that confer radiation sensitivity has already begun across head and neck, central nervous system (CNS), prostate, and genitourinary cancers (16,17). The studies have discovered unique genetic markers whose importance has previously gone unrealized within the field and have led to further research by radiobiologists to corroborate findings within the lab. As genetic sequencing becomes more cost-effective and accurate, radiobiologists will have the opportunity to analyze larger groups of patients to better personalize the field of radiation oncology. Genetic information is only one aspect in which large data analysis can have an impact on radiobiology. The ability to apply similar techniques to the fields of proteomics, metabolomics, and other aspects of systems biology is rapidly emerging within the field of radiobiology (18).

## Big Data Within Clinical Research

Within clinical practice, radiation oncology has seen the rise of large data analysis to answer important questions previously difficult to ascertain. Although the foundation of clinical decision making is prospective randomized clinical trial evidence, data analysis of large retrospective cohorts has increased in prominence within clinical research. The rise of big data within clinical research is largely because of the challenges of randomized clinical trials within modern medicine. Randomized clinical trials have become increasingly regulated, time-intensive, and costly (19). This unfortunately can lead to clinical trials that lose clinical relevance upon completion or whose results are not applicable to a wide range of patients.

Big data analysis has supplemented traditional clinical trials in a variety of ways. Analyzing large clinical data sets allows us to corroborate results from randomized clinical trials. Specifically, big data studies have enabled us to investigate the applicability of clinical trial findings to a broader range of patients beyond those studied in a clinical trial. Moreover, research on large retrospective studies has affirmed trial findings that trended toward statistical significance but, because of limited power or follow-up, were not fully realized. For example, postoperative radiation therapy in N2 non–small cell lung cancer (NSCLC) was not found to improve overall survival in randomized clinical trials and subsequent meta-analyses. However, an analysis of a large retrospective Surveillance, Epidemiology, and End Results (SEER) cohort found an overall survival benefit in the same population attributed to improved radiation therapy techniques (20,21). The SEER analysis prompted further investigation into the utility of radiation therapy in the setting and was a driving force in the decision to open the currently accruing international Lung Adjuvant Radiotherapy Trial (LungART) (22).

Additionally, large retrospective data sets allow the investigation of questions that cannot be studied in prospective clinical trials because of poor patient accrual, difficulty in randomization, and/or disease prevalence. Through a variety of statistical techniques, including propensity score matching, nonparametric regression, and instrumental variable analysis, researchers are able to leverage big data to resemble a randomized clinical trial (23). For example, despite two randomized clinical trials comparing stereotactic body radiation therapy (SBRT) to surgical resection in early-stage NSCLC failing to meet accrual goals, a matched analysis of a similar SEER-Medicare cohort allowed researchers to study SBRT in comparison with surgery (24,25).

A number of leaders within our field have thoroughly described the limitations of large observational studies, and these are an important caveat to any discussion regarding the clinical applicability of big data research (23,26,27). Although the gold standard will continue to be prospective randomized clinical trials, the emergence of big data can improve the efficiency of our clinical research enterprise. Big data analysis can help highlight the most important clinical questions to which we should devote our limited research resources.

## Big Data Within Radiation Physics

The utility of big data to improve the fields of radiation physics and dosimetry has been established for some time. Similar to the analytical principles that led to revolutionary breakthroughs such as intensity-modulated radiation therapy (IMRT), large data have the ability to improve treatment planning and the speed at which radiation therapy is delivered (2). Data-mining techniques have already shown an ability to improve the efficiency of the IMRT quality assurance (QA) process in the treatment of both prostate and head and neck cancers (28). Additionally, big data analytics has improved image guidance to deliver higher doses of radiation such as those seen in stereotactic radiosurgery. Machine learning, specifically, has already emerged within the field of radiation physics and is the basis for *smart contouring* tools such as deformable image registration and auto-contouring (29).

The field of *radiomics* is another innovative area of research relevant to radiation physics. Radiomics aims to use information embedded within radiology exams to draw forth inferences and insights. For example, the shape, texture, and imaging characteristics of different lung or head and neck cancers have been used to predict survival differences between patients (30). As the fields of radiology and radiation oncology often overlap in terms of daily tumor imaging (for image guidance), treatment planning, and the assessment of tumor response, the interest in radiomics within radiation oncology continues to grow (31).

## SOURCES OF BIG DATA WITHIN RADIATION ONCOLOGY

Radiation oncology is a field well suited for large data analysis. Given its technical nature, radiation oncology was among the first fields to employ forms of electronic data storage, which is of emerging utility. Additionally, the robust effort within the greater oncology community to create clinical cancer registries has led to a considerable amount of different data sources available for interested researchers. Table 14.2 describes a number of large data sources that have been used for study within the field of radiation oncology. We will highlight a few of these data sources and their applications in the fields of radiobiology, clinical radiation oncology, and radiation physics.

Much of the large data analysis within radiobiology has centered upon the emerging field of radiogenomics (18). A very robust source of data useful for radiogenomic study is the Cancer Genome Atlas (TCGA) (32). The National Cancer Institute (NCI)-funded TCGA is a publicly available data source with genomic information across 33 different cancer types. Researchers have used big data analysis of TCGA data to identify novel oncogenic drivers of a variety of malignancies. TCGA analysis has led investigators to study genes contributing to functional changes driving cancer development; has established definitions for molecular subtypes of poorly understood cancers; and has identified new biomarkers on the basis of genomic, transcriptomic, proteomic, and epigenomic alterations (15). An alternative data source is genetic information within large cooperative trials. Groups such as NRG Oncology have established central repositories to store specimens for patients enrolled in their clinical trials (33). These programs offer a wealth of possible genetic information that can be used for future large data analyses. Additionally, these organizations lead initiatives that provide opportunities to both clinicians and radiobiologists to combine the benefits of large data analysis to better personalize radiation oncology treatments.

Unfortunately, the large genomic data sets often lack significant subsets of patients who have undergone radiotherapy. Because TCGA and related data sets are composed largely of patients who have undergone surgical resection as the primary therapy for their cancers, the data set has largely been used more for tumor characterization and phylogeny than drawing clinical insights. Further linkages of the data to clinical information or the specific inclusion of radiotherapy patients would be helpful. Other organizations, such as the NCI

**TABLE 14.2** Examples of big data sources

| Data set | Information | Sponsoring institution |
| --- | --- | --- |
| SEER program data set | Clinical, demographic, and outcomes data compiled from multiple cancer registries across the United States | NCI |
| TCGA | Key genomic information across 33 different cancer types | NCI-NIH |
| NRG Biospecimen Bank | Tissue of patients enrolled in NRG (formerly RTOG, NSABP, GOG) trials | NRG |
| NHANES | Clinical, demographic, dietary, and health-related questions from a nationally represented sample of 5,000 patients | CDC |
| HCUP | A collection of multiple data sets that provides hospital-level data regarding quality, cost, and outcomes for multiple conditions across the United States | Agency for Healthcare Research and Quality |
| HMO Cancer Network | A wide variety of clinical data from a network of integrated health delivery sites across the United States | HMO Cancer Research Network |
| Cancer Imaging Archive | A large archive of radiology/medical imaging across multiple cancer types | NCI |
| ASTRO-AANS Stereotactic Radiosurgery Registry | Collaborative registry of patients undergoing SRS | ASTRO-AANS |
| National Cancer Database data set | Clinical, demographic, and outcomes data from a network of hospitals across the United States | American College of Surgeons |
| National Radiation Oncology Registry | Pilot registry comprised of standardized, aggregated radiation oncology data on patients and multiple cancer sites across the United States | ASTRO-ROI |
| Radiation Oncology Incident Learning System | Registry of patient data regarding radiation oncology safety-related incidents | ASTRO-AAPM |

*Note:* AAPM, American Association of Physicists in Medicine; ANNS, American Association of Neurological Surgeons; ASTRO, American Society for Radiation Oncology; CDC, Centers for Disease Control and Prevention; GOG, Gynecologic Oncology Group; HCUP, Healthcare Cost Utilization Project; HMO, Health Maintenance Organization; NCI, National Cancer Institute; NHANES, National Health and Nutrition Examination Survey; NSABP, National Surgical Adjuvant Breast and Bowel Project; NIH, National Institutes of Health; ROI, Radiation Oncology Institute; RTOG, Radiation Therapy Oncology Group; SEER, Surveillance, Epidemiology, and End Results program data set; SRS, stereotactic radiosurgery; TCGA, The Cancer Genome Atlas.

Radiogenomics Consortium, are attempting to build and foster collaboration regarding radiogenomic data sets (34).

A number of data sets are available for researchers to study in the effort to improve clinical decision making. The data range from single-institution registry data to nationwide population-level data resources. The NCI-funded SEER data are some of the most well utilized population-level data sources (27). The SEER program at its core offers a wealth of patient-level clinical information for approximately 25% of the United States. The clinical information provided in the SEER data includes patient demographics, pathologic data, treatment, and outcomes. Over the course of the last 10 years, the number of studies using the SEER data has grown exponentially and provided a wealth of information to inform clinical practice. Moreover, the wide variety of SEER-linked data sources have afforded researchers the ability to study clinical research questions through a different lens. For example, the SEER-Medicare-linked data allows investigators to better study the associated costs of cancer treatment (35,36). Similarly, the SEER-Medicare Health Outcomes Survey (SEER-MHOS) data allow for the study of health-related quality of life issues among patients within the SEER registries (37–39). Some examples of SEER data applications have previously been discussed in this chapter (21,24). The limitations of the SEER data have been well documented and include a lack of data reliability, radiation dose information, and chemotherapy information (26,40). These limitations highlight the imperfect nature inherent to any registry data. However, researchers have been able to creatively overcome some of these limitations using the SEER-linked data sets.

One aspect of the SEER data that has somewhat limited its utility within radiation oncology is the lack of radiation dose information available for study. More recently, the American College of Surgeons National Cancer Data Base (NCDB) has provided a new data source for clinical investigation. Similar to the SEER data, the NCDB is a national patient-level data set that documents demographic, clinical, and outcome data for a number of cancer types. One notable advantage of the NCDB data compared to the SEER data is radiation dose information. NCDB-led studies have highlighted the effectiveness of radiation therapy in the setting of multiple cancer types and represent a wealth of opportunities for big data analyses in the future (1). However, NCDB data are limited by the lack of outcomes beyond overall survival.

Current initiatives in large data collection will represent opportunities for further research. The National Radiation Oncology Registry (NROR) prostate cancer pilot program is an American Society of Radiation Oncology (ASTRO)-Radiation Oncology Institute (ROI) initiative that aims to collect standardized information on cancer care delivery through an automatic abstraction platform (41,42). This initiative, if proven successful, will provide a framework for the expansion to a nationwide electronic registry for radiation oncology.

## OBSTACLES FACING BIG DATA WITHIN RADIATION ONCOLOGY

Along with the additional benefits of big data in advancing the field of radiation oncology are also continued obstacles. The strength of big data relies in the volume of information available for study. Accompanying that strength is data heterogeneity, which is a significant weakness. Critics of large data analysis often cite missing, inaccurate, or uninterpretable data that degrade research studies as a flaw that limits applicability (41). It is important for investigators to be cognizant of the inherent data limitations and take every step to limit spurious results. Although big data research serves as a useful tool to advance the field, the limitations of observational data must be appreciated (26). Investigators must be able to distinguish the statistical anomalies seen in large data analysis from clinically relevant findings (2).

Other significant obstacles facing large data analysis include the increasing resource requirements to maintain and analyze data. As data sources become larger, the amount of storage and computing power needed to effectively study large data increases. Additionally, as data become more complex, the need for training and expertise in computer programming and mathematics becomes more important and serves as a barrier to studies (2).

## ASSURING THE FUTURE OF BIG DATA WITHIN RADIATION ONCOLOGY

The continued improvement of the big data enterprise within radiation oncology is necessary to assure sustained advances within the field. Although randomized clinical trials will continue to be the cornerstones of clinical research, big data will continue to supplement advances in the field of clinical research over the coming years. To ensure radiation oncology is not left behind with the rising wave of big data research, it is necessary to continue the efficient and accurate collection of data to inform clinical practice. National organizations' and professional societies' continued support of cancer registries will be vital. Moreover, clinicians must improve the documentation within the EMR that can reliably be abstracted into future big data repositories. Improvements in natural language software recognition will increase the efficiency of abstracting the unstructured data within EMRs. Software programs that capture clinical data from medical records in real time have already been piloted within radiation oncology with promising results (43). Additionally, the real-time collection of patient-reported outcomes through software programs such as the Apple Health Kit will increase the data that patients can provide to clinicians throughout their treatment course (41).

In addition to continuing to collect data, radiation oncologists must attempt to innovate the types of information we gather in the future. Unique outcome measures such as patient-reported outcomes and health-related quality-of-life metrics will allow us to study patients in different ways and leverage advances in large data analytics. Collaboration across different institutions and disciplines will be critical in testing different outcome measures across various patient populations. Clinicians must continue to encourage patients to participate in registries and large data repositories to further the field.

Lastly, the field of radiation oncology must embrace big data analysis moving forward. Radiation oncologists and trainees must be provided the skills necessary to interpret and study large data as they grow in importance to medical research in the future. A basic understanding of disciplines such as biostatistics, epidemiology, bioinformatics, and computer science must be integrated into residency training. This will create a future workforce of radiation oncologists with an eye for grasping and interpreting big data to answer the emerging clinical questions facing our field.

## References


1. Chen RC, Gabriel PE, Kavanagh BD, et al. How will big data impact clinical decision making and precision medicine in radiation therapy? *Int J Radiat Oncol Biol Phys.* 2016;95(3):880–4.
2. Bibault JE, Giraud P, Burgun A. Big data and machine learning in radiation oncology: state of the art and future prospects. *Cancer Lett.* 2016;381(1):110–117.
3. Jones DE, Ghandehari H, Facelli JC. A review of the applications of data mining and machine learning for the prediction of biomedical properties of nanoparticles. *Comput Methods Programs Biomed.* 2016;132:93–103.
4. Austin PC, Tu JV, Ho JE, et al. Using methods from the data-mining and machine-learning literature for disease classification and prediction: a case study examining classification of heart failure subtypes. *J Clin Epidemiol.* 2013;66(4):398–407.
5. Dipnall JF, Pasco JA, Berk M, et al. Fusing data mining, machine learning and traditional statistics to detect biomarkers associated with depression. *PLoS One.* 2016; 11(2):e0148195.
6. Berger ML, Doban V. Big data, advanced analytics and the future of comparative effectiveness research. *J Comp Eff Res.* 2014;3(2):167–176.
7. Oquendo MA, Baca-Garcia E, Artes-Rodriguez A, et al. Machine learning and data mining: strategies for hypothesis generation. *Mol Psychiatry.* 2012;17(10):956–959.
8. SAS 9.2 Help and Documentation [computer software]. Cary, NC: SAS Institute; 2015.
9. Stata Statistical Software: Release 14 [computer software]. College Station, TX: StataCorp; 2015.

10. IBM SPSS Statistics for Windows, Version 22.0 [computer software]. Armonk, NY: IBM Corp; 2015.

11. JAVA Programming Language [computer software]. Santa Clara, CA: Sun Microsystems; 2015.

12. Python Language Reference, Version 2.7 [computer software]. Python Software Foundation; 2015. http://www.python.org/.

13. R: A Language and Environment for Statistical Computing [computer software]. Vienna, Austria: R Core Team, R Foundation for Statistical Computing; 2015.

14. Das AK, Bell MH, Nirodi CS, et al. Radiogenomics predicting tumor responses to radiotherapy in lung cancer. *Semin Radiat Oncol.* 2010;20(3):149–155.

15. Rosenstein BS, Capala J, Efstathiou JA, et al. How will big data improve clinical and basic research in radiation therapy? *Int J Radiat Oncol Biol Phys.* 2016;95(3):895–904.

16. Meng J, Li P, Zhang Q, et al. A radiosensitivity gene signature in predicting glioma prognostic via EMT pathway. *Oncotarget.* 2014;5(13):4683–4693.

17. Liu N, Boohaker RJ, Jiang C, et al. A radiosensitivity MiRNA signature validated by the TCGA database for head and neck squamous cell carcinomas. *Oncotarget.* 2015; 6(33):34649–34657.

18. Rosenstein BS, West CM, Bentzen SM, et al. Radiogenomics: radiobiology enters the era of big data and team science. *Int J Radiat Oncol Biol Phys.* 2014;89(4):709–713.

19. Yu JB, Lloyd S, Decker RH, et al. Comparative effectiveness research and the surveillance, epidemiology, and end results database: what is comparative effectiveness research (CER) and why is it important? *Curr Probl Cancer.* 2012;36(4):208–215.

20. Postoperative radiotherapy in non-small-cell lung cancer: systematic review and meta-analysis of individual patient data from nine randomised controlled trials.PORT Meta-analysis Trialists Group. *Lancet.* 1998;352(9124):257–263.

21. Lally BE, Zelterman D, Colasanto JM, et al. Postoperative radiotherapy for stage II or III non-small-cell lung cancer using the surveillance, epidemiology, and end results database. *J Clin Oncol.* 2006;24(19):2998–3006.

22. Pechoux CL, Mercier O, Belemsagha D, et al. Role of adjuvant radiotherapy in completely resected non-small-cell lung cancer. *EJC Suppl.* 2013;11(2):123–130.

23. McGale P, Cutter D, Darby SC, et al. Can observational data replace randomized trials? *J Clin Oncol.* 2016;34(27):3355–3357.

24. Yu JB, Soulos PR, Cramer LD, et al. Comparative effectiveness of surgery and radiosurgery for stage I non-small cell lung cancer. *Cancer.* 2015;121(14):2341–2349.

25. Chang JY, Senan S, Paul MA, et al. Stereotactic ablative radiotherapy versus lobectomy for operable stage I non-small-cell lung cancer: a pooled analysis of two randomised trials. *Lancet Oncol.* 2015;16(6):630–637.

26. Jagsi R, Bekelman JE, Chen A, et al. Considerations for observational research using large data sets in radiation oncology. *Int J Radiat Oncol Biol Phys.* 2014;90(1):11–24.

27. Yu JB, Gross CP, Wilson LD, et al. NCI SEER public-use data: applications and limitations in oncology research. *Oncology (Williston Park).* 2009;23(3):288–295.

28. Zhu X, Ge Y, Li T, et al. A planning quality evaluation tool for prostate adaptive IMRT based on machine learning. *Med Phys.* 2011;38(2):719–726.

29. Guo Y, Gao Y, Shen D. Deformable MR prostate segmentation via deep feature learning and sparse patch matching. *IEEE Trans Med Imaging.* 2016;35(4):1077–1089.

30. Aerts HJ, Velazquez ER, Leijenaar RT, et al. Decoding tumour phenotype by noninvasive imaging using a quantitative radiomics approach. *Nat Commun.* 2014;5:4006.

31. Lambin P, Rios-Velazquez E, Leijenaar R, et al. Radiomics: extracting more information from medical images using advanced feature analysis. *Eur J Cancer.* 2012;48(4):441–446.

32. Weinstein JN, Collisson EA, Mills GB, et al; Cancer Genome Atlas Research Network. The Cancer Genome Atlas Pan-Cancer analysis project. *Nat Genet.* 2013;45(10): 1113–1120.

33. Oppitz U, Bernthaler U, Schindler D, et al. Sequence analysis of the ATM gene in 20 patients with RTOG grade 3 or 4 acute and/or late tissue radiation side effects. *Int J Radiat Oncol Biol Phys.* 1999;44(5):981–988.

34. West C, Rosenstein BS, Alsner J, et al. Establishment of a radiogenomics consortium. *Int J Radiat Oncol Biol Phys.* 2010;76(5):1295–1296.

35. Bang H. Medical cost analysis: application to colorectal cancer data from the SEER Medicare database. *Contemp Clin Trials.* 2005;26(5):586–597.

36. Lang K, Menzin J, Earle CC, et al. The economic cost of squamous cell cancer of the head and neck: findings from linked SEER-Medicare data. *Arch Otolaryngol Head Neck Surg.* 2004;130(11):1269–1275.

37. Kent EE, Malinoff R, Rozjabek HM, et al. Revisiting the Surveillance Epidemiology and End Results Cancer Registry and Medicare Health Outcomes Survey (SEER-MHOS) linked data resource for patient-reported outcomes research in older adults with cancer. *J Am Geriatr Soc.* 2016;64(1):186–192.

38. Kent EE, Ambs A, Mitchell SA, et al. Health-related quality of life in older adult survivors of selected cancers: data from the SEER-MHOS linkage. *Cancer.* 2015;121(5): 758–765.

39. Clauser SB, Haffer SC. SEER-MHOS: a new federal collaboration on cancer outcomes research. *Health Care Financ Rev.* 2008;29(4):1–4.

40. Jagsi R, Abrahamse P, Hawley ST, et al. Underascertainment of radiotherapy receipt in Surveillance, Epidemiology, and End Results registry data. *Cancer.* 2012;118(2):333–341.

41. Trifiletti DM, Showalter TN. Big data and comparative effectiveness research in radiation oncology: synergy and accelerated discovery. *Front Oncol.* 2015;5:274.

42. Efstathiou JA, Nassif DS, McNutt TR, et al. Practice-based evidence to evidence-based practice: building the National Radiation Oncology Registry. *J Oncol Pract.* 2013; 9(3):e90-e95.

43. Pan HY, Shaitelman SF, Perkins GH, et al. Implementing a real-time electronic data capture system to improve clinical documentation in radiation oncology. *J Am Coll Radiol.* 2016;13(4):401–407.

CPSIA information can be obtained
at www.ICGtesting.com
Printed in the USA
LVHW02s0055190418
573867LV00001B/1/P